Defining Human Life

Medical, Legal, and Ethical Implications

Defining Human Life

Medical, Legal, and Ethical Implications

Edited by
Margery W. Shaw, M.D., J.D.
A. Edward Doudera, J.D.

Published in cooperation with
the American Society of
Law & Medicine

AUPHA Press
Ann Arbor, Michigan
Washington, D.C.
1983

Library of Congress Cataloging in Publication Data
Main entry under title:
Defining human life.

Papers were presented at a conference held March 11–13, 1982, in Houston, Texas and sponsored by the American Society of Law & Medicine and the Institute for the Interprofessional Study of Health Law.
Includes index.
1. Abortion—Law and legislation--United States—Congresses. 2. Unborn children (Law)—United States—Congresses. 3. Abortion—United States—Congresses. I. Doudera, A. Edward, 1949–   II. Shaw, Margery W., 1923–   III. American Society of Law and Medicine. IV. Institute for the Interprofessional Study of Health Law (Texas) [DNLM: 1. Philosophy, Medical—Congresses. 2. Abortion, Legal—United States—Congresses. 3. Legislation, Medical—United States—Congresses. WQ 440 D313 1982]
KF3771.A75D43 1983   344.73'0419   83-9948
ISBN 0-914904-82-5   347.304419

AUPHA Press is an imprint of Health Administration Press.

Health Administration Press
School of Public Health
The University of Michigan
Ann Arbor, Michigan 48109
(313) 764-1380

Association of University
Programs in Health Administration
1911 North Fort Myer Drive, Suite 503
Arlington, Virginia 22209
(703) 524-5500

Contents

Contributors

CHARLES H. BARON is Professor of Law at Boston College Law School. He received his LL.B. from the Harvard Law School in 1961, and a Ph.D. in philosophy from the University of Pennsylvania in 1972. He was Founding Editor of the *Harvard International Law Journal* and is a member of the Board of Editors of the *American Journal of Law & Medicine*. In addition to various teaching positions and work with law firms, Professor Baron was Executive Director of the Resource Center for Consumers of Legal Services in Washington, D.C. He is the author of numerous articles in the legal literature on medicolegal issues.

RICHARD J. BLANDAU is a Professor Emeritus at the University of Washington Medical School in Seattle where he joined the faculty in 1949. He received his undergraduate degree from Linfield College in 1935, his Ph.D in biology from Brown University in 1939, and his M.D. with honors from the University of Rochester in 1948. He has received numerous awards and honors including, most recently, the Motion Picture Award of the American Fertility Society for the Best Scientific Film and the Brown University Graduate School Citation for Distinguished Contributions to Society. He is a member of numerous professional and honorary societies. Dr. Blandau is the editor or author of a long list of publications and serves as President of the Barren Foundation Board of Directors and as the Chairman of the Post Graduate Policy Committee of the American Fertility Society.

DANIEL CALLAHAN is the Director of the Hastings Center, Institute of Society, Ethics and the Life Sciences in Hastings-on-Hudson, New York. Dr. Callahan received his undergraduate degree from Yale College in 1952, his master's from Georgetown University in 1957, and his Ph.D. from Harvard University in 1965. He is a member of the Institute of Medicine of the National Academy of Sciences and the author of numerous books including *Abortion: Law, Choice and Morality* (1970) and *Ethics and Population Limitation* (1972).

SIDNEY CALLAHAN is Associate Professor of Psychology at Mercy College in Dobbs Ferry in New York. She received her undergraduate degree from Bryn Mawr College, her master's in psychology from Sarah Lawrence College, and her Ph.D. in social psychology from the City University of New York. She has received a number of honors, held numerous teaching positions, and been involved with a number of professional activities. Dr. Callahan, a licensed psychologist, is the author of four books on women, parenting, and birth control and the author of numerous essays and articles.

BERNARD M. DICKENS is Professor on the Faculty of Law, and Professor, Department of Preventive Medicine and Biostatistics of the Faculty of Medicine, University of Toronto in Toronto. He received his LL.B. in 1961 and his LL.M. in 1965 from King's College, University of London. He also received a Ph.D. in the criminology division of law, and his LL.D. in medical jurisprudence from the University of London in 1971 and 1978, respectively. Dr. Dickens was admitted as a Barrister of the English Bar in 1963 and as a Barrister and Solicitor of the Ontario Bar in 1977. He is the author of a long list of publications in the legal literature on medicolegal topics including parental rights and abortion, and serves on a number of advisory panels for the University of Toronto, the Ontario Ministry of Community and Social Services, the Canadian Association of Law Teachers, and Justice for Children.

BENTLEY GLASS is Distinguished Professor of Biology Emeritus at the State University of New York at Stony Brook, New York. He received his undergraduate and master's degrees from Baylor University, in 1926 and 1929, and his Ph.D. from the University of Texas in 1932. He is also the recipient of some ten honorary degrees, and is Director of the History of Genetics Project of the American Philosophical Society. The author of over 300 scientific, professional, and general articles, Dr. Glass has been an editor of the *Quarterly Review of Biology* since 1945 as well as the editor or author of numerous books. He has served as President of the American Association for the Advancement of Science, the American Association of University Professors, the American Institute of Biological Sciences, and the American Society of Human Genetics.

MITCHELL S. GOLBUS is Professor in the Departments of Obstetrics, Gynecology and Reproductive Sciences and of Pediatrics at University of

California Medical Center in San Francisco. He received his undergraduate degree in psychology from the Illinois Institute of Technology, and his M.D. from the University of Illinois School of Medicine in 1963. Dr. Golbus is a Fellow of the American College of Obstetricians and Gynecologists and serves on the Medical Advisory Committee of the National Genetics Foundation, the Scientific Advisory Committee of the National Tay-Sachs & Allied Disease Association, the Clinical Research Grant Review Committee of the March of Dimes Birth Defects Foundation, and the Clinical Service and Program Committees of the American Society of Human Genetics. He has authored or co-authored an extensive list of publications.

CLIFFORD GROBSTEIN is Professor of Biological Science and Public Policy at the University of California–San Diego in La Jolla, California. Dr. Grobstein received his undergraduate degree from the College of the City of New York and his master's and Ph.D. from the University of California, Los Angeles. He is a Fellow of the American Academy of Arts and Sciences and a member of the Institute of Medicine of the National Academy of Sciences. He was dean of the school of medicine and vice-chancellor for health sciences at the University of California–San Diego from 1966 to 1973. He is internationally known for his research in developmental biology and is the author of three books and many publications.

RUTH MACKLIN is Associate Professor (Bioethics) at Albert Einstein College of Medicine, in the Bronx, New York. She received her undergraduate degree in philosophy from Cornell University, and her master's and Ph.D. from Case Western Reserve University. She has co-edited a number of books and authored both books and articles on a wide range of topics. A former staff member and currently a Fellow at the Hastings Center, Institue of Society, Ethics and the Life Sciences, Dr. Macklin has participated in a long list of summer institutes, workshops, lectures, and conferences on bioethical issues.

AUBREY MILUNSKY is Professor of Pediatrics and Obstetrics & Gynecology at Boston University School of Medicine and Director of the Center for Human Genetics, Department of Pediatrics, Boston University Medical Center. He graduated from the University of the Witwatersrand Medical School in Johannesburg, South Africa in 1960, and became a member of the Royal College of Physicians of London in 1965. He is also a Diplomate of the American Board of Pediatrics. He is a past member of the Department of Pediatrics, Harvard Medical School, Director of the Birth Defects and Genetics Clinic at the Massachusetts General Hospital and Director of the Genetics Division, Eunice Kennedy Shriver Center. He is the author, editor or co-editor of ten books including *Genetic Disorders and the Fetus: Diagnosis, Prevention, and Treatment, Coping with Crisis and Handicap,* and *Genetics and the Law, Volume I* (1976) and *Volume II* (1980). He has also published an impressive list of articles in the medical literature.

HARRIET F. PILPEL is of counsel to the law firm of Weil, Gotshal & Manges in New York City. She is also General Counsel to Planned Parenthood Federation of America, special counsel to Planned Parenthood, New York City and one of the general counsel to the American Civil Liberties Union. She received her undergraduate degree from Vassar College and her law degree from Columbia Law School. She has received numerous awards and honors including the Columbia Law School Alumni Association Medal for Excellence and the Allard K. Lowenstein Award for outstanding service in the field of civil liberties.

JOHN A. ROBERTSON is Professor of Law at the University of Texas School of Law in Austin, Texas. He received his undergraduate degree from Dartmouth in 1964 and his law degree from Harvard in 1968. He has also been a Professor in the Law School and the Program in Medical Ethics of the Medical School of the University of Wisconsin, Madison, and has authored numerous articles in the field of health law. He is a member of the Board of Directors of the American Society of Law & Medicine.

LEON E. ROSENBERG is C.N.H. Long Professor of Human Genetics, Pediatrics and Medicine and the Chairman of the Department of Human Genetics at Yale University School of Medicine in New Haven, Connecticut. Dr. Rosenberg received his undergraduate degree in 1954 and his M.D. in 1957 from the University of Wisconsin. He is a member of the American Association for the Advancement of Science, the American Pediatric Society, a past president of the American Society of Human Genetics, and a Fellow of the American Academy of Arts and Sciences.

GEORGE M. RYAN, JR. is Professor of Obstetrics and Gynecology and Professor of Community Medicine at University of Tennessee College of Medicine in Memphis, Tennessee. He received his undergraduate degree from the University of Mississippi and his M.D. from Harvard Medical School in 1953. In 1972, he earned an M.P.H. from Harvard School of Public Health. Dr. Ryan is a member of numerous professional societies and serves on the National Medicine Committee on Planned Parenthood Federation of America, the Rural Infant Care Program Advisory Council of the Robert Wood Johnson Foundation, and the Professional and Technical Advisory Committee of the Joint Commission on Accreditation of

Hospitals. During 1980–1981, he served as President-Elect, and during 1981–1982 as President of the American College of Obstetricians and Gynecologists.

ROBERT M. VEATCH is Professor of Medical Ethics at the Kennedy Institute of Ethics and Georgetown University in Washington, D.C. He received his undergraduate degree in pharmacy from Purdue University, and a Master of Science in pharmacology from University of California Medical Center in San Francisco. He also earned a Bachelor of Divinity degree from Harvard Divinity School as well as a master's and Ph.D. in medical ethics from Harvard University. Before joining the Kennedy Institute, Dr. Veatch was a Senior Associate and Staff Director of the Research Group on Death and Dying and the Research Group on Ethics and Health Policy at The Hastings Center, Institute of Society, Ethics and the Life Sciences. He is a member of the Editorial Boards of the *Journal of the American Medical Association*, the *Journal of Medicine and Philosophy*, and the *Harvard Theological Review*, and Associate Editor of the *Encyclopedia of Bioethics*. He has authored or edited a number of books including *A Theory of Medical Ethics*, *Case Studies in Medical Ethics*, and *Death, Dying, and the Biological Revolution*, as well as an impressive list of articles in the professional literature.

DAVID WESTFALL is John H. Watson, Jr. Professor of Law at Harvard Law School in Cambridge, Massachusetts. He received his undergraduate degree from the University of Missouri in 1947 and his LL.B. from Harvard Law School in 1950. He is the author of *Estate Planning Law and Taxation* and *Estate Planning Cases and Text*, as well as the author of a number of articles in the *Columbia Law Review* and the *Harvard Law Review*.

DANIEL WIKLER is Associate Professor in the Program in Medical Ethics of the Center for Health Sciences and Associate Professor of Philosophy at the University of Wisconsin in Madison, Wisconsin. He received his undergraduate degree from Oberlin College and his Ph.D. from the University of California, Los Angeles. During 1980–1981, he was staff philosopher for the President's Commission for the Study of Ethical Problems in Medicine and Biomedical and Behavioral Research, and was a recipient of a career development award as a Kennedy Scholar in Medical Ethics for 1975–1980. He has published a long list of articles dealing with a variety of bioethical and medicolegal issues.

Preface

The papers contained in this volume were presented at a conference, entitled *Human Life Symposium: An Interdisciplinary Approach to the Concept of Person*, sponsored by the American Society of Law & Medicine and the Institute for the Interprofessional Study of Health Law—a joint venture of the University of Texas Health Science Center at Houston and the University of Houston College of Law. The conference was held March 11–13, 1982, at the Shamrock Hilton Hotel in Houston, Texas, and explored such diverse issues as the continuum of biological life, the changing legal definition of the concept of person, and the essential elements of what it is to be a human being. Societal attitudes toward the regulation of abortion were an underlying theme throughout the discussions.

In part, the conference resulted from a concern by the organizers about the wisdom of legislative efforts, and especially Senate Bill 158 proposed by Senator Jesse Helms (R-N.C.), that sought to define conception as the beginning of each person's life, and, at least by implication, to grant to the conceptus all the rights accorded "persons" under the United States Constitution and other laws. Indeed, on the morning of the first day of the conference, it was reported that a subcommittee of the Senate Judiciary Committee had passed S. J. Res. 110, a constitutional amendment introduced by Senator Orrin Hatch (R-Utah), granting the power to regulate abortion to the individual states. A multitude of similar bills have been proposed, and they are discussed at length in chapters 6, 9, 10, and 11 of this volume. To date, however, none has been, or seems likely to be, signed into law.

Regardless of the success of these bills, the issues associated with them will remain the focus of considerable political and societal debate. As Kathleen Andreoli, Special Assistant for Educational Affairs to the President of the University of Texas Health Science Center, said in her welcoming remarks at the symposium, the topic of personhood for fetuses is one of the most far-reaching and socially significant issues facing our nation, and one that encompasses all segments of our society. The issue of person-hood and its correlate, abortion, has been variously addressed by politi-cians, religious groups, civil rights activists, legislators, and by "pro-choice" and "pro-life" advocates. The symposium was designed to provide a forum for the rational discussion of these divergent views. Consensus on this controversial issue was not expected, but it was hoped that each participant would gain new insights and understanding from the multi-disciplinary discussion. Hopefully, this book will enable many others to learn and benefit from the dialogue that occurred at the conference.

The issues discussed in this volume are societal issues, but they are also personal ones. Robert Knauss, Dean of the College of Law of the University of Houston, highlighted this potential conflict of interest in his welcoming remarks. He asked each of those present, whether physician, attorney, or nurse, to consider whether their professional responses to these issues in individual cases were based on what is best for their patient or client or on what their own personal beliefs supported. While it may be appropriate for individuals to take different positions when acting as policymakers than when acting in professional capacities, it is important that they recognize and deal with the potential conflict of interest.

The importance of and need for a multidisciplinary dialogue on the issues upon which the conference and this text concentrates was evident from the diverse audience that assembled for the conference. Thirty-four states, the District of Columbia, and four Canadian provinces were repre-sented; approximately 36 percent of the attendees were physicians, ten percent biologists or geneticists, ten percent attorneys, seven percent nurses, ten percent hospital or clinic administrators, 14 percent the-ologians, and some ten percent were representatives of various pro-choice or pro-life groups.

The conference papers presented in this book are divided into five parts. In Part One, Clifford Grobstein, a biologist, and Daniel Wikler, a philosopher, discuss their views on personhood and the characteristics that define it. Grobstein asserts that although medicine and scientific inquiry can explain much of the biological process of life, it is not their role to provide the answer to the question of whether or not "human life" is present from conception. Professor Wikler, on the other hand, asserts that medicine and science must provide the answer to what is essentially a medical question. As Brian Zach noted in an editorial in *Science* in July 1981:

> The human life of the scientist's perceptual modeling and the human life whose inviolability the law seeks to ensure are coincidentally the same words used in two entirely different conceptual frameworks. The issue is at what stage of development shall the entity destined to acquire the attributes of a

human being be vested with the rights and protection accorded that status.

The difficulty of the answer becomes even more apparent after we consider the divergent views of Drs. Grobstein and Wikler. The following sections of the book seek to highlight and explore various aspects of the medical, legal, and ethical ramifications of enacting any type of legislation that declares, as S. 158 did, that "present day scientific evidence indicates a significant likelihood that actual human life exists from conception."

Part Two addresses the medical implications of defining human life. An embryologist, a medical geneticist, a specialist in fetal medical and surgical treatment, an obstetrician, and a medical ethicist examine a variety of issues. Richard Blandau not only provides an insightful and moving review of a number of aspects of human reproduction, but highlights what medical science does and does not know about that continuing process. His remarkable and award winning movie depicting the fertilization process unfortunately cannot be captured in the textual material reproduced here. Aubrey Milunsky discusses the recent advances in and current techniques for detection of fetal abnormalities and the counseling of parents whose child is affected by genetic abnormalities. He also examines a number of the existing ethical and medical dilemmas facing couples whose offspring are at risk of congenital abnormalities. Mitchell Golbus briefly traces the advances in the prenatal diagnosis of birth defects and discusses some of the new techniques for fetal treatment. Golbus notes that while most correctable defects which can be diagnosed in utero are best managed by appropriate medical or surgical therapy after delivery at term, a few (and probably more in the future) require in utero correction. Medical guidelines must be developed for the utilization of such techniques, and they must take into account the ethical and legal status accorded the fetus. George Ryan reviews some of the medical implications for pregnant women of bestowing personhood on the unborn and strongly rejects the legislative solutions thus far proposed. And finally, Robert Veatch addresses the question of whether we should require consistency in our definitions of life and death. His chapter provokes new considerations and provides new insights into our views of personhood both at the beginning stages and at the ending stages of the human life cycle.

The papers in Part Three bring into focus the legal implications of defining personhood as beginning at conception, from the perspectives of three law professors and a practicing attorney. As Professor Leonard Riskin of the University of Houston College of Law noted in his introductory remarks as moderator of the session, the law ordinarily reflects community values, albeit occasionally through a distant and distorted mirror. This is especially true where the community is divided about how the law should protect the various values at stake. This lack of uniformity is enhanced by the numerous legal issues involved in the abortion debate. The first chapter, by Charles Baron, provides a historical review of the legal concept of personhood, and urges all those concerned with the abortion question to move beyond their focus on personhood and to examine the individual and personal aspects of a most difficult issue. Harriet Pilpel examines the legal issues involved with the right of privacy, abortion, and personhood, and concludes with a strong preference for preserving the privacy of the abortion decision and for sanctioning personal definitions of what it means to be a human being and a person. John Robertson discusses some of the medicolegal ramifications of bestowing personhood status to the unborn, and argues that the approach of defining the conceptus as a person with the intention of outlawing abortion might not be successful for a variety of legal reasons. David Westfall outlines how proposed constitutional amendments and statutory changes could affect such areas of the law as legislative apportionment, income tax exemptions, estate planning, the scope of tort liability, and the distribution of fiscal benefits. Moreover, he asserts that such laws would cause major alterations in the way health care is delivered, in women's employment options, and in their personal lifestyles.

Part Four of the book concerns ethical, cultural, and religious perspectives on personhood. The three chapters were written by a medical ethicist, a lawyer/philosopher, and a sociologist who described herself as "a feminist, social democrat, anti-abortionist." In her chapter, Ruth Macklin considers the ethical conflict posed by a situation in which there are two persons but only one body. Using analogies to Siamese twins and to the multiple personality syndrome in psychiatric patients, Macklin discusses a number of positions to resolve the abortion issue, and concludes that even granting the fetus the status of a person is not sufficient to warrant a conclusion that the fetus' right to life overrides the rights of the woman who is carrying it. Bernard Dickens presents a detailed and well-documented comparative review of international abortion policies and abortion laws. He reviews the historical perspectives on the commencement of protected life showing the significance of different periods after conception to the definition and punishment of abortion. Dickens notes that the necessity to save life and to protect against grave risks to health are widely recognized legal indications for abortion, and that a number of countries accommodate such grounds as rape, incest, or serious potential handicap of the child. The use of the abortion law as a tool of state population policy in Romania, Czechoslovakia, and Poland is also examined. In the last chapter of this section, Sidney Callahan discusses the impact of religious and other beliefs on our attitudes toward abortion and articulates a position frequently ignored in the abortion debate—that of a feminist who is opposed to abortion as an attack upon a defenseless and "second-class" individual (much like women were thought to be).

Part Five moves the discussion of the issues surrounding personhood, human life, and fetus-person into the future, and examines the direction, capabilities, and political implications of our expanding biotechnology. Part Five starts with a paper by medical geneticist Leon Rosenberg in which he discusses the rapid developments of our knowledge concerning human genetics and how such knowledge is transferred to the bedside to facilitate medical diagnosis and treatment. Rosenberg sees great promise in our ability to correct many genetic defects by enzyme therapy and gene replacement using the newly developed techniques of recombinant DNA. But he also sees the need to retain the alternative of abortion since it remains the only effective "treatment" for many other genetic conditions which will not be treatable in the foreseeable future. Daniel Callahan, Director of the Hastings Center, assesses the role of science in moral and societal decision making, and observes that everyone would like to have science on his or her side of an argument, especially when a difficult question like abortion is involved. There are, however, problems which arise when one relies upon science to provide answers to moral issues. He concludes by asserting that science can provide facts but cannot make normative decisions for society.

In the concluding remarks of the symposium, Dr. Bentley Glass, distinguished professor of biology emeritus at the State University of New York at Stony Brook, offers a moving, sensitive, and insightful summation of the conference presentations, as well as some thoughts to stimulate further reflection on this troublesome question. Perhaps that is the simple objective of this book as well.

A. Edward Doudera, J.D.
Boston, Massachusetts
June 1982

Introduction

Abortion ranks with school busing, school prayer, the teaching of scientific creationism, and sex education as one of the most hotly debated moral issues of the 1980s, both within and outside the federal government. On January 22, 1973, the United States Supreme Court decided, in *Roe v. Wade*,[1] that the constitutional right of privacy encompasses a woman's decision, made in consultation with her physician, whether or not to have an abortion under certain prescribed conditions. Nonetheless, that right has been challenged by individuals, groups, and state legislatures. Even the United States Congress has not been silent. During the middle and late 1970s, many amendments to bills were passed restricting the availability of funds for elective abortions in federal facilities. Although most of the earlier court challenges to the letter and spirit of *Roe v. Wade* went unrewarded,[2] two recent Court decisions suggest the beginning of an erosion of constitutional rights to abortion. In the first, the federal government was not required to fund medically necessary abortions under the Social Security Act,[3] and, in the second case, the Court upheld a state statute requiring that the parents of an immature, unemancipated minor be notified prior to performing an abortion.[4]

With the hindsight of nine years since *Roe v. Wade*, many of these controversies seem like minor skirmishes compared to the more direct assaults being made in Congress today. I am referring to various legislation introduced by Senators Helms, Hatch, and Hatfield.

Senator Jesse Helms (R-N.C.) has introduced various Human Life Statutes (S. 158, S. 1741, and S. 2148) which would legislatively define the term "person" to include the unborn from the moment of conception for the purpose of guaranteeing a right to life under the Fourteenth Amendment. The Human Life Federalism Amendment (S. J. Res. 110), sponsored by Senator Orrin Hatch (R-Utah), would give Congress and the states the authority to legislate on abortion issues and would restrict judicial review. Senator Mark Hatfield (D-Ore.) has introduced a bill (S. 2372) that seeks to prohibit the teaching of abortion techniques in any institution which receives federal funds and prohibits the performance of abortions in these same institutions unless the mother's life is endangered by the continuation of her pregnancy.

Most legal scholars agree that the Helms statutes would serve only as delaying tactics because they would probably not survive Supreme Court scrutiny and would be declared unconstitutional. On the other hand, the Amendment proposed by Senator Hatch would be a perfectly legitimate method of reversing the *Roe v. Wade* decision, but it requires a two-thirds vote in both houses of Congress and ratification by three-fourths of the state legislatures. In the present climate, with a lack of consensus on the abortion issue, this achievement seems highly unlikely. The Hatfield Bill may become moot. As federal funding for human services dwindles, it may be unnecessary to target abortions as a single issue in the appropriations debate.

It is in this climate that we find ourselves today. The abortion controversy is far from settled, and expecting to reach a consensus on this emotional issue would be naive. Perhaps the only solution is the political art of compromise, which requires that all parties be informed of all the competing positions. There must be a willingness to listen to each other's rational and irrational concerns and a readiness to debate, bargain, mediate, conciliate, and negotiate. Only in this spirit can a lasting and peaceful solution be reached rather than simply a temporary cessation of hostilities.

The symposium from which the following papers and discussions were collected represented a first small step in the negotiations. When Edward Doudera and I first began to plan this meeting last summer we asked, "What do we hope to accomplish?" Our hopes were modest. We did not expect the emotionalism of the abortion controversy to wane, nor did we expect agreement on the issues among diverse groups. Rather, we hoped only for rational discussion and a chance for cross-disciplinary education: if a constitutional lawyer learned something from an embryologist, if an obstetrician learned something from a philosopher, then our hopes would be fulfilled.

The conference sought to illuminate the issues in the abortion controversy as viewed from the perspectives of medicine and law. While several philosophical perspectives were included, we did not try to be all-inclusive in a three-day conference. We omitted economic, anthropological, and political considerations because of lack of time. We also omitted in-depth discussions of the religious aspects of abortion attitudes from the perspectives of Roman Catholicism, Judaism (Orthodox, Conservative, and Reform) and the various denominations of Protestantism. Other symposia have addressed this topic.

Our symposium began with a biologist's viewpoint. As Theodosius Dobzhansky once wrote, "A coherent credo can neither be derived from science nor arrived at without science."[5] Thus, science seems to be a good place to start.

Margery W. Shaw, M.D., J.D.
Houston, Texas
March 1982

NOTES

1. Roe v. Wade, 410 U.S. 113 (1973).
2. *See, e.g.*, Planned Parenthood v. Danforth, 428 U.S. 52 (1976).
3. Harris v. McRae, 448 U.S. 297 (1980).
4. H.L. v. Matheson, 450 U.S. 398 (1981).
5. Van Den Hoof, A., *It Has Been Said*, PERSPECTIVES IN BIOLOGY AND MEDICINE 24:67 (1980) (quoting T. Dobzhansky).

Part One

Definition of Personhood

Chapter 1

A Biological Perspective on the Origin of Human Life and Personhood

Clifford Grobstein

Scientific information currently leads to the conclusion that the origin of human life took place a long time ago. Exactly when depends upon the selected definition of human. Humanoid creatures date back several million years, members of our own particular biological species perhaps hundreds of thousands of years. The important point is that by whatever definition, once human life appeared it passed from generation to generation in a continuing line. In fact, all contemporary earthly life has descended in an unbroken, always living lineage that was initiated, by most recent conceptions, not much more than a half billion years after the earth condensed within the solar nebula.

To ask when human life begins in a given life cycle, then, is a confused and confusing biological question. The sperm and egg that fuse in fertilization are living and human by scientific critiera, but their union neither enlivens nor humanizes the resulting fusion-cell or zygote. It does, however, do two other important things. It activates the egg to continue the life cycle and it introduces into the egg a set of chromosomes from the father that, together with the maternally derived set, becomes a new and unique genetic constitution or genotype. If one is asking when a new genetic constitution comes into being, the answer is at fertilization.

However, the new genetic constitution is in a single cell—a unit to which the concept of person does not ordinarily extend. For example, *Webster's Third International Dictionary* takes two and three-quarter inches of small print to convey the several meanings of person without mentioning a cell. The first definition is an "individual human being," further elaborated upon as distinguishable from an animal or thing. One and three-quarter inches later, Webster's explanation refers to the individual personality of a human being and abruptly throws in the term "self." Other meanings cited include a body of persons, as in a corporation, and a being characterized by conscious apprehension, rationality and a moral sense. All this should clarify why a biologist is more comfortable talking about a zygote as a cell and has great difficulty equating it with a person.

On the other hand, the zygote is not an ordinary cell as its subsequent behavior makes clear. It first divides by mitosis, obviously an entirely cellular thing to do. Even though the cells that are produced by early divisions are encased and in close proximity, they do not adhere to each other for several divisions. It is several days before the amorphous cellular mass produced by division begins to reshape and eventually permits a trained eye to discern the beginning of a simple body axis with a forward and a hind end. With still more time this embryo becomes recognizable as an early animal; still later it matures into a human-like fetus and then into a recognizable human infant. Thus, the fertilized egg is an unusual cell that, under appropriate conditions, can turn into a person recognizable by Webster's criteria. It is, therefore, a special kind of cell not because it is living and human but because of its remarkable capability to transform into a recognizable person.

But is this capability to be equated with a later actualized person? Not biologically, from the evidence in nonhuman species. An example of such evidence involves twinning, in which the fertilized egg with its unique genotype can become more than one new individual. In armadillos, in fact, the developing egg regularly splits to give rise to four new individuals—a litter of identical beings with the same genotype but separate individualities. In humans and other species this happens irregularly. The important point is that a unique genotype need not equate with a single biological individual; an identical genotype may be shared among many genetically identical individuals. Secondly, under experimental conditions, a unique genotype may be represented in only part of one individual. An example occurs in the experimental fusion of two mouse embryos of different genotypes at the four-cell stage, producing a single individual whose cells are a mosaic of both genotypes. The whole embryo is genetically derived from four parents. In addition, if four- and eight-celled embryos of some mammalian species are separated into individual cells, single cells that are only one-fourth or one-eighth of the original zygote may give rise to whole individuals, even though they would normally contribute to only a part. All of these observations indicate that establishing a unique genotype at fertilization is not equivalent to establishing a single individual in the developmental sense. The products of early divisions of the fertilized egg remain a collection of cells whose actualization as less than one, one, or more than one individual is strongly susceptible to circumstance.

CELLULAR DEVELOPMENT AND PERSONHOOD

What Webster's dictionary does not say is that a person, in common parlance, is an individual with billions of cells of hundreds of kinds which were derived from a single egg cell, and which are now integrated in their behavior into the singleness we recognize in people—and in ourselves. When is such multicellular singleness that is *sine qua non* for human individuality established? In our own species we cannot provide a precise answer. But if we rely once again on other species that can be studied in ways that humans cannot, the process of achieving singleness is found to be gradual. Eight-cell stages begin to adhere and to establish intercellular communication. At later stages, two different cellular subpopulations can be distinguished—an outer and an inner. It is only the so-called inner cell mass that is the precursor of the later embryo; the outer layer of cells forms external membranes including part of the placenta. At this stage it is still possible to induce twinning by splitting of the inner cell mass; so, fully integrated multicellular singleness is yet to be achieved. Such singleness, however, probably appears soon after, at about the time when the developing embryo implants in the uterine wall.

Does developmentally achieved multicellular singleness satisfy Webster's definition of a person? Hardly, if the requirements include distinction from other animal life, expression of individual personality, or the presence of conscious apprehension, rationality, and a moral sense. At the time of implantation there is still no body form; only an expert could distinguish the human from any other mammal at this stage, and it would be difficult to conceive what individual personality means in such a lowly state of multicellular organization. Yet something important and consequential clearly occurs at implantation. The developing offspring is not only beginning to be integrated within itself, but it is also integrated into a larger system of order—the mother. From this point on the offspring, although usually yet unnoticed, is the subject of maternal nurture and, somewhat later, of maternal and social concern. A mother-offspring unit has been formed, and thereon hangs much of the current debate about the time of origin of personhood. If the developing offspring is a person at this stage then two persons exist in temporary interpenetrating union. The life of one impinges upon the life of the other, and if their interests diverge, there is conflict between the "rights" of the two assumed persons.

Biologically, the offspring at this stage is starting to be characterized as an embryo. The best definition of an embryo is that it is a rudimentary being—the various structures and functions of the adult are making detectable appearance but are not yet recognizable by their definitive characteristics. Rather, rudiments are recognized by premonitory changes occurring at the appropriate place in the forming embryo. A good example are limb rudiments, appearing on the flanks of the embryo at places corresponding to the fore and hind limbs. The first sign is thickening of the surface and the layer of cells below. Initially there is no other hint of what is to come—no muscles, no bones, no fingers or toes. But the presence of what are called limb buds is a typical event in the emergence of body form.

Similarly, a rudiment forms along the midline of the elongating body axis. First seen as an external groove, it closes over and sinks beneath the embryo's surface as the rudiment of the central nervous system, the spinal cord, and the brain. As with the limb bud, the rudimentary central nervous system forms by reshaping part of the earlier proliferating multicellular mass. In its initial stages it shows none of the characteristics of the adult nervous system, no recognizable nerve cells, no synaptic connections among them, no neurotransmitters that are so essential for conduction of nerve impulses from place to place. What exists in the rudiment can be compared to an area of land that has been cleared by bulldozers and roughly shaped so that one may see where streets and individual building sites are expected to be. In community developer language this is site preparation, the result of which is far from achieving the status of a new neighborhood. In the same fashion, the rudiment of the human nervous system at roughly four to six weeks of development can be thought of as undergoing site preparation although it is not yet a nervous system.

This raises some basic issues of the concept of person. As a biologist, I regard what we ordinarily mean by the term as in part biological and in part something else. When Webster's dictionary says that a person is distinguishable from an animal or a thing, it is referring to the biological component of person: to be a person one must be both alive and distinguishable from an animal (other kinds of living things). One must belong to humankind, the biological species Homo sapiens.

NEURAL DEVELOPMENT, SENTIENCE AND PERSONHOOD

Species membership can be established entirely by biological criteria, whether by anatomical examination, chromosome analysis, compatibility of gametes, or sequence of components in proteins and DNA. But these biological criteria are not enough to settle all questions about persons or to include all connotations listed by Webster's dictionary. The level of connotation above the biological has to do with words like personality, self, and consciousness. These terms are not coined or defined by biologists but reach toward a higher level of phenomena that are more often considered in their rational aspects by psychology and philosophy, and in their spiritual and mystical aspects by the arts and religion. However, while the terms are not biological in their origin or essence, personality, self, and consciousness assume a biological substrate in that they are not assigned to nonliving systems and reach their highest level of expression in living human beings. Whatever else the terms may involve, it is a legitimate biological task to define the minimal substrates for states that achieve personality, selfness, and consciousness. Let us call these states subjective awareness.

Biologists, particularly neurobiologists, have been moving toward this task. Communication on these matters has also increased among neurobiologists, psychologists, and philosophers, even if this somewhat incongruous alliance has yet to yield either a bright light of understanding or even general enthusiasm among the disciplines involved. Certain points of agreement have, however, emerged. For example, states of awareness are increasingly regarded as associated with the function of complex neural networks, in particular those occurring in the adult human brain. How complex these networks must be and what organizational patterns they must have is not known, and the determination is complicated by special methodological difficulties. But the networks clearly depend upon large numbers of neurons or rich synaptic connectivity. Moreover, synaptic transmitters and their antagonists exert powerful influences upon subjective awareness, including the capability to modify or extinguish it temporarily or permanently. It appears unlikely, then, that subjective awareness can be present when an adequate neural substrate is absent. This growing recognition is having practical consequence in the current tendency to equate brain death, when adequately documented scientifically, with legal death—that is, the termination of brain function is equated with the termination of a person regardless of what other vital signs may exist.

What bearing does this have on the initiation of a person? While it is clearly relevant, the relationship must be interpreted with caution. Technically, brain death is equated with sustained total loss of electrical activity throughout the brain. There are cases in which electrical activity persists in the brain stem in totally comatose individuals capable of continued autonomous respiration and circulation, such as Karen Ann Quinlan, suggesting that some electrical activity is unrelated to volitional behavior even though it accompanies continued vegetative functions. One may not conclude, therefore, that the onset of electrical activity in developing fetuses is concurrent with sentience or volition, particularly when the electrical activity is far more difficult to detect and is different in pattern from that of the adult.

With these caveats in mind, it is nonetheless reasonable to assume that subjective awareness will not arise before neural maturation, synaptic connectivity, and neurotransmitter activity has reached some critical level. Much more knowledge will be required before the critical level can be specified precisely. Moreover, it will always be desirable to resolve doubt on the safe side and assume subjective awareness is present unless the basis for excluding it is certain. For example, stages prior to appearance of neuronal connectivity and neurotransmitters in some upper level of the brain might be defined to be prior to subjective awareness, even though these criteria are satisfied in lower brain levels. Since, however, we cannot yet specify how low in the brain stem the most primitive mechanisms for sentience may lie, we should err on the side of caution until more clinical information is available from brain-damaged individuals or premature fetal-infants.

A particularly difficult issue is interpretation of the significance of spontaneous and induced fetal movements. These begin at about eight weeks, as judged by direct observation on therapeutically aborted embryos. If such embryos are quickly transferred to a suitable saline solution they respond to tactile stimulation around the mouth by head-turning movements. This behavior implies, and suitable histological observation confirms, that by this time neural connections have been established from the skin to the central nervous system and back out to muscles of the neck. While a neurological substrate has been established for a simple reflex arc, does such an arc provide the essential state for sentience and awareness? Most experts believe that this is not the case. The neural net is relatively simple and lacks connections with the upper brain, particularly with the reticular formation and the cortex. Moreover, similar behavior is observed in decorticate cats, in some comatose humans, and even in severe meningocoele, all presumed to be without sentience.

Such early primitive reflexes become stronger and more diverse as development progresses and are followed by spontaneous movements several weeks later. By 18 to 20 weeks vigorous spontaneous movements are recognized by the mother as quickening. Again we may ask whether this activity represents conscious volition, and here the answer must be more tentative. The cortex is still quite immature at this stage and descriptions provided by observers of prematurely delivered infants are suggestive but far from definitive. Some examples from the technical literature paraphrased in lay language will give the flavor of current opinion.

A recent summary of observations on exteriorized human fetuses concludes that reflex activities displayed up to 18 to 20 weeks involve the spinal cord and lower brain centers but precede formation of the complex functional networks of the upper brain. The neurological situation is roughly comparable to that assumed to exist in the stable comatose state displayed by Karen Ann Quinlan, a state short of the current definition of brain death. If equivalently interpreted, sufficient maturation of the central nervous system is present at 18 to 20 weeks to constitute a gray zone with respect to onset of personhood. It should be noted, however, that at this stage the cerebral lobes, site of the most complex neural nets and the dominant component in the mass of the adult brain, are little more than half of the total brain mass and maturation of their nerve cells has barely begun. The relative mass of the cerebral lobes increases sharply in the second trimester but its still greater enlargement through folding and the complex interconnectedness of its neurons does not occur until the third trimester and continues into postnatal life.

Observations on the behavior of prematurely delivered infants are of interest at this point. Recorded detailed observations on their behavior begin at around 28 weeks, about the beginning of the third trimester. Gesell refers to the behavior at this stage as that of a "loosely articulated mannikin," flaccid in all joints. When disturbed the infant becomes briefly active but soon "dissolves into a limp and torporous desuetude." Torpor is the most conspicuous and consistent behavior with no clear-cut distinctions between activities and rest. The "state is so ambiguous that one scarcely knows whether he is still asleep when he moves or whether he may not actually be awake even when quiescent." There are mild responses to stimuli but these quickly dissolve into drowsy quiescence. Head and facial regions appear to be alive, albeit not attentively alert. Fragmented and uncoordinated facial gestures occur, the frequency and nature of which are such that "one might conclude that Nature is preparing the infant for a histrionic career."[1]

By 32 to 36 weeks the infant shows more forceful and integrated behavior but still "weak, indifferent and unresponsive. There are, however, brief periods of wakeful alertness. Again and again during the day (and night) he pricks the surface of mere being with moments of true wakefulness." Gesell suggests that at this stage the infant is "more than a mere spinal creature," that the subcortical thalamic region of the brain may be sufficiently mature to be the site of primitive awareness. Gesell's impressionistic observations suggest that several weeks before normal term a rudiment of subjective awareness, flickering and fluctuating, may be making its first appearance.

Such a behavioral rudiment of awareness, if it were appearing at about 30 weeks (early third trimester) would be in rough correspondence with microanatomical changes observed in the maturing cerebral cortex.

At 25 weeks a section of the cortex shows scattered neuronal cell bodies with distinct elongating processes but limited branching and very few synaptic connections. By 33 weeks, however, branching of processes is extensive and synaptic connections are numerous. Even at this later stage, of course, the branching and connectivity is quantitatively only a small fraction of the profuseness achieved during the first year or two of postnatal life. It is during the early postnatal period that the professional observer of infant behavior becomes convinced that the developing infant is achieving individual personality, a sense of self and conscious apprehension of surrounding events. Rationality and a moral sense, referred to by Webster as aspects of the definition of a person, do not convincingly appear until later yet—and as products not only of inner maturation but of social interaction.

CONCLUSION

This overly brief and necessarily oversimplified biological account of human developmental history is not intended to suggest a precise point at which the term "person" is properly applied. On the contrary, the account emphasizes that the concept of person is only partly biological and that even those of its components that are biological come gradually into existence. Genetic individuality is a biological component and is established during fertilization at the single-cell level. Multicellularity comes next but singleness at this level is not established for perhaps two weeks, closely associated with fusion of the developing offspring with the tissues of the mother. The offspring now develops within the fusion zone as a rudimentary embryo, with various parts being blocked out but not even its biological parts yet in their definitive form. Among the rudiments is that of the central nervous system and particularly the brain. As this system matures behavior begins, at first quite simple and then increasingly complex. Forceful and integrated behavior such as we associate with persons in the usual context seems to appear first midway in the third trimester, along with maturational changes in the upper brain. Professional behavioral observers have described this behavior as though it indicated a rudimentary and fluctuating subjective awareness, possibly the first appearance of a consciousness of self.

   With the achievement of subjective awareness, the further development of personhood increasingly becomes the scientific province of the social and behavioral sciences. Of course, biological maturation continues to play a role and alterations of the biological substratum can at any time have important consequences for the state of personhood. However, such

Some philosophers use the term person in a purely moral sense. To them, it is simply shorthand for "entity which ought to be given special rights." While the list of special rights may vary from author to author, the right not to be killed for others' convenience is always included. For example, the philosopher Michael Tooley consciously uses the term in this way: "'Person'. . . [shall mean a creature with] a moral right to life."[3]

I call this the *prescriptive* use of person and personhood because the terms do not describe in any way—they merely call for certain kinds of treatment. There is nothing inherently misleading about this usage, but it renders certain sorts of arguments about abortion empty. The statement, "Fetuses should not be killed by abortion because they are persons," becomes true by definition if "person" is used prescriptively.

In the *descriptive* use, the relation of the concept of personhood to ethics is less direct because the term is associated with a group of characteristics typical of entities which we intuitively think of as persons. Examples of these characteristics include being born of human beings and being an organism capable of rationality. Additional steps in the argument are required before any moral conclusion or prescription can be derived. A philosopher might, for example, attempt to demonstrate that capacity for rationality is sufficient reason to ascribe a right to life.

In the balance of this paper, "person" will be used descriptively. The aim will be to contrast the different types of descriptive content which have been expressed by "person" in the literature on abortion and elsewhere.

Preliminary to that, however, I want to distinguish two other topics. First, the sort of personhood of which we speak here is not a legal concept. Corporations and other institutional entities are considered legal persons for certain purposes, but this notion of personhood does not correspond to the moral or philosophical one with which we are concerned. The law creates its own categories according to its own requirements, and there is no good reason to insist that legal persons also be persons in the ordinary sense, or vice versa. In any case, much of the moral debate over personhood is carried on in order to change the law, and the result is intended to be a revision of the prevailing law.

Second, this paper is not concerned with potential personhood. Those who ascribe a right to life to fetuses because they are potential persons implicitly acknowledge that fetuses are not (yet) actual persons. Our subject is, instead, whether fetuses are actual persons—i.e., whether they are persons while they are fetuses.

BIOLOGICAL AND PSYCHOLOGICAL
CONCEPTS OF PERSONHOOD

As one philosopher has suggested,[4] it may be misleading to speak of rival theories of personhood since there is no single subject that such theories seek to describe. Broadly speaking, concepts of personhood can be sorted into two categories. According to the first, a person is a biological organism. According to the second, a person is a psychological entity, a being with mental properties. Obviously these two views are not mutually exclusive.

THE BIOLOGICAL CONCEPT: DOES SCIENCE DEFINE PERSONHOOD?

The biological concept of personhood has figured prominently in the popular debate over abortion. It is this concept which is, perhaps, most often expressed when the phrase "human being" is used in place of "person." However, the exact nature of the biological concept is rarely made clear.

In much of the writing on abortion, the debate is said to center on *when life begins* and the *definition of life*.[5] Right-to-life advocates point to evidence of biological activity in the just-fertilized egg to support their claim that life begins at conception. The implication seems to be that since fertilized eggs are alive, fertilized eggs are persons. These are, of course, the claims of the Human Life Statute being considered by the United States Senate.[6]

However, this line of reasoning is unconvincing. Sperm and egg are also (usually) alive, yet no one suggests that the life in either constitutes personhood. Why, then, should we ponder the life processes of the fertilized egg? Being alive does not itself fulfill the biological sense of personhood.

A second approximation to the biological concept fixes on the notion of being human, in the sense of belonging to the species Homo sapiens. It is pointed out by right-to-life advocates that the fertilized egg is human in its genetic makeup, distinct even at this early stage from all other forms of life. Again, however, it is difficult to show that this fact has much importance in itself. Sperm and egg are also certifiably human in that human sperm are different from sperm of other species. So, for that matter, are skin cells and all other cells making up a human body. The fact that the fertilized egg is both living and human does not distinguish it from the unfertilized egg or other cells. Since ordinary cells are never considered persons, we may conclude that the biological sense of person is not defined by these two characteristics.

We arrive at the biological concept by adding a third element: individuality. The biological concept of personhood is that of an entity which is not only alive and of the species Homo sapiens, but is an individual in its own right. It is not merely a part of any other individual, nor is it simply material from which an individual will sometime arise.

This three-element analysis of the biological concept of the individual permits the right-to-life advocate to respond to certain common objections. One of these, pressed by several biologists, attacks the right-to-life position by insisting that life, far from beginning at conception, actually predates conception. Dr. Joshua Lederberg, for example, states:

> There is no single, simple answer to ["when does life begin?"] . . . In contemporary experience, life in fact never begins—it is a continuum from generation to generation.[7]

Lederberg correctly suggests that the fertilized egg is alive only to the extent that the sperm and the unfertilized egg and all which preceded them are also alive. But the argument does not succeed in its goal of showing that personhood does not date from conception. The argument's insistence that life is continuous across generations is consistent with the claim that new individuals come into and then pass out of existence. Life may be continuous over eons, but individuals are not. The right-to-life position, interpreted as concerned with the advent of living human individuals, is left unscathed.

The right-to-life position is not, however, made secure by this reply, for there are other views of the point at which living human individuals commence. Several other milestones of human development (including implantation, time of possible twinning, attainment of a recognizably human form, heartbeat, quickening, viability, and birth) have all been meant to count as the beginning of biological individuality. Viability and birth, for example, are each thought to mark the "moment" when the fetus ceases to be a part of the mother and becomes a creature in its own right. Detection of the heartbeat may be thought of as evidence that the component parts of an individual (the major organ systems) have at least been assembled into a functioning individual organism. Proponents of recognizing these later milestones as the moment when personhood begins claim that the fertilized egg is not yet a biological individual.

How might we choose between these claims? Is there an objective answer to the question of when biological individuality begins? Right-to-life advocates often state that science, particularly genetics, decides the issue for us. This claim, however, has been strongly denied by scientists of late. For example, in his Senate testimony on the Human Life Statute, Leon Rosenberg said:

> [I] know of no scientific evidence which bears on the question of when actual human life exists; . . . I believe that the notion embodied in the phrase "actual human life" is not a scientific one, but rather a philosophic and religious one.[8]

He also quotes Dr. Lewis Thomas:

> [It] is therefore in the domain of metaphysics: it can be argued by philosophers and theologians, but it lies beyond the reach of science.[9]

Similarly, the membership of the National Academy of Sciences passed a resolution that the beginning of human life is "a question to which science can provide no answer."[10] It should be noted that these scientists are not merely stating that science does not yet have all answers to every question, but denying that the question, "What is a person?" is a scientific one at all. Further, this suggests that scientists have criteria for deciding what is science and what is not. Rosenberg, in fact, offers such a rule:

> The scientific method depends on two essential things—a thesis or idea and a means of testing that idea. Scientists have been able to determine, for instance, that the Earth is round or that genes are composed of DNA because, and only because, experiments could be performed to test these ideas. Without experiments there is no science, no way to prove or disprove any idea. I maintain that concepts such as humanness are beyond the purview of science because no idea about them can be tested experimentally.[11]

This argument was crucially important in the hearings on the Human Life Statute. The legislative strategy of the right-to-life forces depended on obtaining a Congressional declaration that the dating of human life from conception is a scientific fact. There was, as it happened, hardly any disagreement over the (other) scientific facts concerning human development. The only issue was whether the claim that personhood dates from conception was one of these facts. This is an issue of philosophy of science, and Rosenberg's criterion for deciding what is and what is not science is in fact a claim within philosophy rather than science.

The definition of science is as difficult an issue as the definition of personhood and cannot be argued in depth here. It may be noted, however, that Rosenberg's criterion would disenfranchise much of what is universally regarded as basic science. It is particularly unacceptable when applied to scientific work involving classification. The periodic table of the elements, for example, is one of the great accomplishments of chemistry; is there any experiment which can "prove" that its classification of boron with carbon is correct? And what experiment confirms the criteria used by the zoologist in support of the claim that whales are mammals? These classifications, definitions, and taxonomies are a vital part of science, yet they cannot be proved or disproved in the laboratory. They are accepted or rejected on other grounds, particularly in regard to their utility in ordering other scientific data, permitting useful generalizations and inferences.

I do not have a definition of science to propose in place of Rosenberg's. It does seem to me, however, that the definition of "individual

Homo sapiens" may be compared to the scientific definitions and classifications just mentioned. It is up to the scientist to tell us whether whales are mammals and to tell us what lead and silicon are. We will also be likely to rely on zoologists to speak with authority on what counts as death for a virus or bacterium. Why, then, should it be different in determining what qualifies as a new human individual? Why should it be unscientific for a zoologist to propose, for example, that newly fertilized human eggs, or newly implanted ones, or newly born ones be classified as new individuals for our species; and, further, for this zoologist to attempt to argue for his or her new classification scheme in the same manner that other taxonomies, definitions, and classifications are defended?

These questions challenge the widely-aired view that personhood is obviously not definable by science. My suggestion is that if personhood is understood as being a living individual Homo sapiens, then defining personhood is not obviously different from defining "whalehood" or "goldhood." We do not challenge science's authority to define these latter classes. If the definition of personhood were perfectly analogous with these, we should indeed regard it as a scientific matter and should not accuse scientists who testify in the Senate of passing off their personal, moral, or religious opinions in the guise of scientific expertise.

Thus, "living individual Homo sapiens" is the sort of concept which biology might define. Whether it actually does so or not is, I believe, an open question at present. At issue is whether any particular definition, precise enough to date the advent of individuality to a specific point of fetal development, has the kind of scientific utility which mandates its acceptance as a fact of biological science. To establish the claim that biology dates personhood (in this sense) back to the moment of fertilization would require an exercise in biological theory showing that important generalizations and concepts of the science do in fact define "individual living Homo sapiens" in this way. Moreover, the investigation must show that the generalizations must thus define the concept––that is, that this definition is not adopted merely for ease of exposition, or because of tradition, or (we should now add) in order to make science seem to support a certain position on the abortion question.

There are some reasons to doubt that biology does furnish us with a definition meeting this test. For one thing, the definition of "individual of the species" to which we would look for help in the abortion debate would be drawn from biology as a whole. Yet there are numerous organisms which exist (or should we say, "parts of which exist"?) for long periods in the haploid state. To call these "individuals" of the species would suggest doing so for human sperm or egg—not the result we seek. Further, the various disciplines within biology may define "individual" differently. To the geneticist, a new generation of chickens begins when the new genotypes are formed. Perhaps the ecologist starts counting heads only when the eggs hatch and interaction begins, thus raising the possibility that biology defines "individual living member of the species" in more than one way. A multiplicity of biological definitions would make a scientific defense of conception as the starting point for personhood more difficult to mount.

These considerations do not, however, eliminate the possibility of discovering within biology a precise and univocal definition of the individual living member of the human species. My remarks concerning the possibilities of haploid individuals and a multiplicity of definitions are only conjectures. Fetuses seem to be treated as individuals (as opposed to parts of individuals, or materials from which individuals will be formed) in a lot of biology. I regard this as a topic worthy of further research, and leave it to another occasion (and to other hands). Our short discussion supports only the claim that, even though it may be entirely appropriate to look to biological science for a definition of individual living Homo sapiens, we have no guarantee, before engaging in some demanding work in biological theory, that biology has a definition to give.

BIOLOGY AND MORALITY

My discussion thus leaves open the possibility that the right-to-life forces win one round: it may be a fact of biology that, as they insist, "life begins at conception," where this phrase is understood to mean that a living individual Homo sapiens comes into existence at that point. If sustained, these conclusions would support the right-to-life position against a certain class of its critics. These critics hold, first, that the morality of abortion largely depends on whether the fetus is a person; second, that "person" means living individual Homo sapiens; and, third, that fetuses become living individual Homo sapiens at some point later than conception, such as viability or birth. Some of those who hold these positions insist that their views are purely personal, moral, or religious, but my argument suggests that they may be mistaken on this point. If biology supports a definition of the individual living Homo sapiens as beginning at conception, then alternative definitions are simply wrong. Analogously, a man who classified fool's gold as gold would be objectively wrong even if he did so for personal, moral, or religious reasons. If, as I believe, many of those who date the onset of personhood at implantation, first heartbeat, viability, or birth are appealing to the biological conception of personhood, they will have to submit their claims to the same biological arbiter to whom the right-to-life forces have appealed; and they may lose.

A much stronger argument for dating personhood later than conception begins by abandoning the biological concept altogether. The fundamental claim is that the biological definition of person, whatever it may turn out to be, does not determine the outcome of the moral debate, and in fact is nearly irrelevant to it.

From the importance which it attaches to the biological conception of personhood, we may presume that the pro-life argument rests on an implied claim that membership in our species is reason enough to ascribe a right to life. The plausibility of this thesis derives, for most who accept it, from religious belief—particularly the belief that God made a covenant with humans and not with other species. Whatever its origin, the principle seems to be assumed or embedded in much of our ordinary thinking about morality. So-called "human rights," for example, are rights ascribed to humans on no other basis than membership in our species. We demonstrate our respect for these rights in countless ways (though they are, of course, often violated). For example, profoundly retarded humans are protected from the same dangerous medical experiments that we routinely perform on relatively intelligent animals.

Nevertheless, and perhaps surprisingly, the thesis that humans should be ascribed rights simply for being human has received practically no support from philosophers.[12] Indeed, the thesis has come under attack from an articulate group of philosophers who, in arguing for better treatment of animals, brand the thesis "speciesism," an ethical sin akin to racism.[13] According to these philosophers, both speciesism and racism attempt to justify discrimination on the basis of morally irrelevant criteria—i.e., membership in a species and membership in a race. Evaluation of this argument cannot be attempted here, but it should be noted that most of their philosophical opponents avoid speciesism and argue the case for humans and against animals on some basis other than mere membership in the species.

From these arguments, it follows that efforts to resolve the abortion dispute by seeking to define biological personhood are not so much erroneous as they are misdirected. The precise moment at which one becomes an individual living member of our species has no moral importance because being a member of our species, in itself, is not important. Thus, in this view, the argument with which we began—that abortions are wrong because fetuses are persons—cannot be accepted if "person" is understood in its biological sense. No moral conclusions would flow from the fact, even if it were a fact, that "fetuses are persons" in this sense. The task then becomes to find what *is* relevant in determining who has a right to life and to other benefits of primary moral status. This motivates our consideration of psychological concepts of personhood.

PSYCHOLOGICAL CONCEPTS OF PERSONHOOD

Daniel Dennet, a leading contemporary philosopher, begins a recent paper on personhood with these lines: "I am a person. So are you. I'm a human. So *probably* are you."[14] This passage goes part of the way toward stating a concept of personhood which is quite different from the biological one. Dennett's lines reflect his prior knowledge, as an author, that any beings who can read his essay with comprehension (all of whom would be addressed in his use of the second person) will be thinking and perhaps rational creatures. Dennett cannot be sure, however, that his reader is an individual living Homo sapiens, since he believes it is possible that some nonhumans are, or will be, thinking, comprehending beings. Who might these be? Perhaps someday they could be aliens or computers. It does not matter that such thinkers have not yet presented themselves; the philosophical point requires only that we admit the conceptual possibility that such entities could think.

The psychological concepts of personhood, then, share the requirement that persons have the capacity for thinking or, at a minimum, possess awareness or consciousness. Some sort of psychological concept of personhood seems to be involved in several milestones which have been claimed to mark the advent of personhood, such as onset of brainwaves, sentience, and development of the concept of self. It is not involved, so far as I know, in any of the definitions of person used by those who date actual (as opposed to potential) personhood from the moment of conception.

"Thing which thinks" is, however, too simple a definition of psychological personhood. Even when restricting attention to psychological versions, the term person covers a wide range of concepts in philosophical writing. Mere consciousness may be sufficient for the purposes of investigating the mind-body question, in that one can pose the question, "Is the person something over and above the body?" with respect to a near-comatose individual capable of only simple awareness. A philosopher interested primarily in the problem of personal identity might use other criteria, such as Locke's notion of a thing with a concept of self and knowledge of its history. Moral philosophers differ among themselves, depending on the content of their moral philosophy. At one extreme, the hedonistic utilitarian (concerned primarily with maximizing pleasure and minimizing pain) takes an interest in all creatures capable of pleasurable or painful experiences. A Kantian, on the other hand, might exclude from the category of persons a fully conscious, functioning philosophy professor if he happens to be a sociopath incapable of acting on duty.[15] Other theorists seem to have requirements falling between these poles.

We are left, then, in an undesirable state. We find in philosophical writing not one but many distinct psychological concepts of personhood.

This unwelcomed variety would not matter for the abortion debate if the several versions implied similar starting points for development of personhood in fetuses. This, however, is not quite the case. The utilitarian version, for example, includes the fetus after it develops the capacity for pleasure or pain, while most of the others appear to exclude fetuses at any stage and, for that matter, newborns. A pro-choice advocate who wished to defend the morality of abortion might respond by noting that the utilitarian concept reported above is less that of "person" than "object of moral concern," and that the status of the fetus as a person seems dubious in most of the other concepts. The response might conclude, then, that most philosophers' uses of "person" are inconsistent with the proposition that fetuses are persons early, or even later, in their development.

Such a response is correct as far as it goes, but it does not offer us a road to progress in the abortion debate. First, few philosophers and almost no lay writers on abortion have declared themselves in favor of infanticide. Yet, the conclusion of the psychological concepts of personhood (that most fetuses are not persons) may be extended to infants. The pro-choice advocate cannot simultaneously use a psychological concept of personhood to declare fetuses to be nonpersons, yet abandon that same concept when applied to infants. Some philosophers, it should be noted, accept the implication for infanticide;[16] others state opposition to infanticide for reasons having little to do with personhood. The link between the psychological concept of personhood and the moral approval of infanticide, then, constitutes more of an embarrassment than a refutation of those who rely on the former to argue for the morality of abortion.

A second, more fundamental objection to the pro-choice argument is that it seems to use majority rule to decide philosophical issues. If there is a range of respectable opinion on what a person (in the psychological sense) is, it is unimportant whether "most" of the versions have or lack a certain property. What is needed is a convincing defense of one particular version. The pro-choice advocate must state why some particular version of the psychological concept of personhood should be recognized as uniquely valid or appropriate to determine the outcome of the abortion debate.

This, however, is not an easy task. One reason is that many of the versions of personhood are not really rivals. They are simply distinct concepts used in different contexts and making, in themselves, no particular claims. There need be no contradiction in asserting that fetuses are persons according to one concept, and that fetuses are nonpersons according to a different concept. The closest this comes to a contest is in the comparison of notions of personhood embedded in moral theories. Moral theories certainly do contradict each other, and they all cannot be right. If one of those theories could somehow be determined to be correct, perhaps there would be a sense in which the concept of personhood embedded in or presupposed by that theory would be validated. We could then carefully apply the concept to embryological data and determine when, if ever, fetuses are persons.

We should not, however, derive from these observations any optimism about the possibility of resolving the abortion debate by the use of reason. The relation of concepts of personhood to moral theories has not been clearly worked out by philosophers, and so it is not at all certain that the establishment of one theory over its rivals would give us a unique concept of personhood. More importantly, there is absolutely no agreement on which moral theory is correct. It is clear, I think, that there will not be any such agreement in the forseeable future.

CONCLUSIONS

It is clear that "person" is used differently by the various parties to the abortion debate. While some use the term synonymously with "living individual Homo sapiens," there are two reasons for doubting the usefulness of this concept. First, it remains to be seen whether biological science requires a definition of living Homo sapiens which dates it from conception; and biology is the only appropriate source. Second, it is difficult to find secular reasons for attaching such great moral importance to biological personhood (although admittedly, this moral attitude is a very common one).

The term person also involves reference to some sort of psychological entity—a being which has, at a minimum, capacity for consciousness. However, there are many significantly distinct concepts in philosophical and other writings. Fetuses may be persons according to some of these and nonpersons according to others. To choose among these versions of psychological personhood may be as difficult as determining which moral theory is the true one. Many have doubted that any moral theory can be proven to be uniquely correct; in any case, no one has yet come up with such a proof.

I conclude, then, that the concept of personhood does not offer a promising avenue for resolution of the abortion dispute by rational means. Biology may not give us a definition; perhaps it would not matter if it does. Moral theories may or may not offer definitions, but theories differ and the dispute over the theories is at least as intractable as the dispute over abortion. If we are to arrive at a resolution of the abortion issue through reasoned debate, then other concepts and arguments must be found.

However, my own guess is that if any consensus on abortion is reached, it will not be through reasoned debate.

Notes

1. Tooley, M., *Abortion and Infanticide*, Philosophy and Public Affairs, 2(1):37, 62-63 (1972).
2. Unger, P., *Why There Are No People*, Midwest Studies in Philosophy 4:177-222 (1979).
3. Tooley, *supra*, note 1, at 40.
4. Danto, A.C., *Persons*, in Encyclopedia of Philosophy (6):110 (Cromwell Collier and MacMillan, Inc., New York).
5. *See, e.g.*, Gordon, H., *Human Life Bill: Hearings on S.158 Before the Subcomm. on Separation of Powers of the Senate Comm. on the Judiciary*, 97th Cong., 1st Sess. 7,11-24 (1982).
6. S.158, 97th Cong., 1st Sess. (1982).
7. Lederberg, J., quoted in Rosenberg, J., *Human Life Bill: Hearings on S.158 Before the Subcomm. on the Judiciary*, 97th Cong., 1st Sess. 48, 50 (1982).
8. Rosenberg, *supra* note 7 at 49.
9. Thomas, L., quoted in Rosenberg, *supra* note 7, at 50.
10. Reprinted in testimony of Thomas, L., *Human Life Bill: Hearings on S.158 Before the Subcomm. on Separation of Powers of the Senate Comm. on the Judiciary*, 97th Cong., 1st Sess. 74 (1982).
11. Rosenberg, *supra* note, 7, at 50.
12. *See* Wertheimer, R., *Philosophy on Humanity*, in Abortion: Pro or Con (Schenkman Pub. Co., Cambridge, MA)(R.L. Perkins, ed., 1974) at 107-28. For an account of the divergence of ordinary and philosophical ethics on this point *see also* P.E. Devine, The Ethics of Homicide (Cornell University Press, Ithaca, New York)(1978) at Ch. 3. (Philosophers who accept this thesis).
13. *See, e.g.*, P. Singer, Animal Rights and Human Obligations (Prentice-Hall, Englewood, N.J.) (T. Regan, ed. 1976).
14. D.C. Dennett, Brainstorms (Bradford Books, Edward Bros., Inc., Ann Arbor, MI) (1978) at 267.
15. J.G. Murphy, Retribution, Justice and Therapy, Studies Series in Philosophy, (D. Ridell, No. 16, 1979).
16. *See, e.g.*, Purdy, L. & Tooley, M., *Is Abortion Murder?* in Abortion: Pro or Con (Schenkman Pub. Co., Cambridge, MA),(R.L. Perkins, ed. 1974) at 129, 150.

Audience Discussion

CAROLINE WHITBECK, PH.D. (Institute for the Medical Humanities, Galveston, Texas): I would like to make two points. First, I agree that existing philosophical discussions of personhood are not much help in illuminating the moral issues involving pregnant women and fetuses, but it does seem to me that a different philosophical approach could be taken that would illuminate those issues. One question that is raised in debates about the morality of abortion is whether feticide is homicide. That question, I submit, would be answered differently if philosophers, instead of discussing personhood, addressed the extent to which fetuses are like newborns in morally relevant respects. I take it that newborns do not have rights in the strict sense since they are not capable of choosing to waive or exercise rights and they do not have the capacity for moral responsibility, i.e., they are not moral agents. Nonetheless, there are moral requirements upon us in our treatment of newborns. In particular, infanticide counts as homicide and hence it is at least prima facie wrong.

This brings me to my second point, which is that there is no simple ordering of moral statuses so that one status, say that of a normal adult, is "highest" in the sense that the moral requirements that govern our behavior toward other beings are a strict subset of those toward the individual of this status. Instead I think that there are a number of different moral statuses and the moral requirements that govern our treatment of some of those who are not themselves moral agents; these requirements are different from, but not simply fewer than, those that govern our treatment of others who are themselves moral agents and have moral rights in the strict sense. The moral requirements that govern our treatment of infants are in some ways similar and in many ways different from the requirements governing our treatment of adults. What we need is some systematic treatment of the requirements governing our treatment of fetuses and the way to do that is to examine the scope and limits of the analogy between the moral status of fetuses and the moral status of newborns.

DANIEL WIKLER (Conference Faculty): Your remarks seem to presuppose that we have a coherent account of our moral obligations concerning newborns. I attribute this assumption to you because there would otherwise be little utility in making an effort to assess the moral significance of the similarities and differences between fetuses and newborns, as you suggest we do. I do not see that the assumption is warranted. There is little agreement among moral theorists on the grounds for abhorring infanticide, though nearly everyone joins in the abhorrence. Indeed, your own remark concerning newborns' rights is an instance of this lack of consensus. As you know, there is a stock answer to your claim that newborns, not being moral agents, cannot have any rights. It is that newborns, along with young children, the temporarily insane, and others, have interests which ought to be protected by rights, exercised on their behalf by guardians. Those who oppose your position insist that an ascription of rights in such cases remains a special moral claim.

You may be correct in holding that the various moral statuses do not constitute a neat hierarchy. I say "may" because I feel that it is not possible to determine this in the absence of an acceptable, well worked-out account of these statuses. I conjecture that any such account as might emerge will, however, incorporate one hierarchy, however vaguely defined, which separates those beings who must not be slaughtered or otherwise abused for the convenience or use of others from those who may be. This is the division summarized in Nozick's slogan, "Kantianism for people, utilitarianism for animals."[1] In my opinion, both sides of the abortion debate accept the idea of such a division. Their disagreement is over which category fetuses belong to. I think that this is what the notion of personhood is supposed to capture. I agree with you that the real moral question is whether or not newborns and fetuses should be treated in the same way, one as well as the other. My claim, with which I think you would agree, is that it is fruitless to search for a philosophical concept of person which we can then use to decide. But, of course, if you have a moral view that one ought to be treated better than the other, or they both ought to be treated well, or neither well, one expects to have arguments in favor of that position. The notion of personhood simply will not provide a satisfactory back-up for our moral arguments.

ALBERT S. MORACZEWSKI, O.P., PH.D. (Pope John XXIII Medical-Moral Research and Education Center, St. Louis, Missouri): My question is addressed to Dr. Grobstein. While I would like to question several points about your presentation regarding embryological development, because of time constraints I will restrict myself to one point. Somewhere in your lecture you mentioned, I believe, that oneness, or individuality, was not established until about two weeks (or more) after fertilization. Presumably until that time, from your viewpoint, the "embryo" is not really an embryo but a mere collection of cells.

Yet as one of your slides beautifully illustrated, the first cell division after fertilization results in two daughter cells still enveloped by the zona pellucida. As cleavage continues through the four-cell stage and on through the 12- and 16-cell stage, the individual cells (blastomeres) become smaller and smaller, all the while remaining enclosed in the zona pellucida. Shortly before implantation this covering is shed and studies have shown that the blastocyst seems to emerge by an active process. Furthermore, there is already some differentiation as some cells (the inner cell mass) eventually become the embryo proper while the remaining cells (the outer cell mass) eventually contribute to the formation of the placenta and membranes.

I claim the evidence argues that there is already from the time of fertilization a oneness, a true individual, because there is present that degree of organization commensurate with its stage of development. This is not a mere collection of individual cells; they are related to one another in a special manner so that cell division does not result merely in an increase in the number of cells—as in a tissue culture—but results in cells which differ from one another, for there is evidence of the beginnings of cellular differentiation.

Because the one-cell zygote does not have a truly homogeneous cytoplasm, the sequential cleavages of the zygote result in a qualitatively unequal partitioning of its cytoplasm among the blastomeres. The consequence is that the nuclei of the blastomeres are situated in different cytoplasmic environments. The significance of this fact is that because the cytoplasmic milieu has an influence on gene function there will result a differential expression of genes in different cells. Thus, from the first cleavage onward the resulting cells become differentiated and contribute, as it were, their differences to the functioning of the multicellular organism.

Furthermore, the zygote as it undergoes subsequent cleavages has taken the initial developmental steps toward what will be ultimately the adult stage. While at the two- or four-cell stage individual cells may still be plenipotential, clearly at the 12- or 16-cell stage (about day three) only the centrally located cells (the inner cell mass) have the ability to develop into the embryo proper. Hence, there is sufficient unity of structure and coordination of function among the multiplicity of cells to constitute an authentic organism, an individual.

The fact that in the earliest stages several individuals can apparently develop from one zygote (e.g., twinning, or "cloning" such as has been done by artificially separating the cells of the cleaving mouse zygote at the four-cell stage) does not militate against the unity of the original. Furthermore, the claim for the possibility of cloning an existing adult does not impugn the fact that the adult is a true individual. The normal reproductive process involves the formation of new individuals by the fusion of the reproductive cells of existing individuals. Hence, the fact that other individuals may form from the living cells of an organism does not militate against the fact that it is an organism, an individual.

The phenomenon of recombination does not present a convincing argument against my position as the phenomenon could be seen as a process by which, let us say, two initial individuals become fused at a very early stage, within three or four days after fertilization. This could be interpreted as one of the individuals dying and the cells (some or all) becoming part of the remaining individual. Several examples of apparent human recombination have been documented with the help of chromosomal studies.

CLIFFORD GROBSTEIN (Conference Faculty): The evidence for mammalian embryos, particularly extensive studies on mice, indicates that at the eight-cell stage it is possible to separate the cells so that one or more cells will give rise to a single individual; therefore, multiple individuals may result from a single zygote. Whether or not there is any degree of integralness in the collection of cells—and I do not mean to suggest that there can be no interaction—whatever there is can be disrupted without prejudicing the subsequent rise of one or more individuals depending upon circumstance. A stable, single individual (unity in a cell collective) has not been established. The same argument applies to the embryo corresponding to the human stage at approximately two weeks. Although if all other things remain equal such an embryo will give rise to one individual, if suitably disrupted it can give rise to more than one individual. Therefore, without denying the possibility that there already may be interactions taking place, they are not interactions that cannot be interrupted and reversed if circumstances are changed. In that sense, a single, stable multicellular individual has not yet been biologically determined up to the human stage at approximately two weeks of gestation.

WARREN M. HERN, M.D., M.P.H. (Boulder Abortion Clinic, Boulder, Colorado): I have a couple of comments about Dr. Grobstein's paper. I believe that Dr. Grobstein mentioned the competing needs of the developing embryo and the woman carrying it who may be opposed to efforts to save the fetus. He mentioned that the survival needs of each may impinge upon one another.

In this context, I would like to refer you to a couple of papers I have published on this subject. Essentially, I have argued that pregnancy is or can be considered an illness requiring various forms of medical treatment.[2] As you develop this theme, you begin to see that there are, in fact, very clear consequences for medical treatment. The interests of the woman, the risks she experiences as the result of the pregnancy, and her survival may be in conflict with the concept of the fetus as a person.

In my view, this question has clear implications for medical practice. If pregnancy is defined as an illness, the question is not "How do you justify an abortion?" but "What is the appropriate treatment for this pregnancy?" Since pregnancy is a biosocial event and a woman's attitudes toward it might have an important effect on her risks, abortion might be the appropriate treatment under some circumstances. If Dr. Grobstein has some thoughts as a biologist on the consequences of defining pregnancy as an illness, I would be interested in his comments.

Also, I thought Dr. Grobstein's summary statement was extremely interesting when he said that "what we choose to accept as a person depends not only upon scientific fact but upon our purposes, our values, and our wisdom." I would add to that list our political purposes as well. The consequences of our acceptance of the fetus as a person might define, for example, who wins elections and who runs your life. I think that those are important consequences.

CLIFFORD GROBSTEIN: Let me comment first on the reference to the possible conflicting needs of fetus and mother. I certainly do not mean to suggest that the needs of the embryo and the mother are basically competitive. It is obvious that the two depend upon and cooperate with each other in very important ways. My purpose was only to note that if two persons are interdependent their interests can nonetheless diverge. For example, if the mother seeks to terminate the pregnancy at three months, the offspring, under present circumstances, must die. Under these circumstances, the interests of two interpenetrating persons are in competition. The issue, of course, is whether and when the offspring becomes a second person. A similar ambiguity arises with respect to pregnancy as an illness. I would not ordinarily view pregnancy as an illness, but it does have certain parallels and there might be circumstances under which it would be advantageous to emphasize those parallels. I do not at the moment visualize such circumstances for a healthy maternal-fetal unit.

UNIDENTIFIED PARTICIPANT: Why do you think that the definition of personhood in its biological sense is a scientific issue? To ask what a person is has the logical form of asking what happens when you sail off the edge of a flat earth. In other words, it is not a good question and that is why we cannot give it a good answer.

DANIEL WIKLER: I do not believe that "Are whales mammals?" is a bad question. I do not think that the question "Does this batch of fertilized fruit fly eggs constitute a new generation of fruit flies?" is a bad question. Therefore, I do not see any reason why the question "What constitutes an individual living Homo sapiens?" is a bad one either. I gather, from listening to scientists, that there is no one scientific answer to that question; still, I regard it as a question for scientific judgment and not for philosophical or moral judgment.

CLIFFORD GROBSTEIN: It seems to me that we need to distinguish the reasons for which we are asking the question. The question that is being proposed has two possible meanings that need to be separated. The first question is "Did human life begin in the sense of human life as a unique phenomenon first becoming recognizable on earth?" The second is "When does an individual human being come into existence, and what does human life mean in the sense of the life that we think of as being our own? When does our own particular human life begin?" I think those two questions are confused when the question asked is "When does human life begin?" I try to make clear that under the first interpretation, the answer is certainly scientifically nonarguable—human life simply does not begin today. In those terms, we do not have a problem; there is no question as to whether or not human life begins during a given life cycle. It does not; human life is continuous.

In the second sense, we have a problem: when does the life of each individual begin; when is each of us identified as a person? That is a separate and different question, and it really ought to be kept so; it is important that we recognize two quite separate and distinct questions.

LEWIS H. KOPLIK, M.D. (La Mesa Medical Center, New Mexico): Dr. Grobstein, does the concept of fetal anomalies or fetal monstrosities contribute anything in the discussion of personhood? Specifically does the anencephalic fetus represent a person or does a monster where twinning has begun but has not been completed, one with one head but four legs or two heads but only one lower torso? Does this bizarre anomaly represent one or two persons?

CLIFFORD GROBSTEIN: Well, I guess the simplest, if not the most satisfactory answer, is that it contributes even greater complexity to the problem. If one is talking in the first sense, even though severely abnormal, all fetuses are Homo sapiens and should be accorded biological status as such. On the other hand, if one is talking in the second sense, depending on the criteria selected as diagnostic of a person, the extremely defective human embryo may or may not achieve the status of a person, or may receive it only partially or at a much later stage. This is where the problem gets very tough and where much more knowledge is needed.

ELLEN KRAMER, J.D. (Planned Parenthood Federation of America, New York, New York): My question is for Dr. Grobstein. Much of the proposed legislation states explicity that human life begins at conception, but as it is a medical term, I am not sure precisely when conception occurs. Can you tell me, as a biologist and also from the standpoint of medical practitioners, whether keying the determination of life to "conception" would add further confusion to the argument; in other words, are we talking about fertilization or implantation?

CLIFFORD GROBSTEIN: It adds confusion unless the word is defined. As far as I'm aware, the term conception does not have a scientific definition. As used in the proposed legislation, it appears to refer to fertilization, which conforms to what I understand to be ordinary usage. If it means implantation, it should say so. At neither time, however, has a new, stable biological individual come into existence by the developmental criteria I have described. Implantation is very close to the critical point and in humans, we do not have definitive information to say exactly how close. What I'm talking about, of course, is biological individuality; individualness in the sense of the establishment of a multicellular collective that is committed to function as a multicellular individual. That occurs during or just beyond the time of implantation—a process which itself is not sharply delineated, particularly as to its ending.

NOTES

1. R. NOZICK, ANARCHY, STATE AND UTOPIA (Basic Books, New York)(1974) at 39.
2. Hern, W.M., *Is Pregnancy Really Normal?* FAMILY PLANNING PERSPECTIVES 3:1-6 (1971); Hern, W.M., *The Illness Parameters of Pregnancy*, SOCIAL SCIENCE AND MEDICINE 9:365-72 (1975).

Part Two

Medical Implications

Chapter 3

The Complexity of Embryonic Development from Fertilization to Implantation

Richard J. Blandau

To appreciate the complexity of embryonic development from fertilization to implantation one must begin with the origin of germ cells, the ova and spermatozoa, and follow their course of development and maturation within the gonads and their continued maturation within the ductular system of both male and female. I will briefly describe how the ovulated ova and spermatozoa are transported to the site of fertilization, the process of fertilization itself, and the subsequent stages in the development of the embryo until it becomes implanted in the maternal endometrium (the lining of the uterus).

Oögenesis

The ovum is the primary cellular link between the ongoing generations. It is a remarkable cell in that it has stored within its protoplasm the genetic memory of all past generations. The original oögonia, or primordial germ cells, originate outside of the embryo. They arise in the region of the yolk sac stalk in the 23- to 25-day-old embryo (Figure 1). From here they migrate by means of active ameboid movements to the region of the germinal ridges, the future gonads.[1] The gonads arise as epithelial thickenings along the medial-ventral aspect of the developing mesonephros (primitive kidneys). The characteristic ameboid movements of the primordial germ cells have been recorded in vitro on motion picture film.[2]

After the oögonia have seeded the gonads that will become the ovaries, they continue to multiply until approximately 7,000,000 are formed. All except 300,000 or 400,000 of these will degenerate and disappear, even before the baby is born. The mechanism and significance

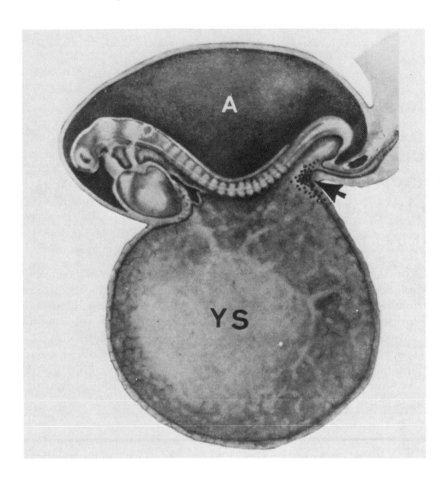

Figure 1:   A 23-day old human embryo showing the original location of the primordial germ cells (arrow); A = amnion; YS = yolk sac. (After Witschi, Carnegie Contrib. to Emb., 1948)

of this large loss remain a biological mystery. Of the hundreds of thousands of ova present at birth, only 420 to 480 may be ovulated during the human female's reproductive life. The number of ova that will be fertilized and develop into a mature living baby is astonishingly small. It is probably appropriate to point out that the human being is very inefficient in its reproductive process.

The oögonia have a tendency to locate in the cortical areas of the gonads. The spermatogonia, which seed the gonads in the same manner, aggregate primarily in the medullary areas. The oögonia are soon encompassed in a flattened layer of epithelial cells that restrict their further movements (Figure 2). The spermatogonia, the progenitors of all sperm cells, are rapidly confined within the primitive seminiferous tubules. They multiply by mitotic division but retain their position on the basement membranes of the seminiferous tubules. They remain more or less dormant until puberty when they begin to multiply rapidly and proceed to undergo spermatogenesis and spermiogenesis to give rise to mature sperm.[3] The significance of this process will be detailed later.

MATURATION OF THE EGG IN PREPARATION FOR FERTILIZATION

The meiotic process (reduction in the number of chromosomes) in the oögonia begins during the fetal period and is completed only after ovulation and sperm penetration. The oögonia seeding the ovaries contain 22 pairs of autosomes and a pair of sex chromosomes. In the human species the female is homogametic (XX), whereas the male is heterogametic (XY). Before fertilization can be accomplished, it is necessary that the number of chromosomes in both oögonia and spermatogonia be reduced by one-half to establish the haploid number in the egg and sperm.

To effect chromosomal reduction in the oögonia, the homologous chromosomes replicate, each forming a pair of chromatids. The pairs of homologous chromatids juxtapose, synapse, and exchange chromosomal or genic material to effect the shuffling of genes. In the human, synapsis (or pairing of the chromosomes) begins at about the fifth month of fetal life in some oögonia; in others at a later time. By birth, the majority are in the diplotene or dictyotene stage (thread stage) of meiosis when the paired chromosomes separate and the bivalents are held together at only those points where crossing-over has taken place. These areas of attachment are called chiasmata (Figure 3). The oögonium is now called an oöcyte and has completed the prophase stage, the first division of meiosis.[4]

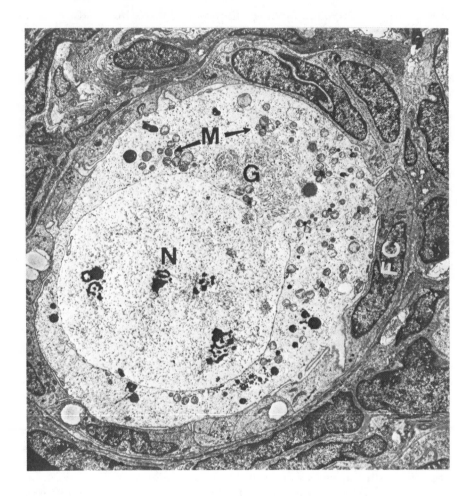

Figure 2:   A low-power electron micrograph of an oöcyte within the late fetal ovary. Note that the ovum is completely surrounded by a single layer of tightly packed follicular cells. (N = nucleus; G = Golgi complex; M = mitochondria; FC = follicular cells)

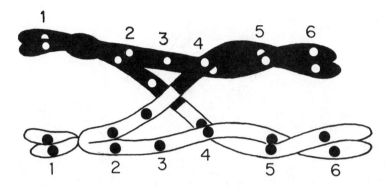

Figure 3: A diagram of an homologous chromosome pair in which crossing-over, or interchange of chromosome segments, has taken place. The points of cross-over are called "chiasmata."

    It is important to recognize that the egg nucleus now contains double the normal amount of DNA because that double amount may subject the ovum to a number of environmental hazards.

    The ova will remain in the prophase stage of meiosis for 12 to 50 or more years or until a few hours before ovulation, when the process of chromosomal reduction, to attain the haploid condition, is continued.

    If an oöcyte becomes selectively reactivated in an enlarging pre-ovulatory follicle the following changes occur. The nucleus (also called "germinal vesicle") moves from the center of the cell to assume an eccentric position just below the egg membrane (Figure 4). The nuclear membrane disappears and the first meiotic spindle forms, paratangential to the surface of the egg membrane. The dictyotene threads begin to condense into thick spiral chromosomes. The condensed tetrads line up on the metaphase plate of the spindle and attach to the spindle fibers by their centromeres. The first meiotic spindle now rotates 90° to the egg surface and a clear bleb of egg cytoplasm is extruded during the rotation (Figure 4: 3). Simultaneously, one-half of the chromosomes (dyads) move into the extruded vesicle. The first polar body is pinched off. It contains a diploid number of chromosomes (one-half of the tetrads) (Figure 4: 4). Almost immediately the second meiotic spindle appears beneath the egg membrane and the condensed diploid chromosomes left behind in the egg immediately arrange themselves upon its metaphase plate (Figure 4: 5). Each of these 23 pairs of chromosomes is held together by a single centromere. The haploid phase of the ovum continues to develop when the spermatozoön penetrates the egg. Since the chromosomes are already split longitudinally, all that must take place to complete the second meiotic

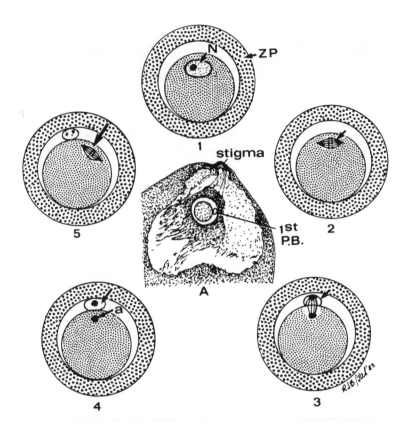

Figure 4:   The sequence of events during the first polar body formation. "A" is the preovulatory follicle. The "Stigma" is the site at which
follicular rupture is beginning. The first polar body is invariably abstricted (arrow) before ovulation. The important steps in first polar body
formation are illustrated in figures 1 through 5. In No. 1 the nucleus (N)
moves from the center of the cell toward the surface of the egg membrane.
This nucleus contains 92 chromatids. No. 2, the nuclear membrane
disappears, the first meiotic spindle forms paratangential to the egg
membrane and the 92 chromatids arrange themselves on the metaphase
plate. In No. 3 the spindle rotates 90°, a clear bleb of cytoplasm is
extruded from the egg and one half of 92 chromatids move into the bleb.
The remainder remain with the egg. No. 4, the first polar body is abstricted and the remaining chromatids are clumped in the egg. In No. 5,
the second meiotic spindle forms immediately and the remaining 46
chromatids arrange themselves on the metaphase plate. This is the condition of the egg before it is penetrated by a sperm.

division is the duplication of centromeres; this is exactly what happens. The chromosomes, attached to the spindle by centromeres, migrate to the opposite poles of the spindle. The spindle then rotates 90° to the surface. A bleb of egg cytoplasm containing the haploid number of chromosomes is pinched off to form the second polar body (Figure 5: 1–3). The ovum has now attained the haploid condition. The haploid chromosomes remaining within the egg will, within two to three hours, form the female pronucleus. The compacted haploid chromosomes contained in the sperm head, which are now embedded within the egg cytoplasm, separate to form the male pronucleus (Figure 6: 1–3). As the male and female pronuclei move toward the center of the ovum the haploid chromosomes replicate and the first mitotic spindle appears. The chromosomes from the male and female pronuclei arrange themselves upon the metaphase plate of the first mitotic spindle where they remain for a brief period of time before separation and movement to the opposite poles. The egg divides into two blastomeres of approximately equal size (Figure 6: 4–5). Each blastomere now contains the diploid number of chromosomes. The time required for the fertilized egg to attain the two-cell stage in the human is approximately 26 hours.

THE DEVELOPMENT AND MATURATION
OF THE SPERMATOZOA

The development of mature spermatozoa capable of fertilizing ova is even more complicated[5] than the development and maturation of ova.

Spermatogenesis is the total cellular process in the formation and development of spermatozoa. Spermiogenesis is the final stage of spermatogenesis in which the spermatids are transformed into spermatozoa.

The production of spermatozoa by the testes of normal adult males is a continuous and dynamic process involving differentiation and cell division—both mitotic and meiotic. No other cells in the body, except ova, undergo meiotic division. When meiosis has been completed both eggs and sperm contain the haploid number of chromosomes, i.e., 23 chromosomes rather than 46.

In 1941, von Kolliker discovered that spermatozoa develop from specialized cell types in the seminiferous tubules of the testes. This discovery led to the morphologic description and classification of various germinal epithelial cells (spermatogonia, spermatocytes and spermatids) in the various subdivisions of the seminiferous tubules. Approximately 20 different cell types can be recognized in the germinal epithelial lineage. To the casual observer the seminiferous epithelium may present a picture of

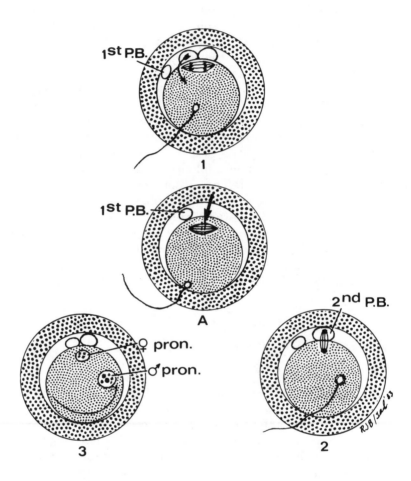

Figure 5:   The sequence of events during second polar body formation. In A, second polar body formation is initiated only if an egg is penetrated by a sperm. No. 1, upon sperm penetration, 23 of the remaining 46 chromatids migrate to each pole of the spindle. Two clear cytoplasmic vesicles appear just above the spindle. As the spindle rotates 90° to the surface, one of the vesicles (arrow) is reabsorbed into the egg carrying 23 chromatids with it. No. 2, the second polar body (2nd P.B.) is abstricted and comes to lie free in the perivitelline space. No. 3, the male and female pronuclei appear, each containing 23 chromosomes, the haploid number.

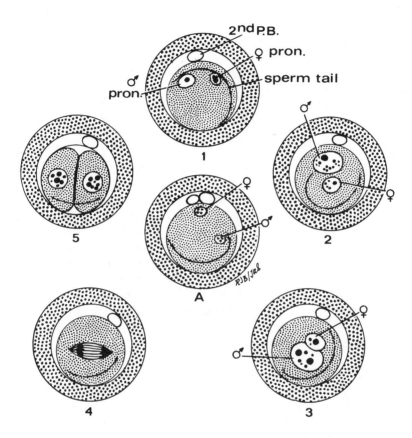

Figure 6: The sequence of events in the formation of the male and female pronuclei and the first segmentation division. In A, the male (♂) and female (♀) pronuclei are forming, each containing 23 chromosomes. No. 1, the sperm tail has been completely absorbed. The first polar body usually disintegrates; the second polar body (2nd P.B.) persists. No. 2, the male (♂) and female (♀) pronuclei increase in size and begin to move toward one another. During this time the 23 chromosomes replicate in preparation for the first segmentation division. No. 3, the pronuclear cytoplasm fuses; No. 4, a mitotic spindle forms and the diploid chromosomes separate to form the two-cell stage, No. 5. During stages 1 through 5 the sperm flagellum gradually disappears.

disorder and chaos. It has taken a large effort by many investigators to clarify the dynamics of spermatogenesis, principally because of the significant variations in this process from species to species.

As we have mentioned earlier, the spermatogonia remain more or less dormant until puberty, when they begin to multiply rapidly and proceed to spermatogenesis. At puberty three types of spermatogonia may be recognized on the basement membrane: (1) A or dark type (often labeled AD)—so called because of the condensation of the nuclear material, which stains darkly; (2) A or pale type (often labeled AP), an intermediary stage (Type A spermatogonia undergo mitosis to perpetuate themselves whereas others differentiate into Type B cells); and (3) Type B cell, in which the nucleus stains much less darkly (Figure 7).

The three types are all derived sequentially by mitotic division and represent the sequence of stages from the older to the younger cell.

The Type B cells divide sequentially two to four times before they differentiate into spermatocytes. The primary spermatocytes are thus produced from the last mitotic divisions of the Type B spermatogonia. These primary spermatocytes pass through the various stages of meiosis, and it is during this stage that DNA is synthesized for the last time. I reemphasize that the meiotic process occurs only in spermatocytes and oöcytes and is the mechanism by which exchange of genic material is accomplished and the chromosome number reduced by one-half (Figure 7).

Perhaps because of the complex and dramatic changes that occur in the homologous chromosomes during meiosis, the time required to complete the prophase stage of the first maturation division is quite long. Each primary spermatocyte divides into two secondary spermatocytes. Following a brief interphase stage, the secondary spermatocytes proceed through the second meiotic cell division to yield haploid spermatids. To repeat, the transformation of the spermatids into spermatozoa is called spermiogenesis (Figure 7). Because of the presence of intercellular bridges linking them into clusters of eight or 16 cells, they are often referred to as clones.

Spermiogenesis takes place in the following manner.

1) A nuclear cap evolves from the Golgi apparatus that eventually develops into the acrosome. The acrosome is a membranous bag covering at least two-thirds of the sperm head. It contains a variety of enzymes, such as hyaluronidase and several different proteinases.

2) The chromosomes (23–haploid number) become so highly condensed and packaged that the nuclear part of the head stains

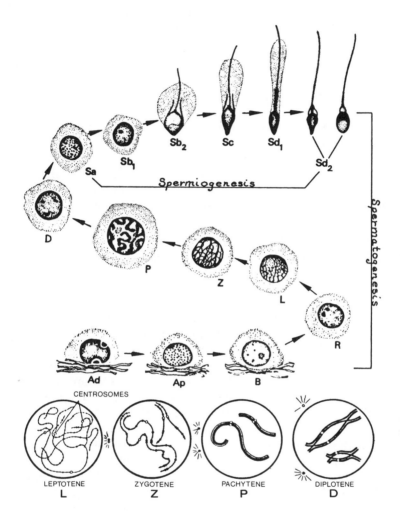

Figure 7:   Drawings showing the evolution of spermatozoa from spermatogonia in man. AD = dark type spermatogonia; AP = pale type
spermatogonia; B = spermatogonia with pale staining nucleus; R =
primary spermatocyte beginning meiotic division; D, P, Z and L = the
four stages of meiosis enlarged below; Sa through S_2 = spermatids in
various stages of spermiogenesis leading to the development of a mature
sperm.

very intensely and the individual chromosomes can no longer be identified.

3) A motile flagellum (sperm tail) forms (approximately 60 micra long) containing a complex axial filamentous arrangement of microtubules and a spiral sheath of mitochondria.

4) Extensive shedding of cytoplasm takes place (Figure 7).

In addition to the spermatogonia that line the basement membrane of the seminiferous tubules mentioned earlier, other cells that have an irregular columnar shape are also anchored on the basement membrane. These are the important Sertoli cells, which are fewer in number and are spaced quite regularly along the basement membrane. They are easily distinguished from the spermatogonial cells and they do not ordinarily undergo cell division. Spermatids in great numbers are embedded in the cytoplasm of the Sertoli cells. It is assumed that the developing sperm cells obtain nutritive substances from the Sertoli cells.

SPERM MATURATION IN THE MALE REPRODUCTIVE TRACT

Spermatozoa removed from the seminiferous tubules, the ductuli efferentes, or the head of the epididymis are incapable of fertilizing mature ovulated ova either in vivo or in vitro. It is well known that mammalian spermatozoa undergo certain changes during their passage through the epididymis that affect their maturation and enable them to fertilize ova. The maturation of sperm is the result of certain physiological, biochemical, and morphological alterations that occur as they proceed through the epididymal tubes.

Transport of sperm from the seminiferous tubules to and through the epididymis is largely passive and is initiated by fluids secreted by the seminiferous tubule epithelium that flow toward the epididymis. It is assisted in its flow by (1) fluid pressures built up in the seminiferous tubules; (2) contractions of the myoid cells in the walls of the seminiferous tubules; (3) contractions of the testicular capsule; and (4) the action of long and very active cilia within the ductuli efferentes that beat in the direction of the epididymis. Spermatozoa remain immotile throughout their passage within the epididymal duct. Their transport depends on the contractile activity of the epididymal wall and possibly the increasing number of cells that affect cellular pressure. Both hormones and neural components are probably factors in transport, but just how they operate is still unknown.

In man, the transit time of sperm through the epididymis is calculated to be about 12 days. While frequent ejaculations may have only a slight influence on the transit time, they will deplete stores of sperm and result in diminished density of spermatozoa in the ejaculate. This must be kept in mind when evaluating sperm output for clinical purposes in patients with suspected infertility.

THE FATE OF UNEJACULATED SPERMATOZOA

As has been suggested earlier, sperm are formed continuously in the seminiferous tubules and are discharged in a continuous stream into the epididymis. In some animals (rat, guinea pig, cat) sperm have been found almost constantly in the urine. It is suspected that in these animals there may be a constant slow discharge of sperm into the urethra. No such leakage of sperm into the urethra has been demonstrated for man as a normal phenomenon.

Although the fate of spermatozoa in the tail of the epididymis has not been precisely determined, the best evidence indicates that they have a limited life span. The older, devitalized ones are broken down, cytolized, and phagocytized. The kinetics of the disposal of sperm from the ductus deferens is still baffling.

SPERM TRANSPORT THROUGH THE CERVIX

The cervical mucus is the first barrier through which spermatozoa must pass to ascend to the site of fertilization within the ampullae of the oviducts. The penetration of spermatozoa through the cervical mucus is controlled by (1) the rheological properties of the cervical mucus at varying times in the menstrual cycle; (2) the rate of flagellation of the spermatozoa passing through the mucus; and finally, (3) the interaction of the spermatozoa and the mucin macromolecules within this hydrogel.

The cervical mucus has its origin in a single layer of columnar secretory cells that line an intricate system of cervical crypts. These epithelial cells contain large numbers of cytoplasmic granules of varying electron density. Their cytological and histochemical characteristics differ in different parts of the cervix. Cervical mucus is a concentrated solution of glycoproteins rich in carbohydrates. The glycoproteins contain 70 to 80 carbohydrates in the form of numerous side chains. It is a colloid that exhibits the rheologic characteristics of viscoelasticity, which implies that it possesses both solid and fluid-like properties. In totality, cervical mucus is a voluminous hydrophilic gel composed of a high viscosity component (gel phase) and a low viscosity component that consists of a variety of electrolytes and organic compounds, such as glucose, amino acids, and soluble proteins. At midcycle in the human, cervical mucus is approximately 99.5 percent water that is bound within the complex of the mucin macromolecules.

There is still contradictory information as to the manner in which spermatozoa move through the cervical canal in the human. It is well-known that in man most of the spermatozoa are contained in the first portion of the ejaculate. One may assume that at the moment of ejaculation the cervix is bathed in a high concentration of spermatozoa. Human semen is deposited in the vaginal vault as an opaque coagulum that liquefies within five to 15 minutes. The abundant midcycle cervical mucus comes into intimate contact with this coagulum; therefore, spermatozoa may enter the cervical mucus without coming into contact with any part of the vagina. Sperm begin to enter the cervical mucus of the human female within one and one-half to three minutes after they are deposited at the os of the cervix. On the basis of all available evidence, there are no scientific data to support the concept that contractions of the uterus or vagina in women play any role in effecting active sperm transport from the vaginal deposits into and through the cervix at the time of ejaculation or for any time thereafter. The best evidence indicates that spermatozoa move through the cervical mucus by their own innate motility.

The cervical canal may then be looked upon as a "receptaculum seminis" through which platoons of spermatozoa migrate with no help from the musculature of the reproductive organs. When sperm penetration into the cervical mucus is observed in vitro, they appear to move along the micellar strands following the path of least resistance. Current data indicate that ejaculated spermatozoa enter midcycle cervical mucus rapidly and in a unidirectional fashion (Figure 8). Subsequent migration through the cervical canal is accomplished principally by their own intrinsic motility. The cervical mucus is a very favorable medium for sperm survival and some believe that it may provide sperm cells with energy substances required for their motility.[6]

When the spermatozoa have passed through the cervical mucus and entered the uterine lumen, they still have a long distance to travel to the site of fertilization.[7] How spermatozoa traverse the uterine lumen to reach the narrow entrance into the oviduct is largely unknown. Two possibilities exist: (1) they move from the cervix to the uterotubal junction by their own flagellation; or (2) they may be assisted by more active uterine contractions at the time of insemination initiated by either oxytocins or prostaglandins. How the spermatozoa are transported through the narrow bottleneck of the uterotubal junction to enter the oviduct is also unknown. Various functions have been ascribed to the uterotubal junction: (1) it may act as a filtering or selective site for sperm entering the oviduct; (2) it may be a

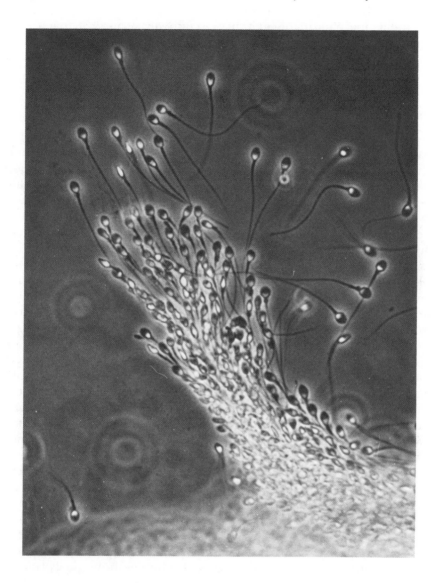

Figure 8: Human spermatozoa entering human midcycle cervical mucus. Note the unidirectional movement of the spermatozoa.

controlling mechanism for egg transport into the uterus; (3) it may act as a mechanism that prevents retrograde transport of endometrial tissue, especially during menstruation. All of these are reasonable speculations but none has been tested.

SPERM TRANSPORT THROUGH THE ISTHMUS

How spermatozoa are transported through the isthmus of the oviduct to reach the site of fertilization in the ampulla has intrigued investigators for many years. The primary problem in resolving this dilemma is a technical one, since it is impossible to see the very small motile spermatozoa within the thick-walled tube by any procedure that has been developed to date. Oviducts have the paradoxical facility of propelling eggs from the ovary to the isthmoampullar junction, the site of fertilization, and simultaneously moving spermatozoa in the opposite direction through the isthmus.

It is fairly well established that spermatozoa do not travel through the isthmus exclusively by their own flagellation. We now know that the cilia lining the mucosa of the isthmus in the human all beat in the direction of the uterus. This seems to present an almost impossible impediment for the upward movement of sperm through this segment. Recently, new insight has been gained into this mystery in several different species, including humans, by observing that in the preovulatory period the muscle contractions of the isthmus are programmed to contract segmentally in an antiperistaltic direction, squeezing the luminal contents in the direction of the ampulla of the oviduct, the normal site of fertilization. Thus, stained materials that could be visualized by transillumination may be transported through the isthmus to the site of fertilization in approximately 25 seconds in women. These preovulatory antiperistaltic contractions have now been observed in the isthmi of rabbits, rats, pigs, and humans.[8] We are confident that the segmental, antiperistaltic muscle contractions are involved in no small way in transporting spermatozoa directly through the isthmus to the site of fertilization during the preovulatory period. We emphasize that the antiperistaltic pattern of contractions seen in the isthmus during the preovulatory period changes during the postovulatory period to a segmental, to-and-fro pattern of contraction that buffets the luminal contents backward and forward. Thus the fertilized eggs are moved from segment to segment during the 36 to 48 hours they reside within the isthmus. How the eggs are finally transported into the uterus is unknown for any animal.

OBSERVATIONS ON IN VITRO FERTILIZATION

We have recently been able to develop a technique by which the entire process of sperm penetration through the zona pellucida, the perivitelline space and into the vitelline membrane in mice could be observed continuously and recorded on film. A total of 7,754 eggs from 585 female mice were inseminated in vitro and the complete process of sperm penetration observed, timed and filmed in more than 150 eggs.[9] No similar observations are available for any other mammal, including humans.

The following statements summarize the technique and the process of fertilization that have been observed and recorded on motion picture film.

1) Sperm capacitation was accomplished by submerging epididymal sperm in a special culture medium. The sperm were obtained by killing the male, dissecting out the cauda epididymis and ductus deferens, and mincing them into a culture medium. It required approximately two to three hours to accomplish capacitation.

2) Mature female mice were induced to ovulate by an intraperitoneal injection of pregnant mare's serum PMS (which is high in follicle-stimulating hormone, FSH), followed 48 hours later by an intraperitoneal injection of human chorionic gonadotropin, HCG (which is high in luteinizing hormone). The females ovulated ten to 12 hours after the last injection and the eggs were recovered from the dilated ampullae and placed immediately in Toyoda's medium.

3) The cumulus oöphorus was removed from ovulated eggs by suspending them in a dilute solution of hyaluronidase.

4) Eggs and sperm were brought together on a slide in the culture medium and quickly covered with a cover glass supported by six pillars of a vaseline-paraffin mixture. Evaporation was controlled by immediately surrounding the egg-sperm suspension with a highly purified, oxygenated mineral oil.

5) The egg and sperm suspension was observed under a phase microscope, the field being illuminated with a Zirconium arc lamp, a cold light source which does not affect living cells.

6) The spermatozoa that penetrated the zona pellucida and eventually fused with the vitellus began their penetration 15 to 60 minutes after the initial insemination (Figure 9). In other words, sperm had to be attached to the zona pellucida for at least 15 minutes before they began penetrating the zona pellucida.

7) Sperm penetration of the zona was at an angle nearly perpendicular to the surface in the great majority of penetrations observed, recorded, and timed by use of a stopwatch.

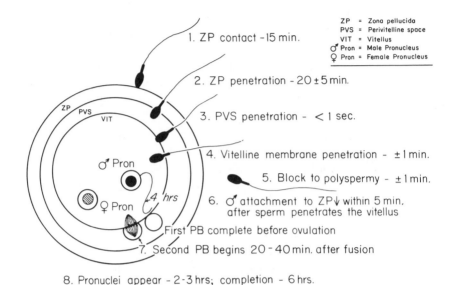

Figure 9:   The time sequence of events of in vitro fertilization as observed and photographed in 150 mouse eggs.

8)   The sperm heads appeared to develop a channel within the zona as they moved forward. Active flagellation was an important and essential component of zona penetration.

9)   The mean time required for the sperm head to penetrate the zona was 20 minutes, with a range of 15 to 26 minutes (Figure 9).

10)   When a sperm penetrated the inner surface of the zona it dashed across the perivitelline space in less than one second and plunged into the vitelline membrane of the egg.

11)   Flagellation ceased within a few minutes after the head had penetrated the vitellus.

12)   After the head became embedded in the oöplasm it soon lost its contrast and began to be transformed into the male pronucleus. The remainder of the flagellum was gradually drawn into the egg cytoplasm. The incorporation of the flagellum was completed in four hours (Figure 9).

13) Penetration of the vitelline membrane was the signal for two events: (a) release of the cortical granules that are located just below the vitelline membrane into the perivitelline space, which somehow "tans" the zona pellucida and vitelline membrane so that no additional sperm may enter; and (b) setting in motion the final steps in second polar body formation.

SECOND MEIOTIC DIVISION AND POLAR BODY FORMATION IN VITRO AS RECORDED ON FILM

The second meiotic division, resulting in the formation of the second polar body, is a dramatic event that follows penetration of the vitellus by a sperm and begins 20 to 40 minutes after sperm head fusion with the vitellus.[10]

Again, there is very little information on second polar body formation from direct observations of this process in any animal except the mouse.

At the time of ovulation the first polar body has been abstricted. It contains one-half of the tetraploid chromosomes; thus, the remaining diploid number of chromosomes are aligned on the metaphase plate of the second maturation spindle. This, then, is the condition of the egg as it awaits sperm penetration. The second maturation spindle lies paratangential to the surface membrane. Twenty to 30 minutes after the sperm fuses with the egg vitellus, the chromosomes on the second spindle begin to move toward the poles of the spindle. It takes, on the average, five minutes for the chromosomes to reach the poles.

During this time, two clear, cytoplasmic blebs appear on the surface of the egg just above the spindle, followed by a furrow directly in line with the equatorial plane of the spindle. As it deepens, the blebs closely resemble half of the cleavage process in normal mitosis. Within ten to 20 minutes after the start of the furrowing, one bleb is gradually absorbed into the vitellus and disappears completely. During this process the spindle rotates 90° to the surface and the second polar body becomes abstricted.[11] When this happens the haploid condition is attained, and the normal fertilization process proceeds in the formation of male and female pronuclei. As the pronuclei move toward the center of the cell, the haploid chromosomes replicate. The cytoplasm of the pronuclei fuses; a mitotic spindle forms; the chromosomes line up on the metaphase plate and the first division occurs to form the first two blastomeres.[12] The impregnated oöcyte at the stage of the first mitosis is properly named the zygote. The zygote contains a new combination of maternal and paternal genes. From the genetic point of view, zygote formation represents the most important period in the individual's life.

The Complexity of Embryo Attachment to the Endometrium and Implantation

When the embryo reaches the uterine lumen in about three days after fertilization, it comprises a ball of 60 to 80 cells called the morula (Figure 10). Within 24 to 36 hours the number of cells will have doubled and are still confined within the zona pellucida. Some of the cells will form a continuous single layer lining the inside of the zona pellucida. The remaining cells (60 to 80 of them) aggregate at one pole to become the inner cell mass from which the embryo and its immediate membranes are developed (amnion, yolk sac, allantois). The cells lining the zona pellucida will become the trophoblast or nutritive layer—a part of which eventually develops into the fetal portion of the placenta. During the entire time that the morula is transformed into a blastocyst, the zona pellucida remains intact and any vital materials entering or leaving the embryo must traverse this selective membrane (Figure 10). Several hours before the embryo attaches itself to the endometrium, the cells of the trophoblast in the region of the inner cell mass begin to proliferate and form a syncytium, the "attachment cone" or attaching trophoblast (Figure 11). It is at this juncture that the zona pellucida eventually thins out sufficiently to allow the remainder to slough off as a grape skin off a grape. The embryo literally appears to "hatch" from its confining zona pellucida. This phenomenon has never been seen in the human but has been recorded in various laboratory animals.

The manner in which the blastocyst orients itself for attachment and accomplishes invasion of the maternal endometrium is unknown for the human, but from observations in several different mammals it appears that this process is accomplished in a series of steps. The trophoblast cells lying above the inner cell mass are transformed, by rapid cell multiplication, into a syncytium (a syncytium is a mass of protoplasm containing numerous nuclei that are not separated by cell membranes). The syncytium forms the attachment cone that becomes so sticky that it adheres to the uterine epithelium. Complex interdigitations of the plasma membranes of the syncytial trophoblast and endometrial epithelial cells may assist in maintaining the attachment (Figure 11). Stickiness of the embryonic trophoblast is a factor in orienting the embryo so that invasion of the endometrium occurs in a very precise manner. When firm attachment has been accomplished, the cells of the attachment cone either force their cytoplasmic processes between the epithelial cells, thus further anchoring the blastocysts, or they secrete proteolytic enzymes that kill and erode the endometrial tissues (Figure 11). The syncytial trophoblast develops very rapidly and forms a thick trophoblastic shell that covers the cytotro-

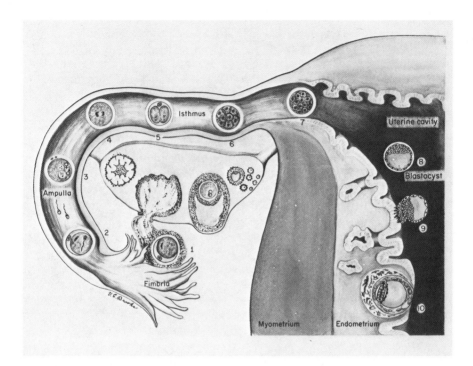

Figure 10: The sequence of development from fertilization to implantation. No. 1, the ovulated egg, in cumulus, is picked up by the cilia on the fimbria of the oviduct and transported into the ampulla of the oviduct. No. 2, sperm penetration of the ovum. No. 3, formation of the pronuclei. Nos. 4 and 5, beginning segmentation. No. 6, formation of the morula. No. 7, morula enters the uterus. No. 8, transformation of the morula into the blastocyst. No. 9, embryo attachment to the endometrium. No. 10, interstitial implantation.

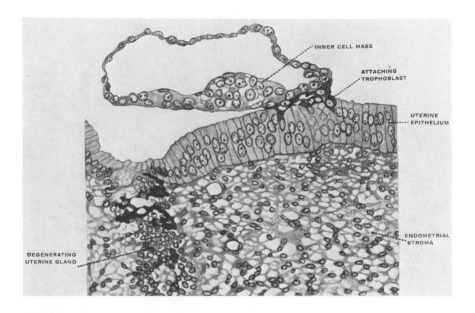

Figure 11:   The early attachment of the syncytial trophoblast to the uterine epithelium in the monkey blastocyst. No similar stage has been observed in the human. (Courtesy of Carnegie Institution of Washington)

phoblast and invades the endometrium. The formation of an extensive implantation cavity is not seen in the human. It appears that after implantation has been accomplished, subsequent expansion of the chorionic sac involves the displacement of the adjacent endometrial tissue without much evidence of endometrial tissue damage.[13]

The youngest known attached human blastocyst was recovered approximately 7.5 days after fertilization (Figure 12). It already was partially embedded in the endometrium; thus, it is usually stated that implantation in the human begins on the sixth day and is completed on the seventh. The human embryo undergoes interstitial implantation—i.e., it sinks into the endometrial connective tissue stroma, is enclosed by it, and comes to lie outside the lumen. Interstitial implantation is almost completed by 9.5 days and the uterine epithelium is now covering over the implantation site (Figure 13).

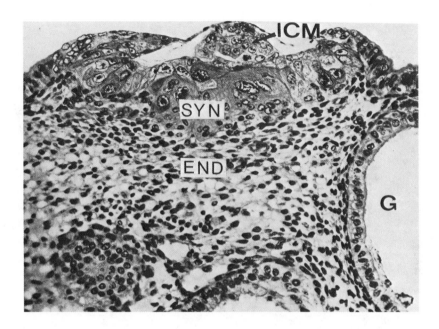

Figure 12:   A 7.5-day implanting human embryo. Note that the syncytial trophoblast (SYN) lies in close apposition to the maternal endometrium (END). The embryonic pole or inner cell mass (ICM) projects
slightly into the uterine lumen. G = endometrial gland. (Courtesy of
Carnegie Institution of Washington)

It is not possible to cover all the changes that occur during implantation and placenta formation here. An excellent description may be found
elsewhere.[14] The following is a brief outline of some of the important steps
in the development of the placenta.

1)   The inner layer of trophoblast is the cytotrophoblast, composed
      of individual cuboidal cells that proliferate at a remarkable rate
      to form the syncytial trophoblast. To repeat, the syncytial
      trophoblast differs from the cytotrophoblast in that it has no cell

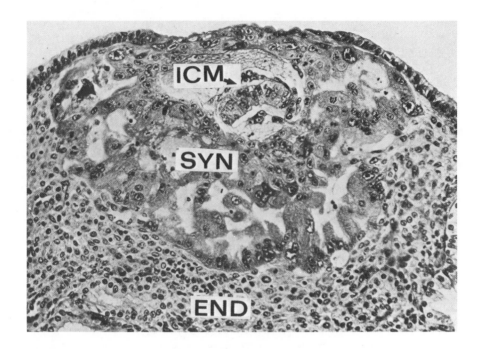

Figure 13:   A 9.5-day human implanting embryo. The syncytial trophoblast (SYN) is encroaching upon the endometrium (END) rapidly. ICM = inner cell mass. Note that the embryo now lies almost completely within the maternal endometrium. (Courtesy of Carnegie Institution of Washington)

boundaries, and the nuclei and cytoplasm all flow together in a manner similar to the mycelium of a fungus.

2)   The syncytial trophoblast kills the maternal tissues, perhaps by secreting proteolytic enzymes that digest the tissues, and encompass the digested material in lacunae, or "little lakes," from which the digested material is transported by cells to the growing embryo in a "bucket brigade" fashion (Figure 13).

3) Cords of trophoblast (i.e., both cyto- and syncytial) extend outward from the surface of the chorion to form the primary villi. On gross examination they appear much as an elm tree with its numerous and fine branchings (Figure 14).

4) Mesenchyme forms in these cores; the cores become vascularized to form the secondary villi, some of which eventually will form the true placenta.

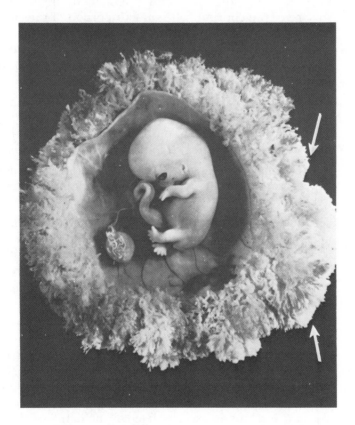

Figure 14:   A seven- to eight-week-old human embryo within its gestational sac. The chorionic villi to the right (arrows) will develop into the fetal placenta; those to the left will disappear.

5) During the first 40 days of development the villi extend over the entire surface of the chorion, which then is called the "chorion frondosum." There appears to be a direct relationship between the extent of villi formation, the establishment of blood circulation within them, and the metabolic needs of the growing embryo (Figure 14).

6) As the placenta forms, all of the villi except those specifically involved in the formation of the placenta disappear from the surface of the chorion. The smooth portion of the chorion is now called the "chorion laeve." The villi that formed the chorion laeve do not become vascularized; thus they differ significantly from those forming the chorion frondosum or the future placenta.

7) The structural and functional unit of the placenta is the villus. As the villi differentiate, they become longer and highly branched, and resemble a complex root system in the chorionic plate with their branches extending into the intervillous spaces.

8) The circulation of maternal blood into the villiated spaces begins toward the close of the third or beginning of the fourth week.

9) The maternal blood flows through the large intercommunicating spaces that were formed by the confluence of the lacunae mentioned above. These spaces are lined by the primitive syncytium and are referred to as the intervillous spaces. From what has been said it should be obvious that the syncytial trophoblast is bathed directly by circulating maternal blood.

10) The circumferential expansion of the placenta as pregnancy proceeds is effected by columns of cytotrophoblast that grow out and penetrate deeply into the endometrium. During this expansion the cytotrophoblast is continuously transformed into syncytial trophoblast. The development of the placenta is so complex that there are few who fully understand it. Full placenta development is completed by the sixth month of pregnancy. It is estimated that at term approximately 12 square meters of surface area have been established by the placental villi.

By the ninth and tenth weeks of development the human fetus is in reality a facsimile of the adult (Figure 15). The primary components of form are present, but there remain significant developmental processes that will continue even for several years after birth. For example, although

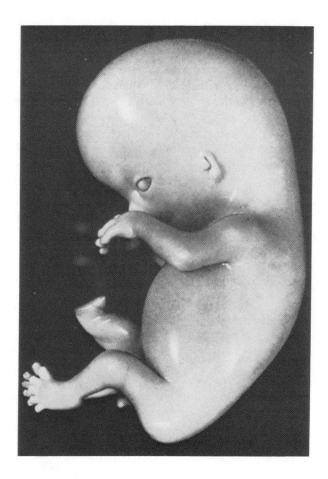

Figure 15: A 60-day-old human fetus recovered from a spontaneous abortion.

by the tenth week five or more billion neurones have populated the cortex of the brain, there remains the complicated process of establishing the innumerable axons and dendrites that form connections between the various neurones and the isolation of the nerves by the deposition of myelin. Another example is the lung, which at this stage has a glandular appearance, and even at the time of birth will not have fully developed the terminal alveoli.[15]

It should be clear, even from this brief examination, that development of a human embryo and fetus is indeed a complexity so intricate as to be almost unimaginable.

Notes

1. J.D. Biggers, A.W. Schuetz, Oögenesis (University Park Press, Baltimore)(1972).
2. Blandau, R.J., White, B.J., Rumery, R.E., *Observations on the Movements of the Living Primordial Germ Cells in the Mouse*, Fertility and Sterility 14(5):482 (1963).
3. A.F. Holstein, E.C. Roosen-Runge, Atlas of Human Spermatogenesis (Gross Verlag, Berlin)(1980).
4. Moor, R.M., Warnes, G.M., *Meiosis in Mammalian Oöcytes*, British Medical Bulletin 35(2):99 (1979).
5. Ladman, A.J., *The Male Reproductive System*, in Histology, (R.O. Greep and L. Weiss, eds.) (McGraw-Hill, New York) (4th ed. 1977); *see also* Holstein, Roosen-Runge, *supra* note 3.
6. Gaddum-Rosse, P., Blandau, R.J., Lee, W.I., *Sperm Penetration into Cervical Mucus In Vitro, Comparative Studies*, Fertility and Sterility 33(6):636 (1980).
7. Settlage, D.S.F., Motoshima, M., Tredway, D.R., *Sperm Transport from the External Os to the Fallopian Tube in Women:A Time and Quantitation Study*, Fertility and Sterility 24(9):655 (1973).
8. Blandau, R.J., *Gamete Transport in the Female Mammal* in Handbook of Physiology , Vol. II,§7 (R.O. Greep and R. Geiger, eds.) (American Physiological Society, Washington, D.C.) (1973) at 153.
9. Sato, K., Blandau, R.J., *Time and Process of Sperm Penetration into Cumulus-Free Mouse Egg Fertilization In Vitro*, Gamete Research 2(4):295(1979).
10. Sato, K., Blandau, R.J., *Second Meiotic Division and Polar Body Formation in Mouse Eggs Fertilized In Vitro*, Gamete Research 2(4):283 (1979).
11. *Id.*
12. Yanagimachi, R., *Mechanisms of Fertilization in Mammals*, in Fertilization and Embryonic Development In Vitro (L. Mastroianni and J. Biggers, eds.) (Plenum Press, New York) (1981) at 81.
13. J.D. Boyd, W.J. Hamilton, The Human Placenta (W. Heffer & Sons, Cambridge) (1970).

14. *Id. See also The Human Placenta,* in HISTOLOGY, *supra* note 5.
15. Boyden, E.A., *Development of the Human Lung*, in PRACTICE IN PEDIATRICS, Vol. IV (Harper & Row, Hagerstown, MD) (1975) at 1.

Chapter 4

Fetal Abnormalities: Detection, Counseling, and Dilemmas

Aubrey Milunsky

The advent of prenatal genetic diagnosis in the mid-50s set the stage for what has become a critically important diagnostic tool. Indeed, this technology now represents the most significant advance thus far in the prevention of serious or fatal genetic disease, or disease characterized by severe and irrevocable mental retardation.[1] While almost 3,000 Mendelian genetic disorders have been recognized and catalogued,[2] only a few hundred can be detected or managed prenatally.

The fundamental philosophy of prenatal genetic diagnosis is to help parents at risk have offspring unaffected by specific genetic disorders. This has largely meant prenatal diagnosis followed by elective abortion of the affected fetus(es), except in rare instances (e.g., methylmalonic aciduria, where treatment of the affected fetus in utero is possible). Despite the continuing need to consider pregnancy termination of the defective fetus, prenatal diagnosis is clearly provided as a life-giving and not a life-taking technique. Four times as many women with genetic risks now undertake pregnancies because of the availability of prenatal diagnosis compared to those faced with the consideration of ending a pregnancy because of a seriously defective fetus.

Although many genetic disorders have been catalogued, the opportunities for prenatal diagnosis continue to be relatively limited.[3] Thus far, prenatal diagnosis is possible for all recognized chromosomal disorders, for the management of all sex-linked disorders through fetal sex determination, for about 100 biochemical genetic disorders of metabolism, neural tube defects, and a few other selected congenital malformations. In fact, three of the most common birth defects/genetic disorders (Down syndrome, neural tube defects, and the fragile-X syndrome) are diagnosable prenatally. However, there is a sobering realization that we have no idea of the cause at present for the condition of at least one-third of the patients with severe mental retardation and perhaps as many as two-thirds of those with mild mental retardation.[4]

About one in 161 newborn infants will have some kind of chromosomal anomaly, while 25 to 30 percent of admissions to children's hospitals in western countries are for birth defects, genetic disorders, or mental retardation.[5] Indeed, more than 10 percent of western populations either have or will develop overt genetic disease while many others will undoubtedly be affected by disorders which reflect environmental/genetic interaction. Except for very rare disorders treatable in utero, prenatal diagnosis must still unfortunately result in elective pregnancy termination in those few cases where serious fetal abnormality is detected. Clearly, the desirable goal would be to selectively prevent the conception of a seriously deformed or defective fetus rather than to avoid such births by selective abortion. However, the pursuance of this goal is hindered by antiabortion groups that seek the enactment of legislation barring fetal research.[6]

OPTIONS FOR PREVENTION

Most babies with congenital malformations or genetic disorders are born to couples without prior warning. However, in recent years it has become possible to apprise more and more couples of their higher risk of having a defective child, and the increasing availability of carrier detection tests for different genetic disorders will steadily continue to facilitate this as a preventive measure.[7] Vasectomy or tubal ligation may also be important measures. Couples at risk for autosomal dominant disorders with paternal transmission are now routinely counseled (or should be) about the availability of artificial insemination by donor. This same option is also a critical consideration for male carriers of autosomal recessive disorders who have a carrier spouse. For both these categories of disease, even if artificial insemination by donor was fully utilized, only a small fraction of fetal abnormalities or genetic defects would be avoided. Obviously, adoption would be available as another choice for these couples.

Prenatal diagnosis of fetal abnormalities remains the most valuable option for the avoidance of serious or fatal birth defects or genetic disorders, although treatment in utero is feasible in only a few rare instances. Recognition of all available options for the prevention or avoidance of birth defects or genetic disorders should be given in the genetic counseling process.

APPROACHES TO PRENATAL DIAGNOSIS

Prenatal diagnosis through the technique of amniocentesis has been in active use since 1967.[8] The amniocentesis procedure has long been known to be associated with only a very small risk of fetal loss.[9] Amniotic fluid containing cells derived from the fetus is placed in cell culture, and from these cultivated cells it is now possible to make the prenatal diagnosis of all recognizable chromosomal disorders, to determine fetal sex for the management of sex-linked disorders, and to diagnose over 100 different biochemical disorders of metabolism. These biochemical diagnoses are feasible mostly through enzyme assays of cultivated amniotic fluid cells. Biochemical estimations of proteins or other substances in cell-free amniotic fluid enable the prenatal detection of neural tube defects as well as a few other fetal anomalies.

Additional invasive techniques include fetoscopy, in which fetal blood samples can be directly obtained, thereby enabling the prenatal detection of sickle cell anemia, thalassemia, and hemophilia as well as a few other disorders. In addition, fetoscopy has allowed visualization of some fetal defects, especially those in which a physical abnormality is known to be directly associated with serious mental retardation.[10] Newer techniques rely upon the extraction of DNA from noncultivated amniotic fluid cells, which will undoubtedly become a very important dimension in prenatal diagnosis in the future.

Noninvasive techniques now largely depend upon the use of ultrasound. Through this modality, normal fetal growth parameters can be measured (e.g., head circumference, body length, limb length, and certain organ sizes) and the presence of multiple fetuses determined. The placenta can be accurately located and the most optimal site for the amniocentesis needle determined. The increasing sophistication of ultrasound has now largely obviated the use of another technique called amniography. This procedure requires the instillation of radio-opaque contrast into the amniotic fluid allowing for greater clarity in the examination of the fetal profile as well as certain internal organs, such as the fetal esophagus and intestinal tract. Intravenously administered contrast to the pregnant mother has also enabled the demonstration of fetal kidney presence, size, or abnormality.

DILEMMAS, PITFALLS AND ERRORS

Many potential dilemmas, pitfalls, or errors in prenatal diagnosis exist and, not unexpectedly, many have already been experienced; some have even been the subject of litigation.[11] This section provides a circumscribed insight into these problems, which are categorized according to the indications for the original prenatal diagnostic study.

CHROMOSOMAL DISORDERS

From time to time women undergoing prenatal studies for advanced maternal age are confronted by the unexpected finding of a disorder less severe than the feared autosomal trisomies, such as Down syndrome. Prenatal detection of a fetus with XXX or an XYY karyotype leads to dilemmas and difficult decision making. Couples are often left in a quandary because of the insufficient data base needed to provide clear and unequivocal prognostic information especially relevant to intellectual development. Clearly, the couple's perception of the burden relative to the severity of the disorder in question weighs heavily upon the decision-making process.

Among the most difficult and persistent problems in prenatal diagnosis of chromosomal disorders is the finding of mosaicism. The difficulty lies not in the diagnosis of true mosaicism but rather in the inability to be certain about the clinical implications of mosaicism and its phenotypic manifestations after birth. Occasionally prenatal chromosome analysis yields an abnormal karyotype where the clinical implications are not known. A typical example would be detection of an especially small chromosomal fragment in the amniotic fluid cell chromosomes. There has also been the occasional, inadvertent discovery during prenatal chromosome analysis of a paternity discrepancy. This dilemma has arisen when an abnormality of the Y-chromosome was suspected, and not confirmed by examination of the putative father. Clearly, ethical issues emerge, the resolution of which may be guided by the nature of any fetal abnormality that may be associated with a suspected Y-chromosome aberration, e.g., X/Y translocation.

Twin pregnancy represents another example of potential problems. While the frequency of twin pregnancy approximates one in 80, those patients undergoing prenatal diagnosis for advanced maternal age have a slightly higher frequency. Besides the attendant increased technical difficulties of amniocentesis in multiple pregnancy, determination of fetal abnormality is fraught with difficulty. Estimates are that between one in 4,000 to one in 8,000 women who undergo amniocentesis for advanced maternal age will be found to be carrying twins in which one twin has a serious chromosomal anomaly. Parents in this situation face the tortured dilemma of continuing the pregnancy with the realization that one fetus has a congenital disorder, or electing abortion including the normal fetus. Recently, in two separate cases, a twin fetus was found to have Down syndrome and Hurler syndrome respectively.[12] In both cases the parents elected to terminate the pregnancy unless the normal twin could be selectively saved. In order to spare the normal twin in both cases, the defective twin was terminated and both pregnancies continued to term resulting in the live birth of normal infants. The ethical and potential legal dilemma spawned by these difficult cases are self-evident. It should be noted that in the second case, the mother already had a child with Hurler syndrome who suffered from the associated severe mental retardation.

Prenatal diagnosis of chromosomal disorders in the third trimester has been an uncommon consideration. There is, however, increasing awareness that intra-uterine fetal growth retardation or other indicators of fetal abnormality may signal the presence of a serious chromosomal disorder. It is also well-known that cesarean sections are frequently done in those very pregnancies where fetal abnormality is present (fetal distress or failure to progress in labor being the most common reasons). In these pregnancies, determination of a serious fetal chromosome abnormality during the third trimester may well influence the method of delivery. For example, given a situation in which concerns about the child's ultimate intellectual abilities may be in question, cesarean section might be avoided (in order to lessen the morbidity to the mother) if the diagnosis of trisomy 13 or 18[13] has already been made. While some may argue that this imposition of physician and parental values is unacceptable, the fact remains that the decision represents the private interaction of the physician and his or her patient.

SEX-LINKED DISEASES

For the approximately 200 disorders in the sex-linked disease category, there is a 50 percent risk that if the fetus is male, it will be affected. Hemophilia and muscular dystrophy are two of the more common disorders that arise in the considerations of prenatal diagnosis. Unfortunately, it is possible to diagnose only about six sex-linked disorders in the male fetus at the present time. For all the others, fetal sex determination results in the option of selective abortion of a male fetus without knowing for certain whether it is affected.

Couples at risk for having males with a 50 percent chance of an X-linked disease (such as muscular dystrophy or Lesch-Nyhan syndrome) may face a difficult decision when confronted with twins, one of whom is a male. The dilemma is heightened when a specific diagnosis on that male cannot be made. Once again, the parents' perception of the severity and burden of the disease will weigh heavily in their decision making, as will religious considerations.

At least one X-linked disease is amenable to treatment, although it cannot be cured. Specific prenatal diagnosis of hemophilia has now been achieved through fetal blood sampling, and couples facing decisions to continue or abort such pregnancies require expert counseling about the disease as well as the method and implications of treatment. Even with treatment, considerable complications and suffering can be anticipated, and these matters require careful consideration. On the other hand, there are other X-linked disorders (such as Becker muscular dystrophy) where major incapacity may have a late onset and is compatible with a life expectancy to about middle age.

BIOCHEMICAL GENETIC DISORDERS

The prenatal detection of biochemical genetic disorders is almost invariably done for conditions characterized by irreparable mental retardation or serious/fatal disease.[14] On rare occasions such studies are also performed for disorders which are "treatable," such as galactosemia or methylmalonic aciduria. The confounding problem in the latter situations is the inability to predict if treatment started even as early as 16 weeks of gestation might be successful, and if so, to what degree. Fetal or embryonic damage could well occur during the first 16 weeks of gestation, perhaps even in those women known to be at risk who take dietary precautions (e.g., the exclusion of lactose for women at risk of having a child with galactosemia). Prospective parents known to be carriers of certain serious genetic disorders, such as sickle cell anemia and the severe forms of thalassemia, also face difficult dilemmas. Through genetic counseling they learn that the affected child is most likely to survive ten to 30 years (or longer) but with considerable pain and suffering from the complications of these disorders.

As noted earlier, a couple at risk of bearing a child with a serious biochemical genetic disorder such as Hurler syndrome, which is characterized by profound mental retardation and multi-organ involvement, may have a twin pregnancy in which one of the pair is affected. However, such a situation is rare.

NEURAL TUBE DEFECTS

Anencephaly is not compatible with survival, and most infants with this defect die either at birth or within the first 48 hours. However, occasionally they may survive for some weeks, rarely even for some months, despite a vegetative existence. While death in the neonatal period or soon after is certain for anencephalic infants, such is not the fate of infants with spina bifida. Survival into the teens occurs in 12 to 40 percent of the cases, albeit with paraplegia, hydrocephalus or mental retardation in many. The prenatal detection of spina bifida is now routinely done using maternal serum alpha-fetoprotein screening, amniotic fluid alpha-fetoprotein and acetylcholinesterase assays and ultrasound. Over 98 percent of these lesions are detected when these methods are used in combination. Diagnostic difficulties arise when fetal blood contamination of amniotic fluid leads to a spurious elevation of alpha-fetoprotein associated in some cases with acetyl cholinesterase activity in the same fluid. This result makes it impossible to rely upon the biochemical assays, and the ultrasound result would weigh heavily in the parental decision-making process. Rarely, and after complete testing, an apparently normal fetus might be aborted. For example, there have been two such instances in some 20,000 (now 40,000) cases at the Center for Human Genetics, and additional cases where parental decisions prior to the completion of all testing led to abortion of an apparently normal fetus.[15]

Discovery of twins discordant for neural tube defects is not very rare. Parental action in these difficult circumstances is often influenced by the nature of the fetal defect. Faced with anencephaly in one twin fetus and the realization that the outcome for that fetus or child will be fatal, some parents will continue the pregnancy in order to secure the delivery of the apparently normal fetus. For other prospective parents, psychological stress under these circumstances may lead to the decision to abort. Confronted with one twin fetus affected by spina bifida and the attendant realization of the likely burden of severity of this disorder, enormous dilemmas are spawned. A decision to continue with such a pregnancy almost invariably leads to further painful decisons immediately after birth when the question of surgical repair arises in the face of a catastrophic lesion.

The prenatal detection of neural tube defects requires biochemical assays for alpha-fetoprotein and acetylcholinesterase in amniotic fluid. In less than one percent of such studies false positive results are obtained. These would imply that the biochemical studies suggest a neural tube defect—a conclusion which is incorrect but which can usually be corrected by ultrasound study. Nevertheless, there are rare instances (two in 40,000) where an apparently normal fetus may be aborted as a consequence of a truly false positive result. In contrast, 102 serious fetal defects were detected in that same large group of patients studied prospectively.

SELECTED PROBLEMS

Prior to undergoing amniocentesis, it is important for the patient to be informed about the maternal and fetal risks of the procedure and about the potential problems arising in the laboratory. Verbal and written consent should be required for laboratory procedures. Basic to that consent must be the understanding that cell culture may fail and that no results may be forthcoming even after a second and, on rare occasions, a third amniocentesis. Not rarely, a slow-growing cell culture may have allowed no analysis by twenty third weeks gestation, especially in a patient who has undergone amniocentesis later than 18 weeks. Under such circumstances, patients at the Center for Human Genetics are routinely advised to make a decision about continuing their pregnancy based simply on the known risks of the anomaly with which they are concerned. The consent form therefore informs them that if the 23rd week of gestation is reached without a result, they would be faced with a decision without further information. These are of course very unusual instances.

The critical implications of diagnoses made prenatally demand standards bordering between excellence and perfection. Not surprisingly, then, worldwide experience[16] reflects extremely accurate and painstaking work. Nevertheless, error rates between 0.2 and 0.6 percent have been recorded. Such errors have evolved in very specific circumstances, the most common being maternal cell admixture resulting in the determination of either karyotypes or enzymatic assays not reflecting the fetal status. As a consequence, fetal sex determination has been incorrectly reported, and on occasion a fetal chromosomal disorder missed. Of course, this error would be critically important only if prenatal studies were being done for sex-linked diseases. Occasionally, poor quality of the metaphases being analyzed (staining or spreading) has been the reason for a misdiagnosis. Faced with the extreme pressures of obtaining a diagnosis with no time for repeat studies, the inexperienced laboratory may venture a guess resulting in an inaccurate fetal karyotypic assessment, rather than report an inability to make a certain diagnosis. On rare occasions, simple incompetence by the cytogeneticist has resulted in either the failure to diagnose a chromosomal abnormality or the misreading of a normal karyotype. There is at least one such example where a normal karyotype was reported as trisomy 21, resulting in the termination of a normal pregnancy.

Prior to the routine use of ultrasound preceding the introduction of the amniocentesis needle, inadvertent aspiration of urine instead of amniotic fluid occurred in about 0.5 percent of cases. Today, despite the use of sonography, a urine sample is obtained once in about every 400 to 500 cases, to the great dismay of the patient and chagrin of the physician. Some of these instances are due to the patient having the ultrasound done in the x-ray department and the amniocentesis on another table elsewhere in the hospital or physician's office. Changed positions and elapsed time allow for bladder-filling which alters the relative anatomy shown from that in the initial ultrasound study.

While problems with biochemical assays are not common, the potential for error is great. Mistakes have occurred in laboratories without demonstrated technical competence. Misinterpretations of assays performed correctly have also occurred, while a lack of sufficient control has led to occasional erroneous interpretations. More difficult misdiagnoses have occurred when rare or unusual variant forms of a biochemical genetic disorder have been present in the fetus. Careful assessment of the parental carrier status in such disorders (e.g., Tay-Sachs disease or metachromatic leukodystrophy) is required. One clear and overriding message from experience with the biochemical genetic evaluation of the fetus is that these tests should be done only by highly experienced genetic diagnostic laboratories.

While it may be easy in a busy laboratory to have a slide or tube-labelling mix-up, no parent who becomes the victim of such misadventure and suffers the tragic consequences will be comforted by understanding human fallibility. Such reported incidents are rare but nevertheless occur with sufficient frequency as to require the most stringent safeguards in these laboratories. There are examples of normal pregnancies being interrupted because of labelling errors, and a few cases in which a defective child was born despite every precaution taken by the parents. Equipment failure (most commonly incubator malfunction) or deficiencies in consumable materials used for prenatal diagnosis, especially cell cultures, have also contributed to this category of diagnostic failures. Such events have occurred even in the most sophisticated and careful laboratories, resulting in the loss of many cell cultures. Despite the necessary constant vigilance, it is inevitable that such technical mishaps will occur. Consequently, patients should be apprised prior to amniocentesis that cell culture may fail. As apparently benign a procedure as using a particular brand of syringe for aspirating amniotic fluid has been reported a few times as cytotoxic to amniotic fluid cells.

In the days before ultrasound became routine prior to amniocentesis, missed multiple pregnancy was not infrequent. The attendant risks in a mother at high risk (e.g., 25 percent) of bearing an affected child are self-evident in the situations where only one amniotic sac might have been tapped. With ultrasound, there is no excuse today to miss the presence of multiple pregnancy.

GENETIC COUNSELING ERRORS OF OMISSION AND COMMISSION

The legal responsibilities of genetic counselors have been fully considered elsewhere.[17] In essence, errors of omission have largely occurred under circumstances in which physicians have allegedly failed to inform their patients of the availability of diagnostic genetic tests and counseling. More specifically, according to available case records,[18] claims have been made against physicians for not informing about the availability of amniocentesis and prenatal diagnosis, or for not referring to another physician elsewhere, or for deceptively presenting amniocentesis risk figures. Some have erred in not offering patients at risk the opportunity for carrier detection tests, simply on the basis of their ethnic group. Also, physicians have been found liable for not properly communicating the possibility of abnormal results to patients to whom a child with a major birth defect was born. The provision of totally erroneous recurrence risk figures has also been the basis for other litigation.

Notwithstanding the complexities and potential dilemmas of prenatal diagnosis, hundreds of thousands of women have undergone these valuable studies without incident. Thorough professional and public education about the indications and limitations of these procedures will serve to reduce to a minimum adverse medical, ethical, or legal complications. Clearly, we can look forward to the benefits of continuing advances in this field and the reassurance that couples at increased risk can have a child unaffected by a specific serious genetic disorder.

NOTES

1. *See generally* GENETIC DISORDERS AND THE FETUS: DIAGNOSIS, PREVENTION AND TREATMENT (A. Milunsky, ed.)(Plenum Press, New York)(1979) [hereinafter cited as GENETIC DISORDERS]; THE PREVENTION OF GENETIC DISEASE AND MENTAL RETARDATION (A. Milunsky, ed.)(W.B. Saunders, Philadelphia)(1975) [hereinafter cited as GENETIC DISEASE].
2. *See* V.A. McKUSICK, MENDELIAN INHERITANCE IN MAN, 5th ed. (Johns Hopkins Univ. Press, Baltimore)(1978).
3. *See* GENETIC DISORDERS, *supra* note 1.
4. *See* GENETIC DISEASE, *supra* note 1.
5. *Id.*
6. *See e.g.,* MASS. GEN. LAWS, c 112 § 12J.
7. *See,* GENETIC DISORDERS, *supra* note 1.
8. *Id.*
9. *See* C.U. LOWE, *et. al.,* THE SAFETY AND ACCURACY OF MID-TRIMESTER AMNIOCENTESIS (Dept. of Health, Education and Welfare, Washington, D.C.)(1978); Simpson, N.E., et. al., *Prenatal Diagnosis of Genetic Disease in Canada: Report of a Collaborative Study,* CANADIAN MEDICAL ASSOCIATION JOURNAL 115:739 (1976).
10. *See* GENETIC DISEASE, *supra* note 1.
11. *See* GENETIC DISORDERS, *supra* note 1; GENETICS AND THE LAW II (A. Milunsky and G.J. Annas, eds.) (Plenum Press, New York)(1980) [hereinafter cited as GENETICS AND THE LAW II.]
12. Kerenyi, T.D., Chitkara, U., *Selective Birth in Twin Pregnancy with Discordancy for Down's Syndrome,* NEW ENGLAND JOURNAL OF MEDICINE 304:1525 (1981);

Alberg, A., Mitelman, F., Cantz, M., *Cardiac Puncture of Fetus with Hurler's Disease Avoiding Abortion of Unaffected Co-Twin*, LANCET 2:990 (1978).

13. Chromosome disorders in which there is an extra chromosome in each cell are called trisomies. When the extra chromosome is a number 21, the disorder is termed trisomy 21, which in fact is Down syndrome. When the extra chromosome is number 13 or 18, specific syndromes are also recognizable, and characterized by severe mental retardation and serious multiple congenital anomalies.

14. *See* GENETIC DISORDERS, *supra* note 1.

15. Milunsky, A., *Prenatal Detection of Neural Tube Defects: Experience with 20,000 Pregnancies*, JOURNAL OF THE AMERICAN MEDICAL ASSOCIATION 244:2731 (1980).

16. *See* GENETIC DISORDERS, *supra* note 1.

17. Healey, J.M., *The Legal Obligations of Genetic Counselors*, in GENETICS AND THE LAW II, *supra* note 11, at 69.

18. *See*, GENETICS AND THE LAW II, *supra* note, 11, at 64.

Chapter 5

Advances in Fetal Diagnosis and Therapy

Mitchell S. Golbus

The medical approach to a disease or group of disorders routinely has three stages: recognizing that the disease state exists; developing methods for diagnosing the disorder; and finding a prophylaxis or therapy for the condition. The recognition that birth defects exist dates from antiquity, but advancement to the second stage, that of considering the fetus as a patient and prenatally diagnosing congenital defects, began only 15 years ago. The third stage, treatment of the fetus in utero, is only beginning now.

FETOSCOPY

As the name implies, the objective of prenatal diagnosis is to determine whether a fetus believed to be at risk for a particular birth defect is actually affected. The most direct method of examining the patient is to look at him or her through a small bore fiberoptic endoscope which can be inserted transabdominally into the uterus under local anesthesia. While isolated parts of the fetal anatomy may be identified, visualization of the entire fetus is rarely accomplished because of the narrow viewing angle (55°) of the commonly used fetoscope in an aqueous medium. Therefore, unless a flexible instrument with a wide field of vision is developed, there will be very limited use of direct visualization for prenatal diagnosis.

The major use of fetoscopy has been for obtaining samples of fetal tissues other than amniotic fluid constituents. Many genetic defects not reflected in the latter are identifiable from other fetal tissues or cells. The most readily accessible and easily sampled tissue after birth is blood, and the major attempt to sample fetal tissues has concerned obtaining a drop of fetal blood from the fetal inner surface of the placenta and umbilical cord. The principal abnormalities which have come under investigation thus far relate to hemoglobin structure and synthesis by the red blood cells. It is possible to detect Mediterranean anemia (β-thalassemia or Cooley's anemia), a defect causing reduced production of one of the protein components of hemoglobin.[1] This disease is a major contributor to childhood mortality in many countries of the Mediterranean basin. It is also possible to detect structural abnormalities of hemoglobin, such as the one which causes sickle cell anemia.[2] More than 2,000 pregnancies have been monitored by fetoscopy and fetal blood sampling because of a fetal risk for a hemoglobin disorder. This procedure is now available at almost two dozen centers around the world.

If fetal red blood cells can be obtained by fetoscopy, it follows that other constituents of the fetal blood are obtained simultaneously and would be available for diagnostic tests. The major attempt to capitalize on this has been to examine the fetal plasma for factor VIII in male fetuses at risk for hemophilia.[3] Prenatal diagnosis of disorders involving other serum proteins which are synthesized early in development may be feasible via fetoscopy and fetal blood sampling. Additionally, red or white blood cells obtained by fetal blood sampling have been used to detect specific genetic diseases. This area of prenatal diagnosis is expected to expand over the next decade.

FETAL THERAPY

The ultimate goal for prenatal diagnosis is treatment of the affected fetus to correct the defect. For many disorders it is unlikely that effective corrective or preventive therapy will be developed in the foreseeable future. Furthermore, in at least some metabolic disorders, irreversible fetal damage may have occurred by the time the prenatal diagnosis is made. However, therapeutic alternatives for the management of a number of fetal disorders which can be recognized in utero may be outlined. Since experience with the fetus as a patient is still quite limited, such alternatives must be considered tentative—the basis for further investigation and refinement.

Most correctable malformations which can be diagnosed in utero are best managed by appropriate medical or surgical therapy after delivery at term. The full-term infant is better able to tolerate surgery and anesthesia than is the prematurely delivered infant. Examples of abnormalities in this category include the narrowing or absence of part of the gastrointestinal tract, a small spina bifida, or a cleft palate. Prenatal diagnosis may be important because many of these anomalies are associated with an excess of amniotic fluid which may initiate premature labor. Therapy for the excess amniotic fluid or premature labor may allow the fetus to remain in utero longer and to be born at term. Additionally, the delivery can be planned so that the necessary neonatologists, anesthesiologists and pediatric surgeons are available.

There is a subset of fetal anomalies which require correction ex utero as soon as possible after the diagnosis is made. For these, the risk of prematurity must be weighed against risk of continued gestation. Elective premature delivery for immediate correction may be preferable to continued gestation for such disorders as hydrocephalus or for moderately severe Rh isoimmunization. The principle in each case is that continued gestation would have progressive ill effects on the fetus. Recent advances in the ability to decrease the risk of neonatal respiratory distress syndrome, the main cause of death in premature infants, make premature delivery a safer therapeutic tool than allowing continued gestation.[4] Three to five days before the planned premature delivery, the mother is given certain steroid hormones which will cross the placenta to the fetus and induce enzymes in the lung which decrease the risk of respiratory distress in the neonate.

Another subset of fetal disorders may influence the mode of delivery and require that a cesarean section be performed. One indication for cesarean delivery is an anomaly such that the fetus could not fit through the maternal pelvis during vaginal delivery (e.g., conjoined twins or a fetus with a large hydrocephalus). Occasionally, an elective cesarean section may be indicated for a malformation requiring immediate surgical correction in a sterile environment. Examples include a ruptured herniation of the bowel out of the abdominal cavity (omphalocele) or an uncovered meningomyelocele. After delivery by cesarean section, one such neonate underwent immediate surgery in the operating room next to the one in which its mother was having her surgery.[5] Occasionally, infants are delivered who are at risk for a severe immunodeficiency state which would cause them to be unable to withstand infections. In such cases, the infant is delivered by elective cesarean section to protect its sterility, then placed in a laminar flow hood which maintains a sterile environment for the first few days of life while diagnostic tests are completed. If the infant is not immunodeficient, it can be removed from the hood and sent home with the mother. If it is affected, a thymus transplant or other therapy can be instituted prior to exposure to our bacteria- and virus-laden world.

IN UTERO INTERVENTION

There is a subset of fetal deficiency states which may be alleviated by in utero treatment. These are conditions in which something vital to fetal well-being is not present in sufficient quantity, and supplementation of the missing element would constitute medical therapy. The simplest method of supplying the fetus is to give the missing element to the mother for transportation across the placenta to the fetus. For example, vitamins often act as coenzymes—compounds necessary for proper enzyme functioning, the absence of which disrupts the metabolic process. Two fetuses have been diagnosed in utero as having vitamin-dependent enzyme deficiencies and have been treated before birth. The first had a vitamin B_{12} responsive enzyme disorder (methylmalonic acidemia),[6] and the second had a biotin dependent disorder (multiple carboxylase deficiency).[7] Each was treated by giving the mother massive doses of the required vitamin, and both children are now developing normally, albeit taking huge daily supplements of the necessary vitamin. Another example of medicating the fetus via the mother has been the successful treatment of fetal heart rhythm irregularities by giving the mother digitalis, which crosses the placenta and returns the fetal heart rate to a normal pattern.

Some substances, however, do not cross the placenta and cannot be delivered to the fetus by the mother. In such cases, the deficient substance must be placed in the amniotic sac where the fetus, who continually swallows the amniotic fluid, will ingest it; alternatively the fetus must be given a shot in the buttocks. For example, thyroid hormone does not cross the placenta but has been given intra-amniotically in one instance to treat congenital hypothyroidism and goiter.[8]

Even more complicated is the delivery of cells, such as red blood cells, to the fetus. In Rh isoimmunization, the maternal antibodies destroy fetal red blood cells and the fetus may die of profound anemia. Thus, it is accepted practice to treat severe cases by transfusing the fetus in utero.[9] The technique is to place a needle transabdominally into the fetal abdominal cavity and transfer the needed cells directly to the fetal peritoneal cavity. The lymphatic system can engulf these cells and deliver them to the vascular system for correction of the anemia. In a few instances, a fetus too sick or too young to receive an intra-abdominal transfusion has been transfused directly by injecting the blood cells into an umbilical cord vessel through a fetoscope.

The list of substances which can be given therapeutically to the in utero fetus is certain to grow. For example, it may be possible to treat intrauterine growth retardation, in which a normal fetus is not receiving sufficient nutrition, by instilling nutrients into the amniotic sac. Scientists are investigating enzyme therapy for enzyme-deficient children. If such techniques can be developed, supplying a missing enzyme to the in utero fetus would represent only one further technical step, and might prevent an irreversible collection and storage of the enzyme's substrate.

With the age of gene manipulation now upon us, attention has turned to the concept of replacing a malfunctioning gene in the fetus. According to this concept, a virus carrying a functional copy of the specific human gene would be introduced into a fetus that is missing a gene product. It is hoped that the viral carrier would be integrated into the fetal genome and that the good copy of the gene would function in place of the malfunctioning one. Experiments to date have demonstrated that it is possible to place a "foreign" gene into a mouse embryo via a viral carrier. How to integrate the foreign gene, how to achieve normal control of the gene, and the dangers, if any, of this process are problems yet to be resolved.

SURGICAL FETAL THERAPY

The complement of medical therapy is, of course, surgical therapy. Correcting an anatomic malformation will be more difficult than providing a missing substrate, hormone or medication to the fetus. The prenatally diagnosable anatomic malformations which warrant consideration for surgical therapy are those which interfere with fetal organ development and which, if alleviated, would allow normal fetal development to proceed. The first malformations being considered are hydronephrosis secondary to an obstruction, diaphragmatic hernia, and hydrocephalus.

URINARY TRACT OBSTRUCTION

Obstructive fetal urinary tract malformations are being recognized with increasing frequency because fluid-filled masses are particularly easy to detect by sonography. The back-up of the retained fetal urine causes a large distended bladder (megacystis), fluid-filled ureters (hydroureters), and fluid accumulation in the kidneys (hydronephrosis). The increased fluid and back pressure interfere with fetal kidney development and may cause sufficient kidney damage to be incompatible with postnatal life. Uremia, a build-up of toxic waste products, does not occur in utero because the placenta performs the same waste removal tasks as the kidneys. The lack of fetal urine excretion secondarily causes a decrease in the volume of amniotic fluid, which in turn is associated with underdevelopment of the lungs, apparently because the ebb and flow of amniotic fluid in the fetal trachae aids lung growth. There are also skeletal and facial deformities because of compression by the uterine walls in the absence of the buffering amniotic fluid. The severity of the damage depends on the degree and duration of the urinary outflow obstruction.

It has been observed that failure to take action often leads to the delivery at term of an infant who has neither sufficient functioning kidney tissue nor lung capacity to survive. Therefore, the philosophy has developed that it may be advisable to relieve the obstruction at the earliest possible time.[10] The concept is that continued obstruction will result in a kidney whose development is so impaired as to prevent survival, while relief of the obstruction may allow sufficient development to support postnatal life as well as "catch-up" development during early childhood.

There are several alternatives for decompressing an obstructed fetal urinary tract. The fetal bladder or kidney can be aspirated with a needle under sonographic guidance, but this offers only temporary relief since the fetus normally produces a relatively large amount of urine (5 ml/kg/hr). Experience has shown that aspirated urine is rapidly replaced. Continuous drainage of the urine from the bladder into the amniotic sac not only would decompress the urinary tract and allow renal development to proceed, but also would restore normal amniotic fluid dynamics and prevent the sequelae of decreased amniotic fluid volume.

A catheter has been developed which can provide such drainage.[11] Made of polyethylene, it can be stretched onto a needle for placement and will resume its original shape when pushed off the needle. The catheter has a curl like a pig's tail at each end and multiple side perforations along its length to allow easy urine drainage. This 12-centimeter long catheter can be inserted by placing it on a long needle with a separate length of tubing above to act as a "pusher." The needle, guided sonographically, is directed through the maternal abdominal wall, the uterus, the amniotic sac, the fetal abdominal wall, and into the fetal bladder. The mother may have local anesthetic, an epidural, or general anesthetic depending upon specific conditions and her preferences. If the mother has general anesthesia then the fetus also will be asleep; if not, then she is given a tranquilizer which crosses the placenta and sedates the fetus. Once the catheter tip is advanced into the fetal bladder, pressure readings are obtained; then the catheter is advanced off the needle until one pig-tail loop can be seen sonographically in the bladder. The needle is then further withdrawn, holding the catheter steady, so that the second loop will be positioned in the amniotic cavity.

After the procedure the mother is given intravenous medications to prevent labor, and the fetus and mother are carefully monitored for complications. Serial sonograms over the next few days usually demonstrate complete drainage of the bladder and partial-to-complete drainage of the upper urinary tract (ureters and kidneys). Accumulation of fluid in the amniotic sac is also carefully monitored. The mother is usually discharged from the hospital four to seven days after the procedure, and will have careful sonographic monitoring until delivery.

Our inability to test fetal kidney function and to know how much residual reserve remains or whether irreversible damage has already occurred represents a very serious gap in our technology. The destruction of kidney tissue may be so great at the time of the procedure that no amount of successful drainage could help. And the procedure is so new that, at this writing, it has been tried less than a dozen times. Therefore, it should be viewed as unproven even though it is biologically logical that it should work. Only when medicine can compare the outcome of a series of such fetuses treated with this procedure to a series of untreated fetuses will it be possible to evaluate the potential of the procedure.

There has been one instance in which the fetal urinary tract obstruction was found so early in pregnancy and was so severe it was believed that placement of a catheter was unlikely to be of any use.[12] The patient in this case requested a procedure which had never been attempted on fetuses, although often used on neonates. When a neonate with such an obstruction is born, the surgical approach is to make small bilateral flank incisions to open the ureter near the kidney, and to fix the opened ureters to the skin so that they are open pouches providing continuous drainage. This allows decompression of the entire system while the neonate grows large enough for corrective reconstructive surgery. The patient asked to have this type of procedure attempted on her in utero fetus. After much discussion with her, her family, the Committee on Human Research, and bioethicists, the decision was made to proceed.

The mother had general anesthesia and her abdomen and uterus were surgically opened as if for a cesarean section. The lower half of the fetus was delivered through the uterine incision and the ureters opened as described above. The fetus was replaced in the amniotic sac and the sac, uterine wall, and maternal abdominal wall reclosed. The mother was treated with labor-inhibiting medications, first intravenously and then orally. Mother and fetus made uneventful recoveries. There were no significant uterine contractions, the fetal heart rate remained good, and the fetal movement returned within 24 hours after surgery.

The mother was discharged after ten days, returned to full activity and enjoyed an otherwise uncomplicated pregnancy for the next 16 weeks. The previously massively distended fetal bladder, ureters, and kidneys remained completely decompressed, and the fetus grew normally. However, the amniotic fluid volume did not increase significantly, and when the fetus was delivered by cesarean section near term, it had insufficient kidney and lung development to sustain life. In spite of its unhappy outcome, this case is very significant in that it represents the first instance in which a fetus was successfully operated on, replaced in the uterus, and carried to term.

DIAPHRAGMATIC HERNIA

Congenital diaphragmatic hernia is usually an isolated anomaly in an otherwise normal full-term infant. The abnormality is a failure of the diaphragm to form to and separate the abdominal and chest cavities. The bowel and other abdominal contents herniate into the chest. Surgical correction consists of placing the herniated bowel back in the abdomen and closing the defect in the diaphragm. However, 50 to 80 percent of these infants die of lung underdevelopment caused by lung compression during the last half of gestation.[13] The incidence of congenital diaphragmatic hernia is from 1:2,500 to 1:5,000 newborns, so that 700–1,400 affected children are born annually in the United States. Despite marked advances in neonatal anesthetic, surgical, and respiratory care over the last two decades, the mortality rate of this anomaly has not changed.

Models of diaphragmatic hernias have been created in fetal lambs and rabbits with the demonstration of the changes which lead to neonatal demise. A more sophisticated model has been developed by Dr. Michael Harrison and his coworkers at the University of California, San Francisco.[14] An inflatable silastic balloon is inserted into the left chest cavity of a fetal lamb. The balloon is progressively inflated during gestation, simulating the expanding bowel, and produces a clinical and pathologic picture identical to that seen in congenital diaphragmatic hernia. Dr. Harrison has further shown that if later in gestation he deflates the balloon in the chest, the lung will grow normally and the lamb will survive. The next step will be the surgical production of an actual diaphragmatic hernia early in gestation in the lamb or monkey fetal model, and then correcting the defect later in gestation and evaluating the fetal/neonatal outcome. Much experimental work remains to be done regarding correction of this anomaly, but preliminary experiments are exciting and promising.

HYDROCEPHALUS

Hydrocephalus of prenatal origin occurs in 0.2 percent of all deliveries. It represents a failure of normal cerebrospinal fluid dynamics so that this fluid accumulates in the ventricles, causing them to enlarge and cause pressure atrophy of the brain.[15] Prenatal hydrocephalus represents a subset of childhood hydrocephalus, with a significantly poorer outlook. Between one-half and two-thirds of affected fetuses are stillborn. Only one-quarter of liveborn hydrocephalic neonates survive infancy untreated. Of those babies having ventricular drainage for decompression, 45 percent survived, one-third with normal intelligence. This contrasts sharply with the outlook for hydrocephalus developing after birth, when shunting produces 80 percent survival rates with 70 percent survivors having IQs over 75.

A variety of techniques exists to create hydrocephalus in fetal animal models. Many teratogenic agents fed to rats will cause this anomaly in their offspring. In larger animals such as dogs, sheep, and monkeys, irritants have been injected into the fetal ventricular system to cause reactive hydrocephalus. The first attempts at prenatal correction in a monkey model were recently reported. The ventricles of affected fetuses were drained with a stainless steel valve, allowing only one-way flow from the ventricles to the amniotic cavity. Improved survival and neurologic function were noted in the treated animals. Many similar studies need to be conducted to examine the fluid dynamics and fetal brain reaction to such in utero corrective measures.

These experiments are being performed because it is clear that for optimal treatment of progressive prenatal hydrocephalus, in utero drainage of the ventricles may be required. Waiting until after a term delivery to treat may critically delay therapy. Two approaches to solving this problem have been tried recently: one group performed six weekly needle aspirations of the dilated ventricles of a fetus with hydrocephalus; a second group treated fetuses with prenatal hydrocephalus by placing a polyethylene shunt that could drain ventricular cerebrospinal fluid into the amniotic sac. This area of endeavor is new, and much more work remains to be done. Also, a significant question exists as to whether there may be untreatable brain damage in some instances by the time the prenatal diagnosis is made.

COMMENTARY

The potential for in utero correction of some birth defects gives added significance to the rapidly expanding field of prenatal diagnosis. Therapeutic decisions will require us to go beyond the anatomic definition of the malformation being considered for therapy and perform a thorough evaluation of the fetus's condition. Because it is known that malformations often occur as part of a syndrome, a search for associated abnormalities is necessary to avoid delivering a neonate with a corrected anomaly, but nonetheless affected by other unrecognized disabling or lethal abnormalities.

A major issue has been whether it would be possible to open the uterus and operate upon the fetus without jeopardizing the mother and/ or fetus. The threat of precipitating preterm labor and abortion remains the principal barrier to such fetal surgery. Limited experience with surgical exposure of the human fetus for even a minor procedure in the 1960s was so unfavorable that the procedure was abandoned. Yet in the last few years extensive research on fetal surgery in models, particularly monkeys, has resulted in improved techniques of anesthesia, surgery, and labor-inhibition. These advances have now been employed in performing the first successful in utero fetal surgical procedure, and a milestone has been passed.

The benefits and risks of fetal diagnosis and therapy will have to be carefully evaluated and weighed, keeping in mind that two patients are being treated. Assessment for the fetus will be relatively straightforward: the risk of the procedure and/or medication versus the benefit of correction or amelioration of the deleterious condition. This last factor will depend on the severity of the condition and its predictable consequences on survival and quality of life. Assessment for the mother will be more difficult. Her health will not usually be affected by the fetal disorder, but she will have to bear some risk from the attempted therapy. Her risk may be negligible if the therapy requires ingesting vitamins, but her risk will be more significant if therapy involves major surgery on her to gain access to the fetus.

Fetal therapy will undoubtedly raise complex ethical issues, many of which are addressed elsewhere in this volume. One positive aspect will be that prenatal diagnosis of certain conditions may lead to treatment rather than selective abortion. The possibility of diagnosing and treating fetal disorders will raise important questions about the rights of mothers and fetuses as patients. Who will make decisions for the fetus? How will we weigh the risk of intervention against the burden of the disorder itself? What if fetal therapy converts a lethal condition into a chronically disabling one? If one of a set of twins has a disorder, what risk may be imposed on the normal twin for the sake of treating the sibling's disorder? These and many more questions will arise, and medicine and society must join forces to answer them.

Our ability to diagnose fetal birth defects has achieved considerable sophistication. Treatment of several fetal conditions has now proven to be feasible, and treatment of more complicated defects will expand as techniques for fetal intervention improve. The concept that the fetus is a patient, an individual whose disorders are a proper subject for medical therapy, has been established.

Notes

1. *See* Kan, Y.W., *et al.*, *Successful Application of Prenatal Diagnosis in a Pregnancy at Risk for Homozygous beta-Thalassemia*, NEW ENGLAND JOURNAL OF MEDICINE 292(21):1096-99 (May 22, 1975).

2. *See* Kan, Y.W., Golbus, M.S., Trecartin, R., *Prenatal Diagnosis of Sickle-Cell Anemia*, NEW ENGLAND JOURNAL OF MEDICINE 294(19):1039-40 (1976).

3. *See* Mibashan, R.S., *et al.*, *Plasma Assay of Fetal Factors VIIIC and IX for Prenatal Diagnosis of Haemophilia*, LANCET 1(8130):1309-11 (1979).

4. *See generally* Ballard, P.L., Ballard, R.A., *Corticosteroids and Respiratory Distress Syndrome: Status 1979*, PEDIATRICS 63(1):163-64 (1979); Thompson, T., Reynolds, J., *The Results of Intensive Care Therapy for Neonates*, JOURNAL OF PERINATAL MEDICINE 5(2):59-75 (1977).

5. Harrison, M.R., *et al.*, *Prenatal Diagnosis and Management of Omphalocele and Ectopia Cordis*, JOURNAL OF PEDIATRIC SURGERY 17(1):64-66 (1982).

6. *See* Ampola, M.G., *et al.*, *Prenatal Therapy of a Patient with Vitamin-B_{12}-Responsive Methylmalonic Acidemia*, NEW ENGLAND JOURNAL OF MEDICINE 293(7):313-17 (1975).

7. *See* Packman, S., *et al.*, *Prenatal Treatment of Biotin Responsive Multiple Carboxylase Deficiency* (unpublished manuscript).

8. *See* Weiner, S., *et al.*, *Antenatal Diagnosis and Treatment of a Fetal Goiter*, JOURNAL OF REPRODUCTIVE MEDICINE 24(1):39-42 (1980).

9. *See* Queenan, J.T., *Intrauterine Transfusion—A Comparative Study*, AMERICAN JOURNAL OF OBSTETRICS AND GYNECOLOGY 104(3):397-409 (1969).

10. *See* Harrison, M.R., *et al.*, *Management of the Fetus with a Urinary Tract Malformation*, JOURNAL OF THE AMERICAN MEDICAL ASSOCIATION 246(6):635-39 (1981).

11. *See* Golbus, M.S., *et al.*, *In Utero Treatment of Urinary Tract Obstruction*, AMERICAN JOURNAL OF OBSTETRICS AND GYNECOLOGY 142:383-88 (1982).

12. Harrison, M.R., *et al.*, *Fetal Surgery for Congenital Hydronephrosis*, NEW ENGLAND JOURNAL OF MEDICINE 306(10):591-93 (1982).

13. Harrison, M.R., *et al.*, *Congenital Diaphragmatic Hernia: The Hidden Mortality*, JOURNAL OF PEDIATRIC SURGERY 13(3):227-30 (1978).

14. *See* Harrison, M.R., Jester, J.A., Ross, N.A., *Correction of Congenital Diaphragmatic Hernia in Utero, Part I: The Model: Intrathoracic Balloon Produces Fatal Pulmonary Hypoplasia*, SURGERY 88(1):174-82 (1980); *Part II: Simulated Correction Permits Fetal Lung Growth with Survival at Birth*, SURGERY 88(2):260-68 (1980).

15. Epstein, M., *Hydrocephalus*, in PEDIATRIC SURGERY (Year Book Medical Publishers, Chicago) (3rd ed. 1979) at 1573-86.

Chapter 6

Medical Implications of Bestowing Personhood on the Unborn

George M. Ryan, Jr.

The Human Life Amendment recently introduced in Congress states:

> The paramount right to life is vested in each human being from the moment of fertilization without regard to age, health, or condition of dependency.[1]

Senate Bill 158 states:

> Human life shall be deemed to exist from conception, without regard to race, sex, age, health, defect, or condition of dependency; and for this purpose "person" shall include all human life as defined herein.[2]

The passage of either the Human Life Amendment or the Human Life Bill would bring new dilemmas to the provider of reproductive health care to women, especially adolescent women. The intent of proponents of these measures is to integrate the presence of cellular life into a legal definition of "personhood" with all of the attendant rights of citizenry that are protected by the Constitution.

I am not a constitutional scholar nor am I qualified to discuss theology in terms of the relative "rightness" or "wrongness" of abortion, but I am an expert with 25 years of experience in the field of obstetrics and gynecology. As a responsible member of my profession, it is imperative that I offer this expertise for consideration as it relates to the potential impact of the proposed human life legislation on health care for women. Granting the conceptus these constitutional protections of personhood, disregarding the relative and critical factors of health, defect, and condition of dependency, will have an immediate and enduring effect on women's health care.

The Fourteenth Amendment to the Constitution states that no "person" shall be deprived of the right to life or liberty.[3] Thus, abortion for any reason would be declared unconstitutional. Such legislation would declare rights for the conceptus equal to those of the woman who is carrying that conceptus and would create two "persons" in one body. The interests of these individuals may diverge on occasion and result in insoluble problems for the physician. Such legislation would affect not only women seeking abortions, but would have a potential impact upon the even greater number of women who are not seeking abortion. The women who intend to carry their fetuses to term whether the fetus is normal or abnormal, and even women who are not pregnant but who seek contraception, would be affected by the proposed legislation.

Most pregnant women and their families are understandably concerned with maintaining the woman's health and producing the healthiest child possible. The physician offers care and advice to enhance the health and quality of life of the woman, both as an individual and as the bearer of children. In this role, the physician is committed to the best interests of the woman who entrusts herself to the physician's care. One of the major advances of the past decade has been the ability to diagnose intrauterine developmental defects which, in conditions such as Tay-Sachs disease, doom the infant to a lingering and painful death, usually by age four. Such a trauma understandably causes the family to seek an absolute guarantee against this sequence of events recurring in a future pregnancy. With the proposed law, the genetic screening program designed to offer the option of abortion in instances of a repetition would be of no benefit, since the woman would be denied the choice of abortion if the outcome of the test revealed an affected fetus. Other genetic problems, such as Down syndrome, are likely to be seen in increased numbers as the women of this country delay childbearing in order to pursue careers and enter the job market in their early years. Increasing numbers will have their children after the age of 30 and the increasing incidence of Down syndrome with age will be manifested. At the present time, physicians generally believe that all patients over 35 should be offered the option of amniocentesis screening for this disease, and that those over age 40 should receive screening. These programs, too, would be essentially destroyed by the proposed legislation. Should families be forced to undergo these risks rather than be offered alternatives made possible by scientific progress? The denial of family rights inherent in the proposed legislation is anti-family in the extreme and not profamily as the proponents suggest.

One of the basic assumptions inherent in human life legislation is that all fertilized eggs will become persons if left alone—an assumption that is clearly not true. Some eggs will implant in the tubes and some in the abdomen as ectopic pregnancies. Such pregnancies not only indicate that the egg will have little chance of normal development, but also pose a potential threat to the life of the woman. Ectopic pregnancy can usually be diagnosed very early, and current medical wisdom dictates that the physician should intervene at that time and remove the ectopic pregnancy. The wording of the present proposed legislation would prohibit the exercise of what is now considered good medicine in these cases. While some have suggested that any bill passed by Congress would contain an exception for instances where the condition was life-threatening to the woman the question is who would determine this condition. Certainly, the woman is in no immediate and life-threatening danger until the ectopic pregnancy ruptures. However, it would be a tragic encroachment upon the legitimate interests of the family and the welfare of the woman if the physician were to wait until such an extreme danger became clear and present before intervening. Thus, physicians have grave misgivings about language which permits exceptions when the action is "required to save the life of the mother."

Another example of divergent interests of the fetus and mother is appendicitis during pregnancy. Any intra-abdominal surgery poses a risk of miscarriage. If the physician operates on a patient suspected of having appendicitis and she subsequently miscarries, has the physician acted to save the life of the mother? Has he or she violated the civil rights of the conceptus? And what if, as frequently happens, the patient turns out not to have had acute appendicitis? At that point, the physician cannot even prove that the surgery was performed to "save the mother's life."

The proposed law would also clearly impact upon the patient who would have a spontaneous miscarriage early in pregnancy. At the present time, when the physician judges that the miscarriage is inevitable, a dilation and curettage procedure (D & C) is performed to remove the products of conception, reducing the danger to the woman of infection, hemorrhage, pain, and duration of pain and disability. If the human life proposals were to become law, the physician would be extraordinarily vulnerable to charges of early interference and actual abortion when performing a D & C which is now accepted as appropriate treatment. Any disgruntled hospital employee, unhappy patient, or ambitious district attorney could bring charges. Any physician who has been outspoken on the subject of abortion may be at particular risk.

Patients with normal pregnancies in terms of fetal development frequently develop complications of the pregnancy. In addition to intra-abdominal disease such as appendicitis, other conditions like diabetes and toxemia of pregnancy are frequently managed by evaluation of the intra-uterine status of the fetus and early delivery at an optimal time. This will produce a premature infant, and although physicians try their best to save premature infants, many die. As must be apparent, human life legislation leaves little latitude for acting swiftly at the initial, critical stages of complications if the interests of the mother and fetus diverge.

In addition to the impact of this legislation upon women with abnormal pregnancies and women with normal but complicated pregnancies in which current concepts of medical care would be drastically altered, there is a third group of patients who are not seeking abortions and who in fact are not even pregnant, but who would also be affected. Today, over 10 million women use intrauterine devices and oral contraceptives. When I testified before the Senate Subcommittee on Separation of Powers regarding this subject, Senator East, (R-S.C.) said I was raising a "chamber of horrors" and that no one intended to interfere with contraception. He simply wished to return the country to the situation that existed prior to 1973 when contraceptives were not banned.[4] I pointed out that the American Life Lobby, in a hearing before another Senate subcommittee declared their intention to ban the pill and the IUD, and this was echoed by spokesmen for the "March for Life" and others. Dr. Mildred Jefferson, a past president of the National Right to Life Committee, stated exactly the same intention on the NBC Today Show during a discussion with me. The fact is that this bill would not return obstetrical practice to the situation that existed prior to 1973, when the fertilized egg was not considered a "person" and interference with implantation was not considered abortion.

Senator East also stated that he did not believe any state would pass such laws. However, when I was at Harvard Medical School in the 1950s the doors had to be monitored and closed when we, as medical students, were receiving any instruction in contraception because it was illegal in Massachusetts even to teach contraception to medical students, much less to provide contraception to the public. It wasn't until 1965 that the Supreme Court granted the right to married women to receive instruction on contraceptive use in the privacy of the physician's office.[5] It did happen, it can happen, and it will happen again if the citizens of this country do not speak out. In terms of the woman's interest, we are really speaking of the risk-benefit ratio of abortion as compared to that of continuing pregnancy. Since 1973 abortion has become one of the safest of all procedures. The risk of childbirth is ten times greater than abortion during the first trimester. How can a law compel a woman to take such a risk when she doesn't wish to do so?

Another stated goal of the anti-abortion movement is that making abortion illegal will "save the lives of unborn children." It is very clear that abortion has been performed since the dawn of humanity, is being performed now, and will continue to be performed in the future. It is estimated that over a decade ago, one million illegal abortions were performed annually in this country. Considering the smaller population then, that figure is proportionate to the 1.4 million legal abortions performed last year. However, the impact on women's health care is significant in that what was once the largest single cause of maternal death in some urban areas has practically disappeared: the fatal complications of illegal abortion. A return to illegal abortions will surely condemn many women to die as a result, and a legal ban will not eliminate the need for, nor the performance of, abortion. Ideal contraceptives are not yet available. Abnormal and unwanted pregnancies will continue to occur.

Sexually active teenagers are particularly at risk of unwanted pregnancy, largely because of lack of education and lack of confidential health services, as evidenced by the 300,000 teenagers who have abortions each year in the United States. It is unrealistic to expect any significant outcome as a result of the proposed legislation other than a leap in the number of teenage deaths from illegal abortions and of teen pregnancies being carried to term. Opponents of teenage sexuality, contraception, and abortion would draw a picture of teenagers in a frenzy of sexual activity who become pregnant without any thought and get an abortion with no questions asked the way we used to go to the corner for a Coke. Nothing could be farther from the truth. Not only is this an inaccurate description of teenagers, but it totally ignores the fact that the majority of abortions— three to one, in fact—are not performed on teenagers. Most are instances of deliberate choice by adult women in our nation.

CONCLUSION

Thus far, I have presented some of the medical information concerning the impact on women's health care of the proposed right-to-life legislation. The following comments are my own personal views. Clearly, proponents of the anti-abortion movement recognize that they are in a minority according to their own strategy reports, and clearly they are being hurt by their attempts to ban abortion regardless of rape, incest, abnormal fetal development or any other reason. As a result, they are changing their strategy and would like to turn the debate from abortion per se to focus on who should make the law in this regard for our nation. Senator Orrin Hatch (R-Utah) has introduced the so-called Human Life Federalism Amendment,[6] which would allow each state to pass legislation on abortion. We must get the message out loud and clear that this is a diversion. If such a constitutional amendment were enacted, the anti-abortion groups will come right back and try to pass a human life bill which they could do with only a one-vote majority without fear of its being overthrown by the Supreme Court.

I agree with Senator Bob Packwood (R-Oregon) who said:

The overwhelming majority of the American people do not think abortion is murder. The American public disapproves of murder. They would not be likely to support abortion if they thought it was murder. The American Medical Association supports a woman's right to have an abortion. They would not do so if they thought it was murder. The American Bar Association would not endorse the right of a woman to choose an abortion if they thought it was murder. The American Public Health Association would not endorse a woman's right to abortion if they thought it was destructive of our society and that it was murder. The dozens and dozens of religious organizations that have endorsed a woman's right to choose, including Catholics for Freedom of Choice, would not do so if they thought it was murder. I reject the idea that God has spoken to any one of us and said, "You are right and those who disagree with you are wrong." If any one of us thinks that God has ordained us to speak for Him, we are wrong. Worse, if we are in a position of power and we believe we speak for God, we become dangerous.[7]

At stake are two underlying basic issues. The first is whether or not a woman's right to act in her own best interest in reproductive matters is to be violated. The second is whether a well-organized and well-financed minority in this country can enact their personal religious beliefs into law, thus destroying the historic separation of church and state. Abortion is only one in a series of debates reflecting these fundamental questions.

NOTES

1. S. J. Res. 110, 97th Cong., 1st Sess., 127 Cong. Rec. 570, 574 (1981).
2. S. 158, 97th Cong., 1st Sess., 127 Cong. Rec. 287 (1981).
3. U.S. Const. amend. XIV, 1.
4. *The Human Life Bill: Hearings on S. 158 Before the Subcommittee on Separation of Powers of the Senate Committee on the Judiciary,* 97th Cong., 1st Sess. 116 (1982) (statement of Sen. East, chairman) (Washington, D.C.: Government Printing Office, Serial No. J-97-16) [hereinafter cited as *Hearings*]. *See also* Roe v. Wade, 410 U.S. 113 (1973) (recognizing the right to abortion).
5. Griswold v. Connecticut, 381 U.S. 479 (1965).
6. *Human Life Federalism Amendment,* 97th Cong., 1st Sess., 127 Cong. Rec. 10194 (1981) (statement of Sen. Hatch). The proposed amendment reads: "The right to abortion is not secured by this Constitution. The Congress and the several States shall have the concurrent power to restrict and prohibit abortions; *Provided,* That a law of a State more restrictive than a law of Congress shall govern."
   Id. at 10196.
7. *Hearings, supra* note 4, at 157-58 (statement of Sen. Packwood).

Audience Discussion

Sidney Scherlis, Moderator

WARREN M. HERN, M.D., M.P.H. (Boulder Abortion Clinic, Boulder, Colorado): I have several questions for Dr. Golbus. First, simply because something is technologically possible, such as intra-uterine fetal surgery, is it justified? Second, what are the long-term consequences of correcting genetic defects that are incompatible with survival in any significant number of people? Third, if the fetus is a person, and if a fetus has a defect correctable by intra-uterine surgery, does the woman have a choice in the matter of these operations? Fourth, who will pay for these operations, and who will decide who gets them?

MITCHELL S. GOLBUS, (Conference Faculty): Certainly, I am not of the philosophy that because we can do something we should do it. I tried to make it clear that I don't even take a position that this is medically the correct thing to do yet. What I do know is that if we do not try to do a series and do it in a well-controlled fashion so that we get reasonable data, we will never know whether or not this is beneficial. For that reason, I think it should be done.

Concerning the long-term effects, I assume you mean the gene pool of Homo sapiens. You can clearly show that not only prenatal surgery, but prenatal diagnosis in general will not have a negative effect. Regarding the question about personhood and choice, I will go back to the question of whether the fetus is a person, and if it's not, then I would leave that to the lawyers and ethicists to wrestle with. This has not been an issue in our very small series of patients to find out whether something works. The insurance companies have, in general, paid for hospitalization and, because it is done under research auspices, it has been supported.

JEFFREY L. LENOW, M.D. (J.D. Candidate, Temple University School of Law, Philadelphia, Pennsylvania): I have two questions I would like to address to Dr. Golbus or to anybody on the panel. According to the *Roe v. Wade* decision we all know that the fetus was not granted rights under the

Fourteenth Amendment.[1] That was clearly stated. But there have been cases, though few, where the interests of fetuses at term were protected. There is one example in our reading manual—the case from Georgia where a C-section was mandated.[2] There is also a case in Colorado where a woman was ordered to have a cesarean section for fetal distress.[3] I ask this question because of the case in New York, the Kerenyi case of discordant twins,[4] where one was destroyed by aspiration of blood and the normal twin was delivered at term. Otherwise they both would have been aborted (by the mother's choice). An article appeared in the *Journal of the American Medical Association* about the legal ramifications of whether there was a consent problem concerning aborting the fetus.[5] You mentioned that, yourself. What do you do when you have a surgical situation with the fetus beyond viability and legal counsel expresses concern about *Roe v. Wade* and the possibly compelling state interests in the life of the fetus?

MITCHELL GOLBUS: I guess it would be nice if the fetus signed the consent form! Seriously, the parents essentially give consent for a procedure and nobody has seriously challenged the validity of their consent on behalf of their fetus.

THOMAS O'DONNELL (St. Francis Hospital, Tulsa, Oklahoma): Up until now I felt we were really getting some place in our discussions since there had not been too much rhetoric on either side, but I was quite disappointed with Dr. Ryan's presentation. Dr. Ryan, you mentioned that the unborn child would be given rights of personhood under the Fourteenth Amendment, but you did not mention that the Fourteenth Amendment also provides that those rights which it encompasses may not be withdrawn "without due process" of law. Therefore, securing protection for the unborn child would indicate that its life would be no more protected than the protection given to a person already born. The Human Life bill or amendment does not secure for fetuses constitutional rights to vote or anything like that. It simply gives them the due process protection of the Fourteenth Amendment. Exceptions can be made under the equal protection clause for hard case abortions. None of the legislation that has been introduced is going to cause any of the terrible events that you envision. This is an involved process of consensus formation within the country concerning when unborn children ought to be protected and when they ought not.

GEORGE M. RYAN (Conference Faculty): I would simply point out that in the past I have heard this argument over and over: "This won't happen; it just depends upon what the enabling legislation says later." In that enabling legislation, by the way, they have written a nice little thing there that says if the state statute is more restrictive than the federal one then the state statute will take precedence. We are on the firing line everyday and it does seem like a chamber of horrors to us to have to practice in that milieu.

AUBREY MILUNSKY (Conference Faculty): I would just like to point out to the participants that the Massachusetts legislature, in its wisdom, has already passed legislation that has resulted in a total ban of fetal research in Massachusetts.[6] This is the kind of legislation which you are quietly allowing to evolve without recognizing the fundamental dangers. What about patients who would benefit from having an Rh fetus treated by in utero transfusion? I am surprised if you are still beguiled by this idea that you are actually saving lives. You are, in effect, developing a system which would deprive children of getting the treatment they need.

THOMAS L. POTTER (Students for Life, University of Wisconsin Law School, Milwaukee): I came to this conference with the hope that one of the most important goals would be to try to avoid the kind of compassionate rhetoric, euphemisms, and language that we saw in Dr. Ryan's talk. But the thing that shocked me more than anything else was when Dr. Milunsky referred to the twin case as the abortion of one twin. I would just like to hear how Dr. Milunsky can call inserting a needle into the heart of the fetus and withdrawing its blood "allowing to die" rather than "killing." I'd also like Dr. Ryan to explain the legal theory behind his claim that the Senate or the Congress as a whole could pass a human life bill and have no fear of it being overturned by the United States Supreme Court. I do not understand either of these positions.

AUBREY MILUNSKY: What I meant was allowing the other fetus to live.

GEORGE RYAN: At the present time, with the current ruling of the Supreme Court as the existing law of the land, it is generally agreed that even if Congress passed a bill similar to S. 158, and it was signed by the President, such a law would immediately be challenged in the Supreme Court because of the fact that it goes directly against the prevailing law. On the other hand, if you took the next step, and you pass a Constitutional amendment saying that the state and the federal legislatures would have the right to restrict access to abortion, the Supreme Court could not overturn a Constitutional amendment. Congress would then have a right to pass a statute outlawing abortion by only one vote and it would be constitutional. I said in the beginning that I am no constitutional lawyer and I am only telling what the strategists of the movement have said, that they cannot pass that law now but if they could get the constitutional amendment passed giving them the right then they'll come back and they will get that restrictive law passed.

CAROLINE WHITBECK, PH.D. (Institute for Medical Humanities, Galveston, Texas): I have a question for Dr. Golbus. I do not understand why you addressed the subject that you did instead of the topic given in your title. As interesting as your talk was, it seemed to me that it did not address the question of bestowing the status of person on the fetus. Rather the subject you addressed was that of taking the fetus as the object of high technology medical interventions.

MITCHELL GOLBUS: I did not pick the topic in the program as it reads. You will have to take that up with the organizers.

Editor's Note: Our objective in asking Dr. Golbus to discuss the implications of bestowing personhood on the fetus was intended to elicit medical information concerning the fetus as a patient. Clearly, if the fetus were deemed a person, it would be entitled to the full attention and skill of its doctors. Medical and surgical treatment rendered in utero are in their earliest stages of development,[7] and given the time restraints, Dr. Golbus' presentation more than adequately fulfilled our expectations.

ANNE E. BANNON, M.D. (Doctors for Life, St. Louis, Missouri): The statement at the beginning of this afternoon's discussion was that we "bestow" personhood. Personhood is no more something that we bestow than human life is something that we bestow on another human being. It is there because it's innate. At least that's my humble opinion. Dr. Ryan used the term "egg" as if he were talking about chicken eggs when he was talking about the female ovum which Dr. Blandau described so eloquently as a beautiful thing. He also used the term "conceptus." My question is: what does he mean by the term "conceptus?" There are many, many physicians who do not believe in the destruction of an innocent human being for whatever reason.

GEORGE RYAN: Egg is the English word; ovum is the Latin word. I think the English language is appropriate in this country. "Conceptus" refers to the product of conception from the moment of fertilization right up to the time of birth. We are talking about bestowing rights from the moment of fertilization.

I represent the majority of the American College of Obstetricians and Gynecologists (ACOG), that is, 23,000 board-certified physicians in this country. I do not, however, speak for every one of them, and there are 600 in our group who back the right-to-life organization. You might be interested to know that there are several staunch right-to-life individuals on our executive board, which makes the policies of our organization. They joined us in the unanimous condemnation of this kind of simplistic legislation for a very complex problem. I will also tell you that the American Medical Association joined us in testifying against this legislation in congressional hearings this past year.[8] I think that shows that the majority of the people in ACOG support the concept that this legislation is not the way to solve the abortion problem. If you want to pass a bill banning abortion, try to do that. But when you start introducing legislation defining a "person," then you have a lot of other ramifications to consider. If you do not take careful account of those problems you are going to find that even well-meaning legislation is going to have a terribly devastating effect on women's reproductive health care.

ELLEN H. KRAMER, J.D. (Planned Parenthood Federation of America, New York, New York): Dr. Ryan, concerning the proposed regulation requiring parental notification when teenage girls are given contraceptives, I am curious, how you would answer the Schweiker proposal.

GEORGE RYAN: I do not think that is an appropriate topic here. I did say in my presentation, I believe, that abortion was but one of the issues that reflects some very serious underlying debates about women's rights to reproductive control and it comes under that heading, but I'd rather not get into that.

UNIDENTIFIED PARTICIPANT: I want to ask Dr. Blandau for a point of information. I think you said that the oögonia in the very early embryo do not come from inside the body. Where do they come from?

RICHARD J. BLANDAU (Conference Faculty): The oögonia have an origin outside the body of the embryo in the region of the yolk sac and from here they will migrate as amoebae toward the genital ridges. So, originally they do have an extracorporeal origin.

M. SIMONE ROACH (St. Martha's Convent, Antigonish, Nova Scotia): I have a simple question, Mr. Chairman, which has to do with, if you will, a point of order. I was very, very impressed by the announcement of this program, particularly with respect to the theme and with the caliber of speakers. I came here because I felt it was one of the most important issues of our time. I came expecting interdisciplinary, scholarly, and reflective dialogue. I would like to ask you a question. Is this program designed to challenge the Human Life Amendment? If so, then I am afraid that I have come here at great expense for the wrong reason.

SIDNEY SCHERLIS, M.D. (President, American Society of Law & Medicine, Towson, Maryland): Well, the program was designed to educate those who attended and to inform them of the current status of scientific, medical, and other various thoughts concerning this subject. It was not designed to proselytize people to be against the Human Life Amendment nor was it designed to support such an amendment.

MARGERY W. SHAW (Conference Faculty): I tried to say the same thing in the few brief remarks I made this morning during the introductions. I think you are very much on the right track in saying that our purpose was hopefully to illuminate, to discourse in a rational and unemotional manner one of the important issues that we are facing in the 1980s. The amount of emotional reaction that is interjected into the discussion will tend to defeat that goal. I do not believe that it is possible to separate the emotional reactions from the intellectual and rational ones, but I would hope that we could listen to each other and we could, without raising our voices, learn from each other.

JACQUELINE MALONEY, J.D., M.P.H. (Long Island University, Greenvale, New York): My question is addressed to Dr. Golbus. Who is your patient? Is the fetus in utero your patient, is the mother your patient, or do you consider them simultaneously?

MITCHELL GOLBUS: Essentially our current attitude is that both of them are our patients and we are trying to evaluate and explain thoroughly the risks and benefits concerning both the mother and the fetus. One of the problems that I alluded to in my talk was: "Who speaks for the fetus?" I do not have a solution to that question. It is a problem we need to recognize and discuss. We owe a duty to both the mother and the fetus as our patients at this time.

GEORGE RYAN: I'd like to echo that we all, as obstetricians, consider them both our patients. The problem is that there are times when their interests diverge. Then, whom do we act on behalf of? And, that's the essence of the discussion.

MITCHELL GOLBUS: We now seek the review and approval of the human experimentation committee at our institution, and we also look for guidance from Professor Albert Jonsen, our resident ethicist. We have been able to get outside consultations and make sure that everybody's interests are being addressed.

JOHN C. FLETCHER, PH.D. (National Institutes of Health, Bethesda, Maryland): I would like to ask the panel if anyone thinks that the technology itself plays a strong role in our perception of when the fetus is a person. I have been interested, over a number of years, in asking physicians who do a lot of sonography, if they haven't noticed that their patients feel closer to the fetus and feel more identified with the fetus as a person than they did 20 years ago or so when they just felt quickening but didn't see a picture of the fetus. I tried a little experiment myself when I was in Chicago visiting at the Lying-in-Hospital recently. A lady there had been in an accident when she was about five months pregnant. She had undergone an x-ray, and was being sonographed when I happened to be in the room and I asked, "How does it make you feel when you see the fetus move?" She said, "It sure does make you feel different. It tends to make you want to rule out the termination of pregnancy." Although my sentiment is on the side of giving people options about abortion, I think this technology itself has had a tendency to allow us to identify fetuses as persons much earlier if we decide to. My point is that there may be a socio-biological force working here. If you identify with a person when you see the fetus this imprints on you the idea that there is one of us here that we can't neglect. I am also impressed with the statements made by Dr. Golbus and his colleague, Dr. Michael Harrison, on television to the effect that they feel very much that they work on fetal patients. The technology itself has a powerful logical grip in terms of identifying personhood.

MITCHELL GOLBUS: I think that is very, very important and I agree subjectively with that. There is no question that the issue comes up when patients see sonographic pictures and prenatal diagnosis karyotypes and it does have an influence. We have been very aware of that. For instance, you can very easily take Polaroids off of the sonography machine and give people pictures. We take no pictures. We have taken the camera off of the machine that we use for prenatal diagnosis because when you go back and tell a certain proportion of those families that they had an abnormal fetus and they are going to be forced to make certain decisions, one way or the other, we try not to worsen the difficulty of the decision making. But there is no question in my mind that it happens, even with the advancement of technology that doesn't have to do with sight. When I was trained, and in the years before that when Dr. Ryan was trained, our concept of our obligations changed. For instance, when should we do an emergency cesarean section in order to save the fetus? When you look over the past 15 years, you can see that the criteria of age and weight were used to determine the time when we would consider a fetus viable and salvageable. But over the years, the age at which we think that we'd better intervene has been dropping. One of the great things that has added fuel to the argument we are seeing today is the fact that we sort of dropped the age at which we can save infants almost back to the age at which we were allowing termination and it has very much muddied the waters.

GEORGE RYAN: I would like to add that technology has an important role to play. It helps not only physicians, but also patients, to understand the process. We are constantly seeing breakthroughs like those which Dr.

Golbus made. My feeling is that's fine and if that brings the mother closer to the normal fetus developing inside of her, by all means let us support that. I truly and firmly support the mother receiving all the information and all the education possible to help her at that time. And there are occasions that she has to make some very tough decisions. And I think that decision rightfully belongs with her. The physician caring for her must carry out whatever decision she makes. So my interest in technology is not a threat at all and if we come to a point in time where we can save all of the fetuses very early, that would be fine. I am not endorsing, proselytizing, evangelizing, or soliciting people to come in and have an abortion. We are not pro-abortion; we are anti-unwanted pregnancy and we would like to spend all our time and effort trying to look at the etiology of unwanted pregnancy and to seek a solution. If we spent resources and time on that topic instead of on the issues being discussed today, we could stop debating this situation emotionally for a few years, and I suspect we'd be a lot further along in preventing unwanted pregnancies.

RICHARD BLANDAU: I would like to mention that one of our major problems is that we so often place abortion in the same category as the use of various contraceptive devices. What is desperately needed is a major effort in basic research in reproductive biology; research in fertility-related social sciences and in contraceptive research. When one considers that the Western European and United States governments spend more money per year subsidizing tobacco production than is spent on reproductive and contraceptive research, is there any wonder that basic information and education in the area of reproduction is flagging? I suggest that the problem of abortion will not be resolved by symposia, it will not be resolved by law, or by religion. It may be significantly limited, however, by developing adequate information that can be relayed to those who do not understand that abortion is not a safe contraceptive method and offer them appropriate alternatives.

SIDNEY SCHERLIS: I want to thank the questioners for the questions they proposed. I do not intend to apologize for the emotion displayed or implied by some of the questions or some of the answers because I think that is a very real part of the problem. This is not a sterile group. There are emotions attached to interpreting the knowledge that we have and I think this has to be considered in making judgments.

NOTES

1. Roe v. Wade, 410 U.S. 113 (1973).

2. Jefferson v. Griffin Spalding County Hospital Authority, 274 S.E.2d 457 (Ga. 1981); Berg R.N., *Georgia Supreme Court Orders Caesarian Section—Mother Nature Reverses on Appeal*, JOURNAL OF THE MEDICAL ASSOCIATION OF GEORGIA 79(6):451 (1981).
3. Lenow, J.L., *The Fetus as a Patient—Emerging Rights as a Person?* AMERICAN JOURNAL OF LAW AND MEDICINE 9(1):1 (1983).
4. Kerenyi, T., Chitkara, U., *Selective Birth in Twin Pregnancy with Discordancy for Down's Syndrome*, NEW ENGLAND JOURNAL OF MEDICINE 304(25):525 (1981).
5. Fletcher, J., Editorial: *The Fetus as Patient: Ethical Issues*, JOURNAL OF THE AMERICAN MEDICAL ASSOCIATION 246(7):772 (1981).
6. MASS. GEN. LAWS, c. 112 §12J.
7. *See generally* Harrison, M., *The Fetus as Patient*, in LEGAL AND ETHICAL ASPECTS OF HEALTH CARE FOR CHILDREN (A.E. Doudera and J.D. Peters, eds.) (AUPHA Press, Ann Arbor) (Forthcoming); Harrison, M., *et al.*, *Fetal Treatment 1982*, NEW ENGLAND JOURNAL OF MEDICINE 307(26):1651-52 (December 23, 1982); Elias, S., Annas, G. J., Perspectives on Fetal Surgery, AMERICAN JOURNAL OF OBSTETRICS AND GYNECOLOGY 145:807-12 (April 1, 1983).
8. *See The Human Life Bill: Hearings on S. 158 Before the Subcommittee on Separation of Powers of the Senate Committee on the Judiciary, 97th Cong., 1st Sess. (1982).*

Chapter 7

Definitions of Life and Death: Should There Be Consistency?

Robert M. Veatch

On the surface, it is puzzling to consider whether the definitions of two different words in the English language ought to be consistent. In fact, I am not sure how definitions of two unlinked terms could be consistent—or inconsistent. But let me tip my hand: if I understand what the question really means, if I am allowed to reformulate the question in terms I can understand, then the answer must be "yes." Not only that, but by clarifying what is often called the definition of death we may learn a great deal about the problem of when fetuses acquire moral or legal standing.

REFORMULATING THE QUESTION

THE DEFINITION OF DEATH

Let me start reformulating the question by looking at the definition-of-death debate. Dictionaries define death as the permanent cessation of vital or life-giving functions, the end of life. Since death is the negation of life, the definition of death contains the definition of life, and in this sense they must be consistent. Death is nothing more than the loss of that which is essential to being alive.

However, the point of the debate is not a linguistic or conceptual analysis of the term "death." We are not even interested in a theological account of the meaning of death, or a scientific account of the biological events that take place in the brain or the heart when an individual dies. Then what is the point of controversy, and why might it be of some interest to those concerned about abortion, genetic engineering, fetal experimentation, and the rights of postnatal humans?

The definition-of-death debate is really a front for a crucial question in public policy and ethics over when it is appropriate to stop treating certain individuals as if we had a particular set of ethical and legal duties toward them. It is a debate over when we should begin treating them the way we treat the newly dead. It is a debate over what I would call the "social system of death behavior."

Traditionally, certain behaviors are viewed as appropriate only at the point at which we agree to call an individual dead. Important social and cultural changes such as the following are then signalled.

1) We stop treatments that would otherwise continue.

2) We begin mourning.

3) We refer to the person in the past tense.

4) We start processes leading to the reading of the will.

5) We start processes leading to the burial, the assumption of the role of widowhood, or the procurement of organs under the Uniform Anatomical Gift Act.

6) If the individual labelled dead is President of the United States, the Vice President is automatically elevated to the presidency.

There is a radical shift in moral, social, and political standing for someone who is labelled dead.[1] But the public policy question raised by the so-called definition-of-death debate is whether we can continue to identify a single point in time when all of these behavioral shifts ought to take place. As we become more sophisticated in stretching out the dying process, we can stand face-to-face with an individual whose heart beats but whose brain is dead. We are forced to become much more precise in identifying the moment of death—that is, the moment when these behaviors become appropriate. We now face patients whose higher brain centers have decayed to the point of putrefaction, but who continue to breathe either on a respirator, or occasionally, spontaneously because of intact lower brain centers. What we really want to know is precisely when an individual loses the legal and moral standing that we attribute to human beings so that this cluster of behaviors I have called "death behaviors" is appropriate.

It may, of course, turn out that there is no single point where all these behaviors become appropriate. We may decide to remove organs for transplantation when the brain is irreversibly destroyed, read the will when and only when the heart stops, and begin mourning at some point not precisely aligned with either of these. If that turns out to be the case, then the definition-of-death debate will cease to be of interest for public policy purposes. It will no longer be meaningful to say someone has died. Different behavioral events will be triggered at different points in the dying trajectory, and death really will become a process rather than an event.[2]

As a society, however, we are continuing to behave as if all (or at least many) of these death behaviors should be triggered at a single point. We want to continue to call that point the point of death. If we can agree morally, legally, and politically on that point, we shall have recovered for our society a definition of death. We also may have learned something about what it means morally, legally, and politically to be alive and what the rights of fetuses are.

It is interesting to note that some people, as they attempt to define life, have been tempted to conclude that different definitions should be used for different purposes. They are saying, in effect, that different behaviors we associate with those given full standing should be initiated at different points in human development, and that in the various contexts we can call each of those points "the beginning of life." What is striking is that if there is any one point over which there is consensus in the defini-tion-of-death debate, it is that there must be one definition for all pur-poses. Some early definitions implied that a brain-oriented definition of death should be used in cases where organ donation was planned, while older, heart-lung-oriented definitions should be used for other purposes. This raised practical problems, such as what should happen if a person were pronounced dead because he or she was scheduled to donate an organ, only to have the potential recipient die before the donor's organ could be removed. In order to avoid the terrible confusion that different definitions for different purposes might create, a substantial consensus has emerged that one definition should be used for all purposes. (Of course according to this view, some behaviors, such as turning off a respirator, might still be considered appropriate even if someone is not dead.)

It should now be clear that insofar as medicine is a body of knowledge about the human body and a set of procedures that can be applied to a human body, there are absolutely no medical implications of defining life or death. Whatever we can say about a human body—its anatomy, its physiology, our capacities to intervene to affect its functioning—we can say it regardless of whether we decide to call that body dead or alive. Deciding to call a body dead is essentially making a moral, legal, or political decision about how a body ought to be treated. There are moral, legal, or political implications for defining death or life. Such definitions will tell us what we ought to do, including what medical professionals ought to do, but they have no bearing on what can be done medically.

The definition-of-death debate, then, is a debate over when we ought to stop treating an individual as a full member of the human community with moral and/or legal standing, as a citizen with all the accompanying rights.

The question of the definition of life presents a problem precisely parallel to that of the definition of death. We can develop an analytical definition probably beginning with some minimal constellation of features, such as cells containing a fixed genetic material carrying out certain processes essential to life (respiration and motility, for example). Identifying features of this sort, however, has no bearing upon the central focus of this paper— that is, clarifying the point at which moral and/or legal standing should be attributed to this living tissue. The interesting moral, legal, and political question concerns what features of human life imply standing so that the claims of an individual are comparable, at least for most purposes, to those of other living human beings.

There is systematic ambiguity in the project of defining life and death. Sometimes the moral or legal baggage is attached to the definition of life analytically, in that we simply define life to *mean* the point at which full moral or legal standing accrues. Likewise, we define death to *mean* the point at which that standing ceases. In that mode, the terms life and death must have moral or legal policy implications. We know that moral shifts take place when life begins or ends, but it is in principle impossible to determine biologically when those points are. If death means the end of legal standing it cannot simultaneously mean the death of the brain or the stopping of the heart. If it is linked to one of those physiological events, it is linked synthetically. It is linked by argument, intuition, or conviction that legal standing ought to cease when the heart or the brain irreversibly ceases to function.

Alternatively, life and death can be defined without reference to moral or legal evaluations. Life could simply mean the beating of the heart or the capacity of the body to integrate its functions, leaving open the moral or legal question of whether not-yet-living bodies and dead bodies still have the same standing as living ones.

The definition-of-death debate has taken our society far down the road of linking the concept of death to this radical shift in standing *by definition*, that is, analytically. If that is the case, then the argument reduces to a debate over what features of a human are so essential that their loss causes this shift in standing and that, therefore, the body can be called dead.

Unfortunately there is no such clear pattern in the use of language regarding the definition of life. Many people are saying that whatever point we determine to be the commencement of standing comparable to that of other human beings shall be called the beginning point of life.[3] The more dominant notion is that we shall define life independent of the judgment about standing. Life will be said to begin when the genetic code is fixed, or when critical cellular activities begin, or when essential organ system functioning begins.[4]

This suggests an initial inconsistency in the use of the terms life and death. While we may be beginning to use "death" so that it has policy content by definition, "life" continues to be used ambiguously, sometimes having policy content and sometimes not. We could avoid all of this linguistic and policy confusion if we dropped all of the talk about the definition of life and the definition of death and simply talked about the beginning and the ending points of that special moral or legal standing that we attribute to human beings.

THE RELATION TO PERSONHOOD

Our problem is made more complex with the introduction of the term personhood. Some people want to say that the beginning and ending of life can be identified without moral or legal judgment, but that personhood is necessarily linked to questions of standing.[5] This is the move that gives rise to the slogan, "Embryos don't have rights; only persons have rights." Of course, if personhood is defined as all those who possess full standing in the human community, then only persons have full standing. It does not follow from that, however, that embryos do not have standing unless we can establish that independently.

To make matters even more complicated, some define person quite apart from the attribution of rights or standing. Persons are self-conscious entities,[6] those capable of communicating or manipulating symbol systems,[7] or those possessing personal identity.[8] Such nonmoral usage leaves open the question of whether those who are persons (because they are self-conscious entities, etc.) have full moral or legal standing. It also leaves open the question of whether those who are not yet persons or never again will be persons have such standing. One could sensibly say that someone has ceased to be a person, but still has the full standing of a citizen of the human community.

In effect, this means that individuals can be classified in three independent ways: whether they are living, whether they are persons, and whether they have standing. Only the last label is necessarily evaluative. Only that one by definition says anything about whether the individual is a bearer of moral or legal claims of a particular type that we attribute to human beings.

SHOULD THERE BE CONSISTENCY?

According to the preceding reasoning, the question of whether or not definitions of life and death should be consistent may be restated in the following way: if there are some features, the inital presence of which signals the beginning of full moral or legal standing, should the loss of those features correspondingly signal the loss of that standing?

If we can identify some feature about human life—the presence of a fixed genetic code, a beating heart, a functioning nervous system, or the presence of consciousness—which we can agree is the essential feature for treating that individual as a full member of the human community, does it make sense to say that the irreversible loss of that same feature would imply the loss of that standing to be treated as a full member of the same community?

Put that way it is difficult to answer anything but "yes." Some feature is a necessary and sufficient condition for an entity to be included in the category of members in full standing in the human community, although it is conceivable that the feature that brings one into the community would not be the same as that which ushers one out. This would be the case, for instance, if there were two or more features, each of which was sufficient for standing but no one of which was necessary, and these features came and departed in a different time sequence. It is hard to imagine, however, that these conditions would ever be met. It seems that the obvious, most straightforward position is the one favoring consistency: if there is some essential feature that gives individuals moral or legal claims comparable to other members of the human community, loss of that feature implies that one no longer relates to the community in the same way. We can safely begin an examination of the definition-of-death debate with a strong presumption in favor of consistency.

IMPLICATIONS FOR THE DEFINITION OF DEATH AND THE DEFINITION OF LIFE

On the presumption, then, that we may learn something about the point where full human standing begins by examining when it ends and vice versa, let us examine four possible answers to the question of what that essential feature may be.

THE PRESENCE OF A FIXED GENETIC CODE

The first, most striking observation is that one major candidate for this feature is never mentioned in the definition-of-death debate. It is widely held that the critical feature that gives a fetus standing is the development of a fixed genetic code. At some point following the fertilization of the egg, a genetically unique individual is created. In a simpler era this could safely be taken to occur at the "moment" of conception. Now, thanks to the pioneering work of geneticists such as Jerome Lejuene[9] and the application of that work to the question of abortion by people like Andre Hellegers,[10] many argue that a truly unique genetic code is not fixed until the time when twinning can no longer take place—perhaps two weeks after fertilization. This move alone opens the possibility that abortifacient-like procedures (such as the morning-after pill) might be more acceptable morally than abortions after the second week of pregnancy. For our purposes, the interesting point is that people following this line of reasoning—whether they take the genetic code to be fixed at conception or some weeks later—consider the fixation of the genetic material to be critical for full standing. Of course, even prior to that time humans may bear some obligation toward the treatment of human material—eggs, sperm, or zygotes. Full human standing, however, is seen as coming when the genetic code first becomes unique. Individuation, as signalled by fixing of the genetic code, is said to be critical.

What is striking is that nobody is claiming that moral standing ends—that is, an individual is "dead"—when the fixed genetic code is destroyed. It is obvious that many people are pronounced dead (by any definition of death) when their genetic patterns are still intact. In fact living cells survive for minutes, hours, perhaps even days after the point when it is appropriate to treat someone as dead even based on the most traditional definitions related to heart function. The full complement of genetic information about an individual is contained in each of those living cells. It is potentially possible to clone those remaining cells so that a new individual with the identical genetic composition would continue living for years after what we would all agree is the death of the individual. If there is to be consistency in establishing the beginning and end points of human standing, either we must radically change the end point or we must reformulate the beginning point. The mere presence of a fixed genetic code will not do the job consistently.

THE PRESENCE OF THE FLOWING OF FLUIDS

We have traditionally pronounced death based on conditions related to the heart and lungs, which suggests that the critical feature we are seeking might be related to heart or lung activity. At first, one might think that the mere beating of the heart was this feature, and the policy claim could then be, "When and only when a beating heart is present, moral and/or legal standing is present."

Consider, however, the possibility that the heart of a terminally ill patient might be removed and attached to a machine so that it continued to beat, perhaps for weeks or months if we were technologically clever enough. The human heart would be reminiscent of the beating frog's heart that we learned to prepare for study in college physiology labs. Yet even in those labs we knew the difference between a living frog and a beating frog heart.

Those who look to heart and lung activity as definitive probably are not really interested in the beating heart per se, but rather in what that beating normally implies: the flowing of so-called vital bodily fluids—blood and breath. What would be the implication of this focus for the abortion debate?

If cardiac function is critical for standing, significant life could not begin before the appearance of the first cardiac tissues, at approximately the fourth week of gestation. But with only a few specialized cells in existence, full cardiac function does not begin at that point. If we are really interested in the more integrated functioning of the circulatory system, we are identifying a point that comes much later in fetal development—probably no earlier than the twelfth week.

This suggests a problem that those involved in the definition-of-death debate have had to face recently. Whatever function is identified as critical, cellular level function may remain intact long after supercellular, organ system functioning ceases. When we shift our attention to brain-oriented conceptions of when we ought to treat people as dead, we shall see that isolated, perfused brain cells may continue intracellular activity long after organ level brain function stops. Thus electrical activity will remain, even when we say a brain is "dead," meaning that the brain has irreversibly lost its capacity to carry out its traditional organ-level functions.

In principle, there is no scientific way to choose whether the cellular level functions or the supercellular level functions are critical. We simply must make a choice based on philosophical, theological, and other evaluative views of what is important in being a human. Most have reached the conclusion that isolated cellular level function is insignificant—that it is the supercellular level that is critical.[11] If isolated heart or brain cells remain living after the organ level functions of these cells have been irreversibly lost, then the continuing presence of the living cells here and there means nothing.

If that is the answer given in the definition-of-death debate and if we seek consistency, then we have an answer to the question of whether cellular activity per se is critical in deciding when a human first gains human standing. In the case of those who focus on cardiac activity, the mere presence of the first differentiated cardiac cells is no more important than the presence of a few living cardiac cells would be in a patient whose heart has stopped providing its traditional supercellular functions. The crucial process is the flowing of the vital fluids in the circulatory and respiratory system. Those who choose to treat a person as dead when these functions cease would, if they are to be consistent, vest a human with full standing when those more integrated, supercellular functions begin. If my reading of embryology is correct, supercellular cardiac function commences at a point no earlier than the twelfth week. If capacity for lung function is included, this point may be established as late as the twenty-fourth week. If it is the actual flowing of the air in the lungs and exchange of respiratory gases that are critical, then one might consistently adopt the position that "life is breath"—that full standing as a member of the human community begins only at birth when the first breath is taken. This leads to identifying a point essentially identical to that sometimes considered significant in traditional Judaism: when the head has emerged from the womb.[12]

Adopting the view that the critical function has to do with circulation and respiration leaves one in a strange position, because abortion policy implied by this view is somewhat liberal in the context of current debate. One would accept or at least tolerate abortion through the first trimester and maybe up until the beginning of the third trimester. Some lesser moral standing might be assigned to fetuses prior to that time, just as special moral obligations exist in many societies for the care and treatment of a new corpse after the critical moment of death. Compromises with the welfare of the fetus prior to the development of circulation would be tolerated, however, at least if good reasons are offered for what is sometimes viewed as a tragic moral compromise. If breath rather than circulation is critical, then similar compromises up to the moment of birth might be acceptable.

At the other end of the spectrum, those focusing on circulatory or respiratory function represent the conservative rear guard. What we might crudely call the "heart-lung people" are thus simultaneously pushing toward liberal abortion policy and conservative death definition policy.

But they face an even more serious problem. They have adopted a view that the essence of being a human has to do with something as crass, as animalistic, as biological as whether liquids are being pumped through the plumbing and gases are properly maintaining the ventilation system. There is nothing unscientific about such a view; it is fundamentally not a scientific judgment. It represents, however, a very limited view of human nature. It rejects the mainstream of the Western Judeo-Christian tradition that says the human is far more than a mere body. It is even more decisively at odds with the Greek emphasis on the soul as man's essence, temporarily entrapped in the flesh.

THE PRESENCE OF THE INTEGRATED FUNCTIONING
OF THE NERVOUS SYSTEM

Two developments have forced us to rethink what it really means to die—that is, when we want to initiate the range of behaviors I have called death behaviors. These are, first, our new capacity to maintain people with dead brains and beating hearts and, second, our philosophical dissatisfaction with that animalistic view of human nature. This discomfort began in 1968 within months after the first heart transplant made the question of when we can treat someone as dead a crucial and emotionally exciting question. It soon gave rise to the idea that we really should start treating people as dead when their brain function ceases, even if the heart and lungs continue to function.[13]

Supporters of this notion (let's call them the "brain people") say that the essence of human existence is not related to mere fluid flow, but to something far more complicated and subtle having to do with the integration of bodily functions by the nervous system. When that is present, we have a "person as a whole" and not merely a collection of cells, tissues, and organs carrying on independent functions. The President's Commission for the Study of Ethical Problems in Medicine and Biomedical and Behavioral Research adopted this position in July of last year when it adopted its report endorsing a brain-oriented definition of death.[14] It has also been officially adopted by 27 states.

The implications for the abortion debate are less striking than they might at first appear. If one adopts a position that central nervous system functioning is critical for moral standing, a determination must be made about when this activity begins in a fetus. Once again, it will depend upon whether we are interested in cellular activity or supercellular activity. The first signs of nervous tissue cells appear at about the third week, while more complex integrated nervous system functioning does not appear until perhaps the tenth week and becomes substantial at about the twenty-fourth week when integration is sufficiently complete so that the fetus can survive independently of its mother. Assuming that we follow the answer being given by those in the definition-of-death debate, we will identify the later time as the critical point to give full moral standing to fetuses—an answer somewhat later than, but still close to, that which would be given by one who applied a heart-oriented definition of death consistently to the abortion question.

In this case, however, there is more consistency in where one ends up on the public policy spectrum for the two issues. One who adopts the more liberal view on the definition of death, perhaps being willing to run the risk of being philosophically wrong when he treats the irreversibly comatose patient as dead, will also adopt a relatively liberal view on abortion, being willing to run the risk of being morally wrong in treating a midterm fetus as having, at most, only limited moral claims. Thus, one who is willing to apply the brain-oriented formulation consistently to matters of life and death has to reject the "safer course arguments" reminiscent of the probabiliorism of moral theologians.[15] It seems reasonable that if one has seen the way clear to reject the safer course arguments at one end of the spectrum, he or she would be willing to reject them at the other end for similar reasons.

PRESENCE OF THE CAPACITY FOR CONSCIOUSNESS

While the abortion debate seems almost stagnant in the murky confusion of policy debate, the definition-of-death debate has continued to evolve. The "brain people" have recently split into two major camps. What is now the old school continues to insist that integrating capacities are critical and that the entire brain—as the primary organ of integration—must be dead for death behavior to be appropriate. A newer school of brain-oriented advocates of a new definition of death says that the "whole brain people" have not gone far enough.[16] Those who focus on the whole brain and its integrating capacities still see the human as essentially a biological creature.

The test case is the patient who retains substantial capacity to integrate respiration, heart rate, cranial reflexes, and the like, but who has irreversibly lost the capacity for consciousness because all higher brain tissues have been destroyed. To use Henry Beecher's language (which now seems inappropriate for defending the whole brain view),[17] advocates of the newer "higher-brain-oriented" definition of death say that a person should be considered dead when the capacity for consciousness, for thinking, feeling, reasoning, and remembering is irreversibly lost. The real argument today is no longer between heart- and brain-oriented formulations, but between whole-brain and higher-brain or cerebral formulations.

What would a higher-brain-oriented definition of death mean in relation to the beginning of full standing? If one opted for this view, presumably such standing would begin when and only when an individual had some capacity for consciousness. However, determining precisely when this capacity for consciousness begins may turn out to be as difficult as determining when it ends. We have had considerable uncertainty over measuring the irreversible loss of the capacity for consciousness. Stories of patients with "locked syndrome," the condition in which someone is conscious but lacks all motor capacity and therefore the capacity to communicate, abound. As a result, many who in principle favor a concept of death related to loss of consciousness fall back in practice to using the destruction of the entire brain as the clinical point at which we are first really sure consciousness is no longer possible.

A similar practical, clinical, and legal implication may be in store for the abortion debate for those who identify consciousness as critical. There is good reason to think that the capacity for consciousness may be present in some crude way well before birth, but since we may not be able to determine its starting point, we may have to fall back on the first presence of integrated brain activity as the decisive point in establishing full standing. If at some later time, however, we could more accurately measure the capacity for consciousness, the higher-brain and whole-brain people would part company at the practical level as well as the theoretical.

POTENTIAL VS. CAPACITY

The search for consistency between the definition of life and the definition of death leaves us with some insights as well as some confusion. Fixation of the genetic code has no defenders in the definition-of-death debate. All three of the plausible definitions of death (heart-, whole-brain-, and higher-brain-oriented) identify supercellular capacities as necessary for full standing in the human community. Only one of them, the higher-brain formulation, insists on a necessary combination of mental and bodily functions. For that reason, many are beginning to argue that it alone is consistent with our Judeo-Christian and Greek heritage. Regardless of whether that conclusion is accepted, all three of the plausible definitions of death imply a somewhat late point in fetal development as the starting point for full human standing. Circulatory function, nervous system integrating functions, and consciousness are all rather late arrivals in fetal development. The heart-oriented formulation has the unpleasant feature of requiring both a late point for the beginning of standing and an early point for the end of it, while the brain-oriented formulations are at least consistently liberal at both ends of the spectrum.

Why is it, then, that the definition-of-death debate, which seems to have rich practical implications, is relatively uncontroversial while the abortion debate lingers, frustratingly unresolvable? I suggest that it is because the definition-of-death debate is able to finesse a critical question that is both decisive and unresolvable in the abortion debate. When one irreversibly loses the critical capacity—circulatory, integrative, or mental—one simultaneously loses any *potential* for that capacity. It will never return again. However, at the beginning of life the potential for a capacity far precedes the presence of the capacity itself. In fact, as the genetic code becomes fixed many characteristics of those capacities are predetermined. To be sure, they are not completely determined and anyone who follows the sociobiology fight wants to hold on to the idea that social and other factors may be decisive in determining capacities as well as actual performance. Still, at the beginning of life potential predates capacity. In order to know when one should be treated as a member in full standing of the human community, one must know whether the elusive critical feature we have been searching for is a capacity or a potential. Since capacity and potential depart at the same time, we need not have tackled this issue in the definition-of-death debate.

In the debate over when standing begins, however, some choice between the options must be made. As we have witnessed throughout this debate, there is no scientific way to choose. Whether potential counts or only the actual capacities is a fundamental question of choice, just the way we are forced to choose on faith whether there is an external world, or to decide whether rights really are inalienable.

It now appears that there are several plausible positions in the definition-of-death debate that reasonable people may take. I am increasingly convinced that there will never be agreement on any one of these. Some tolerable compromise will have to result, possibly including limited freedom of choice.

In the abortion debate, things are a little different. If capacities are critical, all of the capacities we have identified occur late enough so that substantial policy agreement can be achieved. Supporters of the circulation, integrating capacity, and consciousness theories do not have to fight among themselves. What cannot be agreed upon, however, is whether capacity or potential is critical. On that question the definition of death can tell us nothing, just as medical facts can tell us nothing. We almost certainly will be forced to live with the frustrating and perpetual uncertainty this creates, just as we live with uncertainty over when we should treat people as dead.

NOTES

1. Here, and throughout this paper, I am using the concept of "standing" to refer to a status typically assigned to typical members of a society. It is approximately

the same notion as "prime moral status" developed by Daniel Wikler elsewhere in this volume. The concept is built on the idea that full standing or prime moral status is attributed to members of society when rights and claims of a moral or legal sort are justifiably exercised by such an individual in exactly the same way as they are by others given similar status. In practice this means in law that the rights and responsibilities of the Constitution, statutory law, and common law attach to such individuals. In ethics, moral claims and moral responsibilities attach to them. I am using the term "standing" in this paper in a way that can be interpreted as either moral or legal standing. As long as one is consistent throughout, one could thus apply this analysis to either law or ethics.

2. *See* Morison, R., *Death—Process or Event?* SCIENCE 173(3998):694-98 (1971); Kass, L., *Death as an Event: A Commentary on Robert Morison*, SCIENCE 173(3998):698-702 (1971).

3. *See* S. 158, 97th Cong., 1st Sess., 127 Cong. Rec. 570 (1981); Fletcher, J., *Medicine and the Nature of Man*, in THE TEACHING OF MEDICAL ETHICS (R.M. Veatch, W. Gaylin, C. Morgan, eds.) (Hastings Center, Hastings-on-Hudson, N.Y.) (1973) at 47-58.

4. R. MCCORMICK, HOW BRAVE A NEW WORLD (Doubleday & Co., Garden City, N.Y.) (1981) at 194-95; Engelhardt, Jr., H.T., *On the Bounds of Freedom: From the Treatment of Fetuses to Euthanasia*, CONNECTICUT MEDICINE 40(1):51 (January 1976).

5. Tooley, M., *Abortion and Infanticide*, PHILOSOPHY AND PUBLIC AFFAIRS 2(1):37, 42 (Fall 1972); Becker, L.C., *Human Being: The Boundaries of the Concept*, PHILOSOPHY AND PUBLIC AFFAIRS 4(4):334, 348 (Spring 1975).

6. Warren, M., *On the Moral and Legal Status of Abortion*, MONIST 57 (1): 43, 55 (January 1973); Tooley, *supra* note 5, at 44.

7. Warren, *supra* note 6, at 55.

8. Green, M.B., Wikler, D., *Brain Death and Personal Identity*, PHILOSOPHY AND PUBLIC AFFAIRS 9(2):105-33 (Winter 1980).

9. Lejeune, J., *Wann Beginnt das Leben des Menschen?* PÄDIATRIE UND PÄDOLOGIE 16:11-18 (1981).

10. *See* Hellegers, A., *Fetal Development*, THEOLOGICAL STUDIES 31(1):4 (March 1970).

11. Veatch, R.M., *The Definition of Death: Ethical, Philosophical and Policy Confusion*, in BRAIN DEATH: INTERRELATED MEDICAL AND SOCIAL ISSUES (J. Korein, ed.) (New York Academy of Sciences, New York City) (1978) at 310-13, 315.

12. I. JAKOBOVITS, JEWISH MEDICAL ETHICS (Bloch Publishing Co., New York City) (1967) at 184, 190, 191; *see also* F. ROSNER, STUDIES IN TORAH JUDAISM: MODERN MEDICINE AND JEWISH LAW (Yeshiva University, Department of Special Publications, New York City) (1972) at 65, 83.

13. *See* Ad Hoc Committee of the Harvard Medical School to Examine the Definition of Brain Death, *A Definition of Irreversible Coma*, JOURNAL OF THE AMERICAN MEDICAL ASSOCIATION 205(6):337-40 (1968); Institute of Society, Ethics and the Life Sciences, Task Force on Death and Dying, *Refinements in Criteria for*

the Determination of Death, JOURNAL OF THE AMERICAN MEDICAL ASSOCIATION 221(1):48-53 (1972); Capron, A.M., Kass, L.R., *A Statutory Definition of the Standards for Determining Human Death: An Appraisal and a Proposal,* UNIVERSITY OF PENNSYLVANIA LAW REVIEW 121(1):87-118 (November 1972).

14. PRESIDENT'S COMMISSION FOR THE STUDY OF ETHICAL PROBLEMS IN MEDICINE AND BIOMEDICAL AND BEHAVIORAL RESEARCH, DEFINING DEATH: A REPORT ON THE MEDICAL, LEGAL AND ETHICAL ISSUES IN THE DETERMINATION OF DEATH (U.S. Gov't Printing Office, Washington, D.C.) (1981).

15. C.J. MCFADDEN, MEDICAL ETHICS (F.A. Davis Co., Philadelphia, Pa.) (1967) at 19-20.

16. Veatch, R.M., *The Whole-Brain-Oriented Concept of Death: An Outmoded Philosophical Formulation,* JOURNAL OF THANATOLOGY 3(1): 13-30 (1975); Green, Wikler, *supra* note 8, at 105-33; Engelhardt, Jr., H.T., *Defining Death: A Philosophical Problem for Medicine and Law,* AMERICAN REVIEW OF RESPIRATORY DISEASE 112(5):587 (1975); Brierley, J.B., *et al., Neocortical Death after Cardiac Arrest,* LANCET 2(7724):560-65 (September 11, 1971); Institute of Society, Ethics and the Life Sciences, Task Force on Death and Dying, *supra* note 13, at 53.

17. Beecher, H.K., "The New Definition of Death: Some Opposing Views" (paper presented at the meeting of the American Association for the Advancement of Science) (December 1970).

Audience Discussion

Sidney Scherlis, Moderator

UNIDENTIFIED PARTICIPANT: Do you think that the arguments in the anthropological area concerning identification of human bones vs. prehuman bones might have any bearing on the arguments that you are discussing?

ROBERT M. VEATCH (Conference Faculty): What is at stake is not really an analysis of the definition of life and the definition of death in terms of scientific classification. Rather the question we want to ask is when to start and stop treating people in a particular way. That is a moral or public policy question. I'm really hard-pressed to see how it could be answered directly from evolutionary and anthropological data.

CAROLINE WHITBECK, PH.D. (Institute for the Medical Humanities, Texas): I liked your paper very much, but I have the same problem with your notion of "full moral standing" that I had with Dan Wikler's notion of "prime moral status." It seems to me that if philosophy is going to help clarify the moral issues surrounding abortion, then we have to sort out a number of very different moral standings, not one of which is well described as "full" or "prime" in comparison to the others. In particular we need to examine the moral standing of an adult, the moral standing of an infant, and the moral standing of a fetus and the consequent differences in our responsibilities toward such individuals. I would argue that there are some responsibilities that we have for the welfare of infants, for example, that we do not have for the welfare of adults, and this point is obscured if we call the standing of the adult "full moral standing."

If we are to clarify the moral status of the fetus, one obvious approach would be to compare the status of the fetus to that of a newborn. Unfortunately the philosophical literature contains very little on the moral status of infants and newborns. Indeed, there is virtually nothing apart from some discussion of infanticide. To understand the moral status of a newborn we would need to address issues that are much more complex and subtle than the question of when, if ever, killing an infant is morally justified. I would like to see us give more attention to the question of the moral status of infants and to the scope and limits of the analogy between the moral status of newborns and of fetuses. Perhaps the fact to which Dr. Ryan brought our attention, that there are so few women among the conference participants, will hinder our efforts to accomplish that task here. It seems to me that you have given us at least one important distinction to use in the clarification of the moral status of infants—that is, your distinction between a capacity and a potential. Using the distinction we may ask, "What are the differences in our moral responsibilities toward a being who is very vulnerable to the loss of future capacity but presently has only potential, and our responsibilities toward a being who has well-developed capacities?"

ROBERT VEATCH: Thank you, Caroline. That does seem to be an appropriate agenda for people who are going to continue to work in this area. I plead guilty to using the phrase, "full standing" or "full human standing." These are terms that need more precise definition. What I had in mind is a very widely held view that there is a large cluster of behaviors that are appropriate vis-à-vis people who are in that category: "prime moral status" in Dan's terms; "full standing" in mine. Such individuals, for example, may be the legitimate bearers of legal and/or moral claims that do not attach to others or attach only derivatively. For those within the United States, the Constitution would apply to them. To the extent that moral philosophers are concerned with inalienable rights of human beings, those rights apply to those with full standing, but they do not necessarily apply to others.

There are legal, political, and psychological behaviors that are appropriate vis-à-vis those who are in that category. When they are in that category there is, at least ideally, some notion of egalitarianism. The Constitution applies equally to all, or at least all in certain broad categories, once it applies to anyone. Identifying the dividing lines at the beginning point and the ending point are essentially the agenda that is being sketched here.

UNIDENTIFIED PARTICIPANT: I assume that if some individuals have full moral standing then some have partial standing. Do you think it would be critical to argue for a position that those who have the capacity should have full standing in the sense that the state now has a duty by means of the criminal code to protect these lives, but that until they have full standing such duties would not apply?

ROBERT VEATCH: Possibly. The whole function of a concept of full standing is to distinguish those with full standing from others with partial standing. Whether the separation is based on capacity or potential I view as an open question. Likewise I view it as an open question whether the criminal code should always protect the lives of those with "full standing." It might not "protect the lives" of competent treatment refusers, for instance. It would treat those with full standing differently from those with only partial standing, however.

UNIDENTIFIED PARTICIPANT: Are you against granting standing to those who have only potential?

ROBERT VEATCH: I cannot think of arguments either for or against. People take stands on those issues all the time, but I do not see rational discourse penetrating the controversy between potential and capacity. I suspect if there were a knock-down drag-out rational argument for one position or the other, those of us in this room, being reasonable people, would see things alike and would develop a consensus on the subject. I would like to have rational argument for one of those views or another. I don't see it. In the meantime we have people expressing preferences, intuitions, conscience, or faith statements on whether they see capacity or potential as the critical outlook. I don't see ways of moving beyond that. I can give you my intuition on whether capacity or potential is important, but I do not think my answer is really very important.

SIDNEY SCHERLIS , M.D. (President, American Society of Law & Medicine, Towson, Md.): What is your view of what is important?

ROBERT VEATCH: When I do rounds in hospitals and clinicians ask me, as a so-called medical ethicist, what my opinion is about what ought to be done, I generally do not reveal that opinion unless I'm convinced that those who have asked me are certain as to what my opinion is worth. I am trained to analyze medical ethical positions and claim no expertise in identifying which positions are correct.

UNIDENTIFIED PARTICIPANT: I would like you to comment concerning the language that has developed in the area of the definition of death. If I remember it correctly, the Kansas statute has two definitions of death. Can you make a suggestion as to what we could do to improve that?

ROBERT VEATCH: The new definition of death does, indeed, contain language somewhat reminiscent of the Kansas statute. The two definitions are cardiac-oriented and brain-oriented. The President's Commission was very much aware of the problem of dual definitions in the Kansas statute. I think they have quite satisfactorily avoided this problem. The first formal critique of the presidential report that I have seen, that by Bernat, Culver, and Gert in the *Hastings Center Report,*[1] attacks the Presidential Commission on the grounds that it has called for two definitions. I do not find the attack very convincing.

WARREN M. HERN, M.D., M.P.H. (Boulder Abortion Clinic, Boulder Colorado): I think this is an exceptional paper, which seems to say we cannot come to any firm conclusion as to what definition of death (or the corollary, life) we should use. Therefore, I would have to conclude that the definition that is used in operating our society or any society, until that point is resolved, depends entirely on who controls the political and administrative apparatus of the state. It becomes a political question, then, rather than a question that leads to rational discussion. This is an issue that I struggle with, as a physician providing abortion services. When a woman comes into my office asking for an abortion, I must recognize that, while there may be some debate or some concern about the capacity or potential of the fetus, I have no doubt about the woman's capacity as a person. Therefore, I'm forced to choose in favor of her. As a philosopher, you would appreciate that. But one of the things you alluded to when you talked about moral standing, but didn't mention specifically, is the question of whether the act of abortion is an ending of innocent life. This raises the questions, of course: innocent compared to what? Innocent compared to whom? Does this imply some status with regard to the woman who desires an abortion as to her innocence or guilt? If so, innocent or guilty of what? You mentioned the linguistic controversy in the abortion issue. I think that when we hear about the "unborn baby," we also have a question of whether or not there is an "undead corpse." I certainly hope no one would bury me if I am not a dead corpse.

ROBERT VEATCH: We should be careful to avoid the dangers of concluding that since there is no definitive philosophical argument for or against actions with ethical import such as abortion, that these matters are "merely" political and administrative. In the first place all political and administrative decisions involve ethical judgments. They are impossible to escape. More fundamentally, many other crucial ethical questions having vital public policy significance cannot be resolved definitively by rational analysis, yet it is clear that we must take public stands on these issues. I doubt that it is possible to prove definitively by rational argument that young children have full standing. Some minority of philosophers deny they do. Yet as a society we certainly will act as if they do. I believe your argument based on inability to prove the status of the fetus also could be used against children, women, or ethnic minorities.

I did not refer to the question of the innocence of life, because the question of what characteristics of human beings are so essential that they have full standing seems to me to be far more fundamental. When we are able to identify that characteristic, we shall know when full moral standing begins and when it ends. Then we can go on, if we want, to ask whether guilt or innocence is morally relevant to the way we treat those with full standing. Continuity in understanding of what gives full standing at the beginning and what ends full standing at the end of life seems to me to be fundamental and open to rational exploration.

Note

1. Bernat, J., Culver, C., Gert, B., *Defining Death in Theory and Practice*, HASTINGS CENTER REPORT 12(1):5 (Feb. 1982).

Part Three

Legal Implications

Chapter 8

The Concept of Person in the Law

Charles H. Baron

The focus of the abortion debate in the United States tends to be on whether and at what stage a fetus is a person. I believe this tendency has been unfortunate and counterproductive. Instead of advancing dialogue between opposing sides, such a focus seems to have stunted it, leaving advocates in the sort of "I did not!"—"You did too!" impasse we remember from childhood. Also reminiscent of that childhood scene has been the vain attempt to break the impasse by appeal to a higher authority. Thus, the pro-choice forces hoped they had proved the pro-life forces "wrong" by having had the Supreme Court of the United States decide in *Roe v. Wade*[1] that a fetus is not a person for purposes of the Fourteenth Amendment. Now the pro-life forces are trying to prove the pro-choice forces "wrong" by passing legislation or a Constitutional Amendment[2] that declares a fetus to be a person after all! I believe that there is a better, more productive way to approach the abortion debate, and that is the way the law has historically approached the concept of person.

However, before I examine the law's approach to personhood, I want to explore briefly some likely sources of the tendency to focus the abortion debate on the issue of whether the fetus is a person. One source, clearly, arises from the simple social-psychological fact that people—at least people in today's civilized society—tend to believe that personhood brings with it a certain basic entitlement to life. This is likely to be less true in societies whose members do not perceive a clear difference between human and nonhuman things. Tribes which confer souls—and therefore a kind of personhood—on animals, trees, streams, and so forth, must be very used to the notion that personhood does not protect such "persons" from being eaten, felled, or drunk from. Therefore, it may be an easy step for them to

The author dedicates this article to his wife, Irma Elaine Baron, in appreciation of the humane perspective she has lent to his work and to his life. The author thanks Eric Finamore, a third-year law student at Boston University, for research assistance provided in the preparation of the article.

accept such exploitation of human persons as well. Both types of person may be entitled to respect, apology, and remorse, but both may be seen as naturally subject to exploitation when necessity dictates.[3] However, in a modern, humanistic society such as ours, a clearer dichotomy is established. In one camp are objects or entities inferior to persons and subject to their exploitation without respect, apology, or remorse. In the other are persons, superior beings entitled (at least in theory) to being treated as ends in themselves and not merely as means for achieving other ends.[4]

Against such a social-psychological background, it is easy to see why the abortion battle would seem to hinge on the issue of the fetus' personhood. For one thing, natural predilection would lead people to think in personhood terms. For another, advocates for the opposed positions would assume that the debate could be won or lost in these terms, and they would present arguments and evidence designed to increase or diminish the degree of empathy felt for the fetus. Thus, some pro-choice activists attempt to win acceptance of the view that the fetus is merely "a clump of tissue" that may become inimical to the mother's health or life and, under those circumstances, subject to removal without compunction like any other malignancy. In opposition, many pro-life activists refer to the fetus as an "infant" or "child" and draw attention to how human it begins to look and act at early stages of development.[5] Of course, such efforts to win humane treatment through empathy do not begin with the abortion controversy. A classic example is Shylock's speech in *The Merchant of Venice*:

> [Antonio] hath disgraced me, and hindered me half a million, laughed at my losses, mocked at my gains, scorned my nation, thwarted my bargains, cooled my friends, heated mine enemies; and what's his reason? I am a Jew. Hath not a Jew eyes? hath not a Jew hands, organs, dimensions, senses, affections, passions? fed with the same food, hurt with the same weapons, subject to the same diseases, healed by the same means, warmed and cooled by the same winter and summer, as a Christian is? If you prick us, do we not bleed? if you tickle us, do we not laugh? if you poison us, do we not die? and if you wrong us, shall we not revenge?[6]

As we know, this appeal for empathy gained Shylock no advantage,[7] and history should teach us that such appeals have failed repeatedly to guarantee humane treatment even for human beings. As Sissela Bok has pointed out, "Slavery, witch-hunts, and wars have all been justified by their perpetrators on the ground that they thought their victims to be less than fully human."[8] This is not to say that the argument from empathy is pointless. In close cases, the force of such empathy may carry the day and it ought always to have the virtue of making the perpetrators feel some limiting moral discomfort. However, it ought to be clear that we are perfectly capable of refusing to grant personhood on the basis of empathy where that status would seem to exact a result which we are unwilling to accept. Rather than serving as a criterion for decision making, the ascription of personhood may well be a way of announcing a decision, based on other grounds, to treat something the way we would a person.

A second reason that the abortion controversy has focused on the issue of personhood is that some participants seem to believe that it is simply true that the fetus is a person and therefore entitled to a live birth. This is, of course, an article of faith of the Roman Catholic Church and, perhaps, of some other religious groups.[9] However, in a pluralistic, democratic society such as ours, it is hard to justify imposing the revealed truths of a religious group upon the whole of that society. It is, therefore, to the credit of the pro-life movement that it has largely avoided basing its position on the ground of revealed religious truth. A great many Catholics have opposed recriminalizing abortion because they do not wish to impose their moral views on others,[10] while proponents of recriminalizing abortion have attempted to substitute science for religion as the source of the truth that justifies their position. "Present-day scientific evidence indicates that a human being exists from conception," reads one pro-life bill which has been proposed in the effort to undo *Roe v. Wade*.[11] "The Congress finds that present-day scientific evidence indicates a significant likelihood that actual human life exists from conception," reads another.[12] Yet, many scientists modestly and, I believe, quite properly refuse to accept the responsibility to decide a question that is not one of objective science.[13] Biologist John Biggers has said, "The abortion controversy does involve real and substantial moral issues, for which there seem to be no simple solutions, but by asking precisely when a human life begins, Congress is turning away from these profound and serious problems and raising instead a question that is fundamentally absurd—even meaningless."[14] Hence, science is likely to fare no better than religion as an acceptable basis for objectively deciding whether or not the fetus is a person.

A third and more immediate source of the focus upon personhood in discussing abortion is a legal one. Both the equal protection and the due process clauses of the Fourteenth Amendment to the United States Constitution apply to, and only to, "persons."[15] As a result, when the Supreme Court decided *Roe v. Wade*, the Justices thought they had to grapple with the question of whether the fetus was a person for Fourteenth Amendment purposes. Justice Blackmun, in speaking for the Court, assumed that if the appellee's "suggestion of personhood is established, the appellant's case, of course, collapses, for the fetus' right to life would then be guaranteed specifically by the Amendment."[16] In dealing with the question, the Court purported to avoid looking beyond the four corners of the Constitution itself. The Court explicitly rejected the appellee's invitation to do this, saying: "We need not resolve the difficult question of when life begins. When those trained in the respective disciplines of medicine, philosophy, and theology are unable to arrive at any consensus, the judiciary, at this point in the development of man's knowledge, is not in a position to speculate as to the answer."[17] The appellee had conceded that it could find no legal precedent holding that a fetus was a person within the meaning of the Fourteenth Amendment. The Court was presented with a momentous question of first impression, and incredibly, it chose to answer by merely listing the various places where the word "person" appears in the Constitution, concluding:

> [I]n nearly all these instances, the use of the word is such that it has application only postnatally. None indicates, with any assurance, that it has any possible prenatal application.
>
>   All this, together with our observation, *supra*, that throughout the major portion of the nineteenth century prevailing legal abortion practices were far freer than they are today, persuades us that the word "person," as used in the Fourteenth Amendment, does not include the unborn.[18]

Happily, the Court's seemingly wooden approach to the concept of personhood in *Roe v. Wade* does not typify the approach to that concept in the law generally. The more typical approach—which I want to recommend as a model for helping us out of the rut in which we find ourselves on the matter of abortion—is characterized by flexibility, pragmatism, and common sense.

CORPORATIONS AND SLAVES AS LEGAL PERSONS

Somewhat paradoxically, one of the best examples of the more typical approach of the law to the concept of personhood is provided by a series of earlier Supreme Court decisions. These are the cases in which the Court decided that, at least for some purposes, a corporation is to be considered a person. Of course, the Constitution does not explicitly speak of corporations any more than it does of fetuses. Nonetheless, in a series of decisions rendered in the late nineteenth century,[19] the Supreme Court held that corporations were to be considered "persons" coming under the protection of various provisions of the Constitution—including the Fourteenth Amendment. Thus, by 1898, the Court could observe in one such case that it had become "well settled" that corporations are persons within the meaning of the equal protection clause of the Fourteenth Amendment.[20] And although it was not until the twentieth century that the Court granted due process protection to the liberty interests of corporations,[21] it recognized corporations as persons under the due process clause of the Fourteenth Amendment for the purpose of protecting their property interests as early as 1886.[22] Moreover, the Court has interpreted the word "person" to include corporations when it is used in a great variety of federal statutes, such as early bankruptcy laws, the federal criminal codes, the Federal Power Act, and the Internal Revenue Code.[23]

Why has the Court done this? Is it because the members of the Court have adopted some theory that ensoulment occurs at the moment of incorporation? Is it because they were shown ultrasound images of a corporation that revealed a startlingly human form? Of course not. The real basis, even though the Court may not always be so clear about it, is in the social consequences foreseen as the result of a failure to apply the particular law to corporations. Where those consequences are judged untoward—perhaps because they seem inconsistent with the presumed intent of the law—the Court will interpret the word "person" to include corporations. Where they are not, the Court will not. Thus, a corporation may be a person for some purposes under the Constitution, and it may not be a person for others.

One can see why it would be sensible to accord personhood to corporations for purposes of the equal protection clause. Not all corporations are enormous, wealthy, and powerful, and even the most powerful may be subject to state regulation that we would think arbitrary, irrational, or invidiously discriminatory[24] if it were applied to an individual human being. But then, corporations comprise human beings; when you scratch a corporation, it is human beings who bleed. How are we to protect these human beings from being unconstitutionally injured through the treatment accorded their corporation? We could, of course, just grant each human being a separate claim against the state—refusing to recognize a claim brought by the corporation since the equal protection clause speaks only of "persons." However, forcing each shareholder, officer, or employee to bring a separate lawsuit based upon a discrete interest in the corporation is manifestly inefficient and fraught with potential for producing incongruous and unfair results. Allowing the corporation to bring one suit seems to make much more sense, even though that may mean according it its own rights under the Constitution, and that, in turn, may mean calling it a "person," at least for these narrow purposes.

On the other hand, a glance at the consequences may lead the courts to decide that, for other purposes, a corporation is not a person. This has, for example, been the position of the federal courts with respect to the Fifth Amendment guarantee that "[n]o person . . . shall be compelled in any criminal case to be a witness against himself."[25] In this context, it has been held that a corporation is *not* a person and that, therefore, it may be forced to provide information incriminating to itself.[26] How can this be?

Can it be consistent with the cases holding that a corporation is a person for purposes of the Fourteenth Amendment? It can be if one is less concerned with the words used by the framers of the Constitution than with the consequences one believes its various provisions are supposed to protect against. Assuming that the right against self-incrimination was designed to avoid the disquieting spectacle of forcing a criminal case out of the mouth of the accused—to insulate our developing democracy from the devices of torture which had been central to the armory of the government prosecutor in the old world—it may make sense not to extend that right to corporations as such.[27] After all, it is not the corporation that is being forced to testify against itself. Some individual representing the corporation is being forced to give up papers or testify against the corporation, and that individual is frequently someone who is not subject to the burden of the criminal sanctions involved. It may be that only the corporation will be subject to criminal liability in the form of a fine. And even if some human being may ultimately have to pay a fine or be imprisoned, it may be a person other than the individual who is being forced to supply the evidence. However, in the case where the potential bearer of sanctions is the same person from whom evidence is sought, he or she can be amply protected by exercising his or her own right against self-incrimination. There is no need to protect this individual by extending the constitutional right to the corporation.[28]

Justice Holmes once observed: "A word is not a crystal, transparent and unchanged; it is the skin of a living thought and may vary greatly in color and content according to the circumstances and the time in which it is used."[29] The enterprise of the law is dedicated to goals other than the compilation of a simple dictionary. In that enterprise, words serve as the imperfect medium through which our legal institutions attempt to carry on the business of ordering our society. Where the words employed in a given context and the meanings they may have from outside the law conflict with some important goal of social ordering, it is likely to be the words and those meanings that will be made to give way. Hence, a corporation—which seems very unlike what we would normally call a "person" outside the law—becomes a person, at least for some purposes. And for certain purposes the law is just as capable of treating as nonpersons classes of individuals we would intuitively regard as persons.

Perhaps the most stark example in American law of the latter phenomenon is the status accorded blacks during the slavery era. Although the legal context of slavery did not require the Supreme Court to wrestle with the question of whether or not a slave was a person, the Court did find itself compelled to resolve the question of whether or not a slave could ever become a "citizen" capable of asserting a claim in federal court. In the notorious case of *Dred Scott v. Sandford*,[30] Chief Justice Taney concluded that the answer was clearly no:

> The words "people of the United States" and "citizens" are synonymous terms, and mean the same thing. They both describe the political body who, according to our republican institutions, form the sovereignty, and who hold the power and conduct the Government through their representatives. They are what we familiarly call the "sovereign people," and every citizen is one of this people, and a constituent member of this sovereignty. The question before us is, whether [negroes of African descent, whose ancestors were of pure African blood and brought into this country and sold as slaves] compose a portion of this people, and are constituent members of this sovereignty? We think they are not, and that they are not included, and were not intended to be included, under the word "citizens" in the Constitution, and can therefore claim none of the rights and privileges which that instrument provides for and secures to citizens of the United States. On the contrary, they were at that time considered as a subordinate and inferior class of beings, who had been subjugated by the dominant race, and, whether emancipated or not, yet remained subject to their authority, and had no rights or privileges but such as those who held the power and the Government might choose to grant them.[31]

As the Chief Justice knew, "those who held the power and the Government" had not chosen to grant a good deal to their slaves by way of rights and privileges. And yet, state law had dealt with slaves in much the sort of flexible and pragmatic way in which the courts have dealt with corporations. Thus, although slaves were considered to be the property of their masters—sometimes real property and sometimes personal property[32]— "[t]he master's property in his slave was *sui generis*, the slave being considered in the law in many respects in the light of a human being entitled to the law's protection."[33] Slaves were entitled to the protection of the criminal law, but not to the same extent as whites.[34] And, not suprisingly:

> Slaves were treated as persons by the criminal law, and were legally punishable for their crimes. Slaves were punishable for assault and battery, larceny, mayhem, rape, and homicide. . . . [T]he slave undoubtedly had the natural right of self-preservation or self-defense, although certain facts which as between whites might excuse or mitigate the offense did not so operate in the case of slaves. . . .[35]

Dark and repulsive as the mirror may be, we here seem to have the mirror image of the phenomenon we saw with respect to corporations. Despite the *prima facie* entitlement of blacks to personhood, the law under a regime of slavery was capable of treating them as persons for some purposes and property for others.

THE UNBORN AND THE COMMON LAW

When we move to the issue of the status of the unborn, we find the law generally evidencing the same sort of flexibility and pragmatism in ascribing personhood. For some purposes, the fetus is a person. For some, it is not. The stage at which it is granted personhood varies from one area of the law to another. Thus, the common law of crimes did not recognize the killing of an unborn child as homicide, and the rule in the majority of American jurisdictions continues to be "that there is no homicide of any grade unless the deceased had been born alive."[36] Inducing an abortion was, at common law, a separate crime of only misdemeanor status. It could be committed only upon a fetus which was "quick," that is, one that had already displayed independent movement within the mother—a phenomenon which generally begins somewhere between the sixteenth and eighteenth week of pregnancy.[37] At the opposite extreme is the treatment accorded the fetus by the law of property. For purposes of the law of inheritance of real property, a child has been considered to be a person eligible to inherit at the moment he or she is conceived, although this property interest has been held subject to defeasance if the child has not subsequently been born alive.[38] How can this apparent inconsistency in the law be justified? The justification is a function of the different social policies being advanced by different areas of the law. Prime among the goals of the laws of inheritance is fulfillment of the presumed intentions of the testator. Thus, where a will or the laws of inheritance specify that property shall be inherited by one's child or children, it is presumed that the deceased would have wanted any of his children born subsequent to his death to inherit, even if he did not know of the child's impending existence at the time that he died.[39] In order to assure this consequence, the law confers on the child at the time of conception a type of personhood in which the inheritance can vest if the parent dies prior to birth. On the other hand, the criminal law has different goals. Basic to these is preserving the public peace by publicly punishing those who threaten that peace with acts that society considers to be blameworthy.[40] Clearly, treatment afforded the unborn by the common law of crimes reflects a judgment that the society of the time considered the killing of a fetus to be less blameworthy than the killing of a man, and the killing of a fetus that had not yet displayed a separate personality within the mother to be less blameworthy than the killing of one which had.

In the law of torts, we can see even more clearly the interrelationship between social engineering and ontology. Here, where the question is usually whether money damages are to be awarded a plaintiff for injuries caused by the fault of the defendant, the law was very slow to recognize a cause of action on behalf of an injured fetus. Prior to 1946, there were substantially no cases allowing damages to the child born deformed as a result of injuries sustained while *en ventre sa mere*.[41] *A fortiori*, the courts denied recovery in wrongful death to the child that was stillborn or aborted as a result of such injuries.[42] Among the grounds given for such decisions by the courts was "that the defendant could owe no duty of conduct to a person who was not in existence at the time of his action."[43] In 1946 with the District of Columbia decision of *Bonbrest v. Kotz*,[44] the tide turned with stunning force. As Professor Prosser observed in 1969, that case and its sequel

> brought about what was up till that time the most spectacular abrupt reversal of a well settled rule in the whole history of the law of torts. The child, if he is born alive, is [now] permitted to maintain an action for the consequences of prenatal injuries, and if he dies of injuries after birth an action will lie for his wrongful death. So rapid has been the overturn that after the lapse of a scant 23 years from the beginning, it is now apparently literally true that there is no authority left still supporting the older rule. The last jurisdiction to overrule it was Texas, in 1967.[45]

The process of undoing the earlier rule continues to the present. Thus, as Prosser additionally noted, there was in 1969 still substantial resistance to allowing recovery for injuries sustained prior to viability or at least quickening.[46] There was also resistance to allowing recovery in wrongful death for the child that was not initially born alive;[47] however, since 1969, courts have increasingly recognized a right to sue in wrongful death on behalf of a stillborn.[48] Courts have also recognized rights to sue for injuries sustained at any time after conception and, in some cases, before.[49] Thus, in the 1977 case of *Renslow v. Mennonite Hospital*, the court allowed recovery to an infant for injuries it sustained from the mother's Rh-negative blood having been sensitized many years before with negligently administered Rh-positive blood by way of transfusion. The court stated:

> The cases allowing relief to an infant for injuries incurred in its previable state make it clear that a defendant may be held liable to a person whose existence was not apparent at the time of his act. We therefore find it illogical to bar relief for an act done prior to conception where the defendant would be liable for this same conduct had the child unbeknownst to him, been conceived prior to his act. We believe that there is a right to be born free from prenatal injuries forseeably caused by a breach of duty to the child's mother.[50]

We seem to have reached a point where personhood, for purposes of at least some torts, may be said to begin before conception!

What was the basis for this revolution in the law of torts? Once again, the reasons seem very practical. It was based upon changes of the last several decades in both the facts and values which related to this area of the law. The law of torts is characterized by a concern both for encouraging people to take due care not to harm others and for attempting to "make whole" (through money damages) people who do suffer harm at the hands of others. Because of the increasing availability and acceptance of insurance as a way of covering tort liability and as a regular "cost of doing business," the courts have tended more and more to concentrate on the goal of compensating hapless victims of injury and have worried less and less about whether it could be said that the particular defendant was at fault.[51] It seems clear that the early reluctance to recognize a cause of action on the part of the injured fetus was motivated by concern with the unfairness that might be done a particular defendant in an area where the question of whether the defendant's acts caused the fetus' injuries was not subject to solid scientific answer.[52] But the last few decades have seen such spectacular improvements in the field of perinatology that questions of causation are no longer speculative in most cases.[53] When this development is combined with the trend toward lessened concern for the blameworthiness of the defendant, the case for allowing recovery for the prenatally injured child becomes compelling.

Other examples, from more obscure areas of the law, could be drawn upon to illustrate and confirm the fact that the law has been largely willing to confer personhood upon the unborn when solid policy considerations have suggested that course. Like many other lawyers, I have represented, by court appointment, "unborn persons" whose interests in the disposition of the money in a trust might be adversely affected by a court's approval of actions that have been taken by the trustee.[54] In other situations as well,[55] courts have not balked at appointing counsel for unborn clients when they believed that fair procedure required it. Additional instances are plentiful, and they are not all of recent vintage. As one English judge observed of the fetus in 1798:

> Let us see what this nonentity can do. He may be vouched in a recovery, though it is for the purpose of making him answer over in value. He may be an executor. He may take under the Statute of Distributions. He may take by devise. He may be entitled under a charge for raising portions. He may have an injunction, and he may have a guardian.[56]

THE UNBORN AND THE CONSTITUTION

In light of all this, what are we to make of the decision in *Roe v. Wade* that a fetus is not to be considered a person for purposes of the United States Constitution? From all that has been said, it should now be clear that the key to the decision is in the following language from the Court's opinion:

The detriment that the state would impose upon the pregnant woman by denying [the abortion] choice altogether is apparent. Specific and direct harm medically diagnosable even in early pregnancy may be involved. Maternity, or additional offspring, may force upon the woman a distressful life and future. Psychological harm may be imminent. Mental and physical health may be taxed by child care. There is also the distress, for all concerned, associated with the unwanted child, and there is the problem of bringing a child into a family already unable, psychologically and otherwise, to care for it. In other cases, as in this one, the additional difficulties and continuing stigma of unwed motherhood may be involved.[57]

Clearly, the Court decided to deny personhood to the fetus for purposes of the Fourteenth Amendment because it thought it had solid social policy grounds for doing so. In order to avoid denying to the mother altogether the right to take the life of the fetus through termination of pregnancy, it thought it had to refuse to confer upon the fetus any rights under the Constitution and, at the same time, to recognize in the mother a "right to privacy" that the state could regulate only to the extent that it could show a "compelling interest" for doing so.[58] However, in my opinion, the Court was mistaken and misguided in so concluding.

First, the Court was in error in assuming that the mother would be denied the abortion choice altogether if it held that a fetus was a person for the purposes of the Fourteenth Amendment. The Fourteenth Amendment regulates only "state action"; it does not regulate the action of individuals unless their activity can be linked with that of a state in one or more well-recognized ways.[59] Therefore, a woman who poisons her five-year-old child does not violate the Fourteenth Amendment—although she is most likely to have violated the homicide laws of her state. How, then, did the Court think the Fourteenth Amendment might protect fetuses (considered as persons) from mothers who wished an abortion? The thought must have been[60] that the state would have to treat fetuses the same way it treated five-year-olds. If the state did not prosecute mothers for homicide of fetuses under the same circumstances and to the same extent as it did for homicide of five-year-olds, the state would be found to have violated the Fourteenth Amendment. Thus, mothers securing abortions would have to be treated as murderers under state law.

But the Court's implicit reasoning is simplistic. Not considered, among other things, is the fact that the Fourteenth Amendment permits the state to treat different classes of persons differently if a sufficiently rational and legitimate state ground can be given for so doing.[61] Even if the Court felt compelled to accord fetus-persons a specially protected "suspect classification" status, differing treatment could be justified by a state ground found to be (as protection of the life or health of the mother might) a "compelling state interest."[62] Moreover, the state might protect the mother's interests without even resorting to treating the fetus differently from other persons. The defense of self-defense is available in prosecutions for homicide generally. Of course such a defense to an abortion would cover only the case where the mother's bodily safety was at stake, and self-defense is usually available only where the deceased is thought responsible for some act that threatens that safety.[63] However, it does not seem to me intuitively obvious that it would be unconstitutional for a state to extend the availability of self-defense beyond traditional bounds. Moreover, the state need not do so. A better, though somewhat less established,[64] defense to homicide is already available—the defense of "necessity" or "choice of evils":

> The pressure of natural physical forces sometimes confronts a person in an emergency with a choice of two evils: either he may violate the literal terms of the criminal law and thus produce a harmful result, or he may comply with those terms and thus produce a greater or equal or lesser amount of harm. For reasons of social policy, if the harm which will result from compliance with the law is greater than that which will result from violation of it, he is justified in violating it. Under such circumstances he is said to have the defense of necessity, and he is not guilty of the crime in question—unless, perhaps, he was at fault in bringing about the emergency situation, in which case he may be guilty of a crime of which that fault is an element.[65]

If such a defense can constitutionally justify homicide of the born, it ought constitutionally to justify homicide of the unborn as well. And it does not seem obvious to me that the state would act unconstitutionally if it were to eliminate or dilute the "emergency" requirement[66] or make specific provision for the weighing of evils involved in an abortion.[67]

Second, the Court cannot seriously mean that it is unwilling to treat the fetus as a person for all purposes under the Fourteenth Amendment. Suppose a state statute provided that damages were recoverable in tort to compensate for death or injury caused by prenatal injury to a fetus, *except where that fetus was nonwhite*. Could the Supreme Court hold other than that such a statute was flagrantly in violation of the Fourteenth Amendment's equal protection clause? If you are tempted to resort to the ploy of suggesting that it is the right of the nonwhite parents of the fetus to recover damages that the court would be protecting, consider another case. Suppose a state program paid fees to mothers planning an abortion who agreed to allow experimentation on the fetus prior to and after the abortion—*but only if the fetus is nonwhite*. Should not such a statute be held violative of the Fourteenth Amendment? Would it be because mothers of white fetuses were being cheated of similar benefits? Or would it be because we believed nonwhite fetuses were being treated in a fashion which smacked of "invidious discrimination?"

Unfortunately, cases not unlike my hypotheticals have already come before the lower federal courts, and anomalous results have been produced by the Court's overbroad holding in *Roe v. Wade*. Several times since *Roe*, the question has been raised of whether a fetus is a person for purposes of an action in tort under the federal Civil Rights Act.[68] In every case but one,[69] the answer has been no. Thus, in the recent case of *Harman v. Daniels*,[70] a mother and her infant child brought suit against a police officer who had allegedly injured them both in violation of the Civil Rights Act. The infant claimed

> that she was assaulted by the defendant officer when he allegedly struck her mother in the stomach. Sarah Beth Harman was *in utero* at the time of the alleged assault. Allegedly, she received major injuries as a result of the attack and suffered severe complications at birth which required substantial medical treatment and which will require continued medical care. It is claimed that the defendant knew that Ms. Harman was pregnant when he struck her and that he failed to seek immediate medical assistance for Ms. Harman once she developed severe stomach pains from the alleged blow to her abdomen.[71]

As we have seen, and as the court noted,[72] such a claim could be brought on behalf of a prenatally injured child under modern state law. However, while recognizing a federal Civil Rights Act claim for Ms. Harman, the court refused to recognize such a claim for Sarah Beth. As its reason, the court cited an earlier federal decision where it was stated:

> Roe v. Wade, supra, persuades this court that an unborn child is not included among persons who are entitled to relief under this Act. The Supreme Court states at page 158: "All this . . . persuades us that the word 'person,' as used in the Fourteenth Amendment, does not include the unborn. . . ."
>
> It necessarily follows that if an unborn is not a person under the Fourteenth Amendment an unborn has no right of action under [the Civil Rights Act] and this claim must fall.[73]

"In effect," the *Harman* court concluded, "fetal life has no constitutional rights or protection."[74]

Third, in dealing with the abortion controversy by means of a holding that the fetus is not a person under the Fourteenth Amendment, the Supreme Court masked the real and substantial choice-of-evils problem with which abortion confronts our society and forced the controversy into an all-or-nothing posture that rigidifies positions and blocks the normal legal processes for reaching accommodation between conflicting interests. Whether or not the fetus is called a "person," one cannot escape the sense that its potential for a future life as a person creates problems for the abortion decision that any society ignores at its peril. After all, if any one of us is killed, what is the loss to us? Assume that someone has determined to do away with you in a quick and humane fashion, for example, by means of some instantly effective poison gas under circumstances where you experience not even a moment's anxiety or agony. All you would suffer under such circumstances is the loss of your future life as a person. If this is a loss that our society feels it can visit on fetuses without compunction, what prevents it from being visited on you without compunction? Indeed, why is it not more justifiable in your case than it would be in the case of the fetus? Presumably the average fetus has more future life as a person to lose than you do. But this "slippery slope" rests on a seesaw. It is capable of carrying us backward as well as forward—and producing a *reductio ad absurdum*. For if potential future life as a person is the critical loss incurred, the zygote that is never brought into being suffers that damage as well. Let us call such a potential zygote a "spegg" (that is, a possible combination of sperm and egg). If we may not without compunction deny future life as a person to the born and to the unborn-but-conceived, how can we deny it without compunction to the unconceived spegg? Do we, then, have a duty to realize the conception potential of as many speggs as possible?[75] Of course we could not accept such a duty since it would mean speciesuicide. Even if we restricted ourselves to old fashioned methods of *in vivo* conception and gestation, we would light the fuse on a population bomb that would devastate our planet.

One way off this seesaw is to recognize that more weighs in the balance here than just the stage of development of the potential life involved. On the same side of the balance, there is the matter of how long a potential life is at stake. The anencephalic fetus can expect no future life outside its mother. The fetus with Tay-Sachs disease can expect only a few years. There is also the matter of what the potential life is likely to be worth to the fetus. Is the short life of sickness and gradual decline of the Tay-Sachs child better than no life at all? On the other side of the balance are the interests of the mother, the other members of her family, the other fetuses she might conceive if this one were aborted, and society as a whole. Is the mother likely to die in childbirth or has she just decided that the child would be born at an inopportune time? Is the family threatened with being sapped of emotional, physical, and financial strength by the addition of a severely disabled child or have the parents just decided that they would prefer a child of a sex different from that of the fetus? Do the parents plan other children that they will not have if they are forced to devote all of their resources to raising a severely disabled child? And, perhaps most important, what stake do the rest of us in society have in the outcome of the particular decision? In most cases, the benefit or detriment to society of the particular birth will be insignificant. But patterns and principles that may be produced by many such decisions hold the potential for societal impact of great significance. From the point of view of economics and eugenics, we may not only want to permit therapeutic abortion, we may want to encourage it. From the point of view of preserving a societal attitude of respect for human life, we may want not only to discourage abortion, we may want to forbid it. From the point of view of preserving personal autonomy, we may want not only to leave the choice to the mother, but to provide her with support and protection in exercising that choice.

FINDING A CONSENSUS

If anything should be clear from all of this, it is that there is no one abortion problem. There are as many abortion problems as there are possible combinations of all of the elements that might make a difference in our thinking about whether an abortion would be justified. It is part of the genius of Judith Thomson's fine article on abortion[76] that the author lifts us out of the personhood rut to give us a glimpse of what dialogue on abortion could look like if we began to grapple with the issues raised by a rich range of cases—hypothetical and real. This sort of grappling with particular cases and the principles that they implicate is a process for which the institutions of the law are ready-made.[77] But the prospects for employment of such institutions, with flexibility, pragmatism, and common sense, were cut short by the Supreme Court's precipitate decision in *Roe v. Wade*.

In *Roe*, the Court took note of a few of the many competing elements involved in abortion decisions, worked out its own rough compromise between them, and cast the result in constitutional concrete. It refused to recognize any rights under the Constitution on behalf of the fetus, but it did recognize an interest in the state in protecting "potential life."[78] It then decided that the state's interest does not become sufficiently compelling to override the mother's right to privacy until the fetus reaches the stage of "viability"—that is, the point when it has developed the "capability of meaningful life outside the mother's womb."[79] Only after that stage has begun may the state, if it chooses to do so,[80] protect the fetus from abortion—and then only if no doctor decides that an abortion is necessary "for the preservation of the life or health of the mother."[81] As an attempt at a compromise of interests, the Court's decision is not without virtues. Had I been a legislator asked in 1973 to vote on such a compromise as legislation, I might well have voted for it. But the Supreme Court of the United States is not a legislature and its decisions do not have the force only of legislation.

Courts are supposed to render decisions based upon principles drawn from shared values and interests; compromises worked out on the basis of arbitrary dividing lines (like "viability") are supposed to be left to the legislature.[82] But, more important, court decisions based on constitutional grounds cannot be repealed as legislation can. As a result, the compromise announced by the Court in *Roe* is not one that invites continuing dialogue, experimentation, and fine tuning. It smacks of humiliating fiat. And, not surprisingly, it calls forth from those who are humiliated efforts at counter-fiat, such as the Human Life Amendment.

If only we could find a means for fragmenting the abortion problem into the many different particular abortion problems with which life really presents us, I think we would find a surprising amount of consensus over what ought to be allowed and what ought not. Current public opinion polls indicate a good deal of agreement over cases at the extremes. For example, a poll commissioned by *Life* magazine in 1981 revealed that

> [s]eventy-seven percent of the women who disagree with the statement that "any woman who wants an abortion should be permitted to obtain it legally" state that abortion should be legal for "a woman whose health is at risk," 62 percent, for "a woman who has been raped," and 60 percent, for "a woman who is carrying a fetus with a severe genetic defect." For the sample as a whole [including the 70 percent who agreed that "a pregnant woman should have the right to decide whether she wants to terminate a pregnancy or have the child"] 92, 88, and 87 percent, respectively, say that abortion should be legal for those reasons. . . . Thus, almost all women surveyed believe that abortion should be legal under certain circumstances.[83]

The poll, like others before it, also showed very little difference on these questions between Catholic and Protestant women.[84] On the other hand, there are indications of consensus that abortion should be considered immoral, and perhaps illegal, where it is opted for in the last trimester for reasons that are considered "frivolous."[85]

Of course, it would be naive to assume that widespread consensus could be reached on whether abortion should be legal with respect to every particular choice situation. Thus, if the question of legality were to be returned to state legislatures and courts,[86] the result would likely be varying sets of state laws that represented the varying compromises negotiated in each state. There is patent unfairness in such a situation. But it is remediable, and it is a price we often pay for the benefits of a majoritarian democracy and the rule of law. Where we dislike a law, we are goaded into continuing dialogue for the purpose of winning a majority to support change. Such a dialogue has the potential for broadening understanding on both sides. Even where it fails to create a new consensus, it may at least create better appreciation for the good faith of the other side. Moreover, although failure to win one's own position in one's home state may seem an intolerable injustice, it is one which is simply not seen as such by a majority of the other citizens of the state. And things can change. Consider, for example, the injustice to the disabled infant, until the middle of this century, that resulted from denying him or her recovery in tort for injuries which had been caused before birth.

At this juncture, I feel I ought to share with you the fact that the issue of abortion is not one of only theoretical import for me. Several years ago, I participated with my wife in making a decision in favor of an abortion in the second month of pregnancy for reasons of maternal health and family planning. It was not an easy decision. We have only occasionally and fleetingly since felt that we might have made the decision differently. But we did not make it without compunction. Neither of us can see how such a decision can be made without remorse. I don't think it would have helped us in the long run to have pretended that the decision was easy by telling ourselves that the fetus involved was not a person. I don't think it would have helped us in the long run to have pretended that we had no decision to make by convincing ourselves that the fetus was a person with a right to life that outweighed all other considerations. The result was tragic, but we believed the alternative to be even less acceptable. Life does not always present us with choices between good and bad. Frequently we have to decide which of two options is less unacceptable.

Conclusion

As members of a society, we are frequently confronted with similar sorts of choices between unpleasant alternatives. We are by nature social animals, and few of us are willing to turn our backs on the benefits of society to live the isolated life of a hermit. But those benefits come at a price. Other people may not always want to do things our way, and they may not always be willing to even let us do our own thing our own way. In such conflict situations, it is tempting to think that we can win all that we want—even against a majority—by proving that our own position is "right" and that the opposed position is "wrong." But frequently such proofs are unavailing. Where a majority cannot be brought around to agreement that our position is "right," the best course open may only be that of asking others to understand our predicament and grant us the favor of freedom to do as we wish. Granting us a favor does not exact from them the price of admitting that we were "right" and they were "wrong." Thus, they may be ready to grant us a favor where they would not recognize a right. Of course, accepting a favor does exact a price from us. We will be expected to show appreciation and willingness to grant favors in return. We will have entered into a process of negotiating favor for favor and freedom for freedom.

In their wonderful, small book on negotiation,[87] Fisher and Ury conclude with the following:

> In 1964 an American father and his twelve-year-old son were enjoying a beautiful Saturday in Hyde Park, London, playing catch with a Frisbee. Few in England had seen a Frisbee at that time and a small group of strollers gathered to watch this strange sport. Finally, one Homburg-clad Britisher came over to the father: "Sorry to bother you. Been watching you a quarter of an hour. Who's *winning*?"
>
> In most instances to ask a negotiator, "Who's winning?" is as inappropriate as to ask who's winning a marriage. If you ask that question about your marriage, you have already lost the more important negotiation—the one about what kind of game to play, about the way you deal with each other and your shared and differing interests.[88]

As members of the same society, we are, for better or for worse, married to each other. The acrimonious debate over abortion has caused some strains in the marriage. By focusing argument on issues like personhood, each side has tried to win what it wanted from the other by proving the other side "wrong." Harsh words have been exchanged. But by now we may be ready to see the poverty of this approach. Some of us may be willing to apologize for the harsh words, to retreat from "right" and "wrong," and to ask for and grant accommodations through an ongoing process of negotiation. The marriage is worth saving. If only for the sake of the children— born and unborn—we should do our best to make it work.

Notes

1. 410 U.S. 113(1973).
2. Examples are S.158, 97th Cong., 1st Sess.(1981); S.J.Res.110, 97th Cong., 1st Sess.(1981).
3. For evidence of a renaissance of such attitudes in our civilized society, see (T. Regan and P. Singer, eds.), Animal Rights and Human Obligations (1976) and Stone, *Should Trees Have Standing? Toward Legal Rights for Natural Objects*, Southern California Law Review 45:450 (1972).
4. The reference is, of course, to Kant's second formulation of his categorical imperative: "So act to use humanity, both in your own person and in the person of every other, always at the same time as an end, never simply as a means." Of it, one commentator has said:

   > Strictly speaking, this formula, like all others, should cover rational beings as such; but since the only rational beings with whom we are acquainted are men, we are bidden to respect men as men, or men as rational beings. This is implied in the use of the term 'humanity' — the essential human characteristic of possessing reason, and in particular of possessing a ra-

tional will. It is in virtue of this characteristic that we are bound to treat ourselves and others, never simply as a means, but always at the same time as ends.

H.J. PATON, THE CATEGORICAL IMPERATIVE: A STUDY IN KANT'S MORAL PHILOSOPHY (1947) at 165.

5. As two samples from this widespread genre of debate, consider the following:

Is this human life? This is the question that must first be considered, pondered, discussed, and finally answered. It cannot be brushed aside or ignored. It must be faced and honestly met. Upon its answer hinges the entire abortion question, as all other considerations pale to insignificance when compared with it. In a sense nothing else really matters. If what is growing within the mother is not human life, is just a piece of meat, a glob of protoplasm, then it deserves no respect or consideration at all, and the only valid concern is the mother's physical and mental health, her social well-being, and at times even her convenience.

But if this growing being is a *human* being, then we are in an entirely different situation. If human, he or she must be granted the same dignity and protection of life, health, and well-being that our western civilization has always granted to every other human person.

J.C. WILLKE, HANDBOOK ON ABORTION (1973) at 4.

In newspaper advertisements and direct-mail fund-raising appeals, [the pro-choice groups] stressed that the [human life] amendment (HLA) would affect not only a woman's right to abortion, but to certain forms of birth control as well. The response of the National Right to Life Committee (NRLC) to these onslaughts was mildly schizophrenic.

In his eagerness to dispute the charge that the NRLC was anti-birth control, Bopp was clearly willing to sacrifice millions of fertilized eggs—Dr. Willke's "tiny boys or girls." Under Bopp's interpretation of the HLA, an abortifacient drug or device would be acceptable as long as its action occurred before pregnancy could be detected. The deaths of millions of zygote-people would be acceptable as long as nobody knew when they were killed. Thus, in Bopp's analysis, the notion that a fertilized egg deserves equal protection under the law breaks down completely.

Those who pledge allegiance to the wording of the human life amendment live in a surreal kingdom where the truths and everyday assumptions of life are harsh and demanding. In this kingdom, the life of a zygote produced in a mental institution by a paranoid schizophrenic man and a congenitally incompetent woman is sacred. So is the zygote inside the high school girl gang-raped by twelve college fraternity men, any one of whom could be the father. So is the zygote with Tay-Sachs disease, doomed to die after four years of suffering.

A.H. MERTON, ENEMIES OF CHOICE (1981) at 219-224.

6. W. SHAKESPEARE, THE MERCHANT OF VENICE, Act III, Sc. 1, lines 58-72.

7. Immediately after hearing the speech, Salanio says to Salerio of the entrance of Tubal: "Here comes another of the tribe: a third cannot be matched, unless the devil himself turn Jew." *Id.* at lines 83-85. Perhaps a half dozen times in the play, Shylock is referred to by name. Otherwise he is always referred to and

addressed as "Jew." Incredibly, this holds true even for the man who placed the speech in Shylock's mouth. Thus, Shakespeare begins Act II, Scene Five, for example, with the stage direction: "Enter Jew and his man that was the Clown."

8. Bok, S., *Who Shall Count as a Human Being?: A Treacherous Question in the Abortion Discussion*, in ABORTION: PRO AND CON (R.L. Perkins ed.) (1974) at 91, 97.

9. *See* A.H. MERTON, ENEMIES OF CHOICE (1981) at 91-116, 133-150.

10. One recent public opinion poll revealed that, while 65 percent of the Catholic women polled believed that abortion was "morally wrong," 61 percent of them believed that the law should not prohibit abortion. Henshaw, S., Martire, G., *Abortion and the Public Opinion Polls*, FAMILY PLANNING PERSPECTIVES 14(2):53 (March/April 1982) at 54.

11. Biggers, J., *When Does Life Begin?: Congress Has Asked the Unanswerable*, THE SCIENCES 21(10):10 (December 1981).

12. S.158, 97th Cong., 1st Sess., (1981).

13. *See* Grobstein, C., "A Biological Perspective on the Origin of Human Life and Personhood," Chapter 1.

14. *Supra* note 11.

15. Section 1 of the Fourteenth Amendment reads in its entirety:

> All persons born or naturalized in the United States, and subject to the jurisdiction thereof, are citizens of the United States and of the State wherein they reside. No State shall make or enforce any law which shall abridge the privileges or immunities of citizens of the United States; nor shall any State deprive any person of life, liberty, or property, without due process of law; nor deny to any person within its jurisdiction the equal protection of the laws.

16. 410 U.S. at 156-57.

17. *Id.* at 159.

18. *Id.* at 158-59 (footnotes omitted).

19. *See, e.g.*, Gulf, C. & S. F. R. Co. v. Ellis, 165 U.S. 150 (1897); Covington & Lexington Turnpike Road Co. v. Sanford, 164 U.S. 578 (1896); Charlotte, C. & A. R. Co. v. Gibbes, 142 U.S. 386 (1892); Minneapolis & S.L.R. Co. v. Beckwith, 129 U.S. 26 (1889); Missouri P.R. Co. v. Mackey, 127 U.S. 205 (1888); Pembina Consolidated Silver Mining and Milling Co. v. Pennsylvania, 125 U.S. 181 (1888); Santa Clara County v. Southern P. R. Co., 118 U.S. 394 (1886).

20. Smyth v. Ames, 169 U.S. 466, 522 (1898).

21. *See* First National Bank v. Bellotti, 435 U.S. 765 (1978) (freedom of speech); NAACP v. Button, 371 U.S. 415 (1963) (freedom of association); Grosjean v. American Press Co., 297 U.S. 233 (1936) (freedom of the press).

22. Santa Clara County v. Southern P.R. Co., *supra* note 19.

23. *See* Annot., 56 L. Ed. 2d 895, 899-900 (1979).

24. This is the language used to express the outside limits of the protections of the Fourteenth Amendment. As a minimum, all persons are entitled to such protection with respect to the exercise of any rights. Where "fundamental" rights are involved or special burdens are placed upon persons who belong to "sus-

pect classifications," more strict limits are theoretically placed upon state action. *See* L.H. TRIBE, AMERICAN CONSTITUTIONAL LAW (1978) at 1000-1002.
25. U.S. Const. amend. V.
26. Bellis v. United States, 417 U.S. 85 (1974); United States v. White, 322 U.S. 694 (1944).
27. For support for this theory behind the privilege against self-incrimination, see E. GRISWOLD, THE FIFTH AMENDMENT TODAY (1955).
28.   [I]ndividuals, when acting as representatives of a collective group, cannot be said to be exercising their personal rights and duties nor to be entitled to their purely personal privileges. Rather they assume the rights, duties and privileges of the artificial entity or association of which they are agents or officers and are bound by its obligations. In their official capacity, therefore, they have no privilege against self-incrimination.
United States v. White, 322 U.S. at 699.
29. Towne v. Eisner, 245 U.S. 418, 425 (1918).
30. 60 U.S. 393 (1857).
31. *Id.* at 404-05.
32. 80 C.J.S. *Slaves*, § 4 (1953).
33. *Id.* at 1320.
34. 80 C.J.S. *Slaves*, § 8 (1953).
35. *Id.* at 1325-26.
36. R.M. PERKINS, CRIMINAL LAW (2d. ed. 1969) at 29.
37. *Id.* at 140.
38. *See* Annot., 50 A.L.R. 619 (1927).
39. *See* Shaw, M., Damme, C., *Legal Status of the Fetus* in GENETICS AND THE LAW, (A. Milunsky and G. Annas, eds.) (1976) at 3, 4.
40. Despite pious pronouncements to the contrary, blameworthiness (rather than deterrence or reform) still seems to play the central role in the criminal law. As proof, consider the terms in which debate over the insanity defense is conducted:
    Joseph Weintraub, C.J.: . . . My thesis is that insanity should have nothing to do with the adjudication of guilt but rather should bear upon the disposition of the offender after conviction. . . .
    I think we all agree that society must be protected from hostile acts and when a forbidden act is done, it must be adjudged that the accused committed it before he may be deprived of his liberty. And so the issue is, shall we employ a criminal process or a civil process to determine that he did the act and to determine society's right to commit him, and as long as we have two processes which may be employed to deal custodially with antisocial conduct, one criminal and the other civil, the test for their application must be blameworthiness or the nonexistence of blameworthiness in a very personal sense. . . . No definition of criminal responsibility and hence of legal insanity can be valid unless it truthfully separates the man who is personally blameworthy for his makeup from the man who is not, and I submit to you that there is just no basis in psychiatry to make a differ-

entiation between the two.

    Professor Herbert Wechsler: . . . Chief Justice Weintraub has . . . ventured the suggestion that the whole effort to develop a criterion for determining criminal responsibility as affected by mental disease or defect is a misguided effort. . . . I think it is not a misguided effort. It rests not only on the universal experience of all modern legal systems but I'm tempted to say of all civilized legal systems. . . .

    It is a very important thing for all of us to know that if we should be afflicted and in the course of affliction should be the physical agent of harm to others, that the legal system will conduct an inquiry in which the nature of that affliction can be adduced for an estimate of its bearing on blameworthiness in the ordinary sense.

Insanity as a Defense: A Panel Discussion, 37 F.R.D. 365, 369-71, 380-81 (1964).

41. W.L. PROSSER, LAW OF TORTS (4th ed. 1971) at 335.
42. *Id.* at n.14.
43. *Id.* at 335.
44. 65 F. Supp. 138 (D.D.C. 1946).
45. PROSSER, *supra* note 41, at 336.
46. *Id.* at 337.
47. *Id.* at 338.
48. *See* Annot., 84 A.L.R. 3d 411 (1978); Danos v. St. Pierre, 402 So. 2d 633 (La. 1981); Shirley v. Bacon, 267 S.E.2d 809 (Ga. App. 1980).
49. *See* Jorgensen v. Meade-Johnson Laboratories, 483 F.2d 237 (10th Cir. 1973); Renslow v. Mennonite Hospital, 367 N.E.2d 1250 (Ill. 1977). *Compare* Morgan v. United States, 143 F. Supp. 580 (D.N.J. 1956).
50. *Renslow, supra* note 49, at 1255.
51. PROSSER, *supra* note 41, at 22.
52. *Id.* at 335.
53. *See* Scott v. Kopp, 431 A.2d 959, 962 (Pa. 1981) (Larsen, J. dissenting).
54. *See* MASS. GEN. LAWS ANN. c.203, § 17 and c.206, § 24.
55. For example, I was appointed counsel for a fetus in one case where a maternal grandmother sought authority to consent to an abortion for her daughter who was a long-term inmate of a mental institution. Out of an abundance of caution, the judge wanted the record to reflect advocacy for the fetus in addition to that which was provided for the mother. Ultimately, the court decided that, though mentally ill, the mother should be allowed to refuse an abortion since she was not proved to be incompetent to make that decision. *In re* Culcotta, Middlesex Probate No. 522761 (Mass., November 19, 1979).
56. Thellusson v. Woodford, 31 Eng. Rep. 117, 163 (1798) (Buller, J.).
57. 410 U.S. at 153.
58. *Id.* at 156-59.
59. *See* TRIBE, *supra* note 24, at 1147-74.
60. The Court never makes its reasoning in this regard explicit, but it is suggested in the following:

    When Texas urges that a fetus is entitled to Fourteenth Amendment protection as a person, it faces a dilemma. Neither in Texas nor in any other state are all abortions prohibited. Despite broad proscription, an exception always exists. The exception contained in Art. 1196, for an abortion procured or attempted by medical advice for the purpose of saving the life of the mother, is typical. But if the fetus is a person who is not to be deprived of life without due process of law, and if the mother's condition is the sole determinant, does not the Texas exception appear to be out of line with the Amendment's command?

Roe v. Wade, *supra* note 1, at 157-58, n.54.

61. NOWAK, ROTUNDA, & YOUNG, CONSTITUTIONAL LAW (1978) at 519–22.
62. *Id.* at 522-27.
63. *See* LAFAVE & SCOTT, CRIMINAL LAW (1972) § 53.
64. "While the point has not been free from controversy, it seems clear that necessity has standing as a common-law defense; such issue as there is relates to its definition and extent. The decisions, however, have been rare and legislative formulations most infrequent. . . ."

MODEL PENAL CODE § 3.02 (Comments to Tentative Draft No. 8 1958).

65. LAFAVE & SCOTT, *supra* note 63, at 381.
66. Indeed, the Model Penal Code eliminates the "emergency" requirement altogether:

Section 3.02 *Justification Generally: Choice of Evils* (1) Conduct which the actor believes to be necessary to avoid harm or evil to himself or to another is justifiable, provided that: (a) the harm or evil sought to be avoided by such conduct is greater than that sought to be prevented by the law defining the offense charged; and (b) neither the Code nor other law defining the offense provides exceptions or defenses dealing with the specific situation involved; and (c) a legislative purpose to exclude the justification claimed does not otherwise plainly appear. (2) When the actor was reckless or negligent in bringing about the situation requiring a choice of harm or evils or in appraising the necessity for his conduct, the justification afforded by this Section is unavailable in a prosecution for any offense for which recklessness or negligence, as the case may be, suffices to establish culpability.

MODEL PENAL CODE § 3.02 (Proposed Official Draft 1962).

67. LaFave and Scott see the abortion laws prior to Roe v. Wade as having made just such specific provision:

The defense of necessity is available only in situations wherein the legislature has not itself, in its criminal statute, made a determination of values. If it has done so, its decision governs. Thus the legislature might, in its abortion statute, expressly provide that the crime is not committed if the abortion is performed to save the mother's life; under such a statute there would be no need for courts to speculate about the relative value of preserving the fetus and safeguarding the mother's life.

LAFAVE & SCOTT, *supra* note 63, at 382.

68. *See, e.g.,* Poole v. Endsley, 371 F.Supp. 1379 (N.D. Fla. 1974), *aff'd in part and remanded,* 516 F.2d 898 (5th Cir. 1975); McGarvey v. Magee-Women's Hosp., 340 F. Supp. 751 (W.D.Pa.1972), *aff'd* 474 F.2d 1339 (3d Cir. 1973).
69. Douglas v. Town of Hartford, 542 F. Supp. 1267 (D.Conn. 1982).
70. 525 F. Supp. 798 (W.D.Va. 1981).
71. *Id.* at 799.
72. *Id.* at 802.
73. Poole v. Endsley, 371 F.Supp. 1379, 1382 (N.D.Fla. 1974), *aff'd in part and remanded,* 516 F.2d 898 (5th Cir. 1975).
74. Harman v. Daniels, *supra* note 70, at 800.
75. If the notion of according personhood to the spegg for these purposes seems outlandish, recall the fact that the law has done just this for other purposes in preconception tort cases such as Renslow v. Mennonite Hospital and Jorgensen v. Meade-Johnson Laboratories, *supra* note 49.
76. Thomson, J., *A Defense of Abortion,* PHILOSOPHY AND PUBLIC AFFAIRS 1:57 (1971).
77. I have argued elsewhere the value of the common law courts in seeking answers to these questions. *See* Baron, C., *Medical Paternalism and the Rule of Law: A Reply to Dr. Relman,* AMERICAN JOURNAL OF LAW & MEDICINE 4:337 (1979); Baron, C., *Euthanasia Decisions in the Courts: The Post-Saikewicz Experience,* in GENETICS AND THE LAW II (A. Milunsky & G.J. Annas, eds.) (1980) at 141.
78. 410 U.S. at 163.
79. *Id.*
80. Because some states have not enacted abortion laws to replace those which were struck down as unconstitutional by *Roe v. Wade,* "abortion on demand" is available in those states through the entire period of pregnancy. The occasional abortion of a viable fetus which takes place in such states can produce very discomfiting results. For example, a storm of controversy developed in June, 1982, over a 26 week old fetus which had died 27.5 hours after it was aborted in a Wisconsin hospital. Suggestions were made that the civil rights of the fetus had been violated by peforming the abortion in a facility which did not have facilities for the care of premature infants. *See U.S. Pledges Probe of UW Abortions,* Madison Capital-Times, June 2, 1982, at 4, col.1.
81. 410 U.S. at 165. This is only one of several places where the Court shows a distressing tendency to delegate governmental power to physicians. Here the doctor is given discretion to decide whether an abortion in the third trimester is "necessary" for the preservation of the "health" of the mother. But what degree of diminution of health of the mother will outweigh the life of a healthy, third trimester fetus? Will indications of the necessity for a ceasarean section be enough? *See* Jefferson v. Griffin Spalding Cty. Hosp. Auth., 274 S.E.2d 457 (Ga.1981). What about threatened impairment of mental health where changed circumstances make the mother no longer want the child? Roe seems to leave these "choice of evils" determinations entirely to the medical community. In a later case, Colautti v. Franklin, 439 U.S. 379 (1979), the Court delegates to the individual physician the power to decide whether or not a

particular fetus is "viable"—not only for determining the medical facts regarding probability of survival outside the mother, but also for determining the governmental question of what degree of probability of survival brings in to play the state's "compelling interest" in protecting fetal life.

Id. at 391-96. Too often overlooked by pro-choice advocates is the fact that *Roe* does not recognize a woman's right to an abortion; it recognizes power in the physician to prescribe an abortion for his patient. As the Court says of its holding in *Roe*:

> The decision vindicates the right of the physician to administer medical treatment according to his professional judgment up to the points where important state interests provide compelling justifications for intervention. Up to these points, the abortion decision in all its aspects is inherently, and primarily, a medical decision, and basic responsibility for it must rest with the physician. If an individual practitioner abuses the privilege of exercising proper medical judgment, the usual remedies, judicial and intraprofessional, are available.

Roe v. Wade, 410 U.S. at 166. This is true even for the period of the first trimester:

> . . . For the stage prior to approximately the end of the first trimester, the abortion decision and its effectuation must be left to the medical judgment of the pregnant woman's attending physician.

Id. at 164. This deference to doctors on the part of Justice Blackmun, who wrote the Court's opinions in both *Roe* and *Colautti*, has not escaped the notice of the other members of the Court:

> Blackmun's 1973 abortion opinion had subjected the Court to a great deal of ridicule. It was as if Blackmun had developed a special constitutional rule for handling medical questions. [Justice] White dubbed it Blackmun's "medical question doctrine." It seemed to hold that, under the Constitution, doctors, rather than the Court, had the final authority on certain medical-legal questions. White found that notion ludicrous. Blackmun had created another "political questions" doctrine. The notion that the Court couldn't meddle in the affairs of the other branches of government had been broadened to include the medical profession.

B. WOODWARD & S. ARMSTRONG, THE BRETHREN (1976) at 146. Equally patent was the source of Blackmun's willingness to defer to doctors. Before coming to the Court, he had been for ten years general counsel to Minnesota's famous Mayo Clinic.

> At Mayo, he had watched as Doctors Edward C. Kendall and Philip S. Hench won the Nobel Prize for research in arthritis. He rejoiced with other doctors after their first successful heart bypass operation, then suffered with them after they lost their next four patients. . . . He grew to respect what dedicated physicians could accomplish. These had been terribly exciting years for Blackmun. He labeled them the best ten years of his life.
>
> If a state licensed a physician to practice medicine, it was entrusting him

with the right to make medical decisions. . . . To completely restrict an operation like abortion, normally no more dangerous than minor surgery, or to permit it only with the approval of a hospital committee or the concurrence of other doctors, was a needless infringement of the discretion of the medical profession.

Blackmun would do anything he could to reduce the anxiety of his colleagues except spurn the assignment [to write the opinion in Roe v. Wade]. The case was not so much a legal task as an opportunity for the Court to ratify the best possible medical opinion.

Id. at 174-75. In essence, the doctors whom Blackmun respected so highly were to take over from the state governments the job of making the "choice of evils" decision inherent in abortion. This role they would perform on a case-by-case basis by influencing and, perhaps in some cases, blocking the mother's decision. Thus, after the Court recognizes a right of privacy covering the mother's decision and lists the cost factors the state would impose on the mother if it denied the abortion choice altogether, the Court concludes: "All these are factors the woman and her responsible physician necessarily will consider in consultation." Roe v. Wade, 410 U.S. at 153.

This distressing tendency to want to leave to physician philosopher-kings tough ethical questions which the courts find "too hot to handle" is not restricted to the U.S. Supreme Court or the issue of abortion. In regard to the issue of euthanasia for terminally ill patients, some courts have expressed a willingness to delegate to doctors the power to decide what circumstances justify cessation of life-prolonging treatment. The trial judge in the famous Karen Quinlan case, for example, acceded to medical judgment on the question of whether Karen's respirator was to be turned off, saying: "The morality and conscience of our society places this responsibility in the hands of the physician. What justification is there to remove it from the control of the medical profession and place it in the hands of the Court?" *In re* Quinlan, 137 N.J. Super 227, 259, 348, A.2d 801, 818 (Ch. Div. 1975). For their part, most doctors have seemed eager to have such matters labelled "medical questions" so that involvement of courts in medical practice can be kept to a minimum. See Relman, A., *The Saikewicz Decision: A Medical Viewpoint,* AMERICAN JOURNAL OF LAW & MEDICINE 4:223 (1978). However, like Justice White, some courts have openly rejected Justice Blackmun's "medical question doctrine." Thus, the Supreme Judicial Court of Massachusetts has held that termination of life-prolonging care decisions are to be made by the courts, concluding:

We do not view the judicial resolution of this most difficult and awesome question—whether potentially life-prolonging treatment should be withheld from a person incapable of making his own decision—as constituting a "gratuitous encroachment" on the domain of medical expertise. Rather, such questions of life and death seem to us to require the process of detached but passionate investigation and decision that forms the ideal on which the judicial branch of government was created. Achieving this ideal is our responsibility and that of the lower court, and is not to be entrusted to any other group purporting to represent the "morality and conscience of our society," no matter how highly motivated or impressively constituted.

Superintendent of Belchertown School v. Saikewicz, 370 N.E.2d 417, 435 (1977). *See generally* Baron, C., *Medical Paternalism and the Rule of Law: A Reply to Dr. Relman*, AMERICAN JOURNAL OF LAW & MEDICINE 4:337 (1979); Baron, C., *To Die Before the Gods Please: Legal Issues Surrounding Euthanasia and the Elderly*, JOURNAL OF GERIATRIC PSYCHIATRY 14:45 (1981).

82. *See* H. HART & A. SACKS, THE LEGAL PROCESS: BASIC PROBLEMS IN THE MAKING AND APPLICATION OF LAW (Tent. Ed. 1958) at 665-67. Because the focus of this paper has been on the question of personhood, I have not directly criticized the Court's argument that the *Roe* decision was mandated by the Court's "discovery" that the Constitution protects a woman's choice of an abortion as part of her "right to privacy." For criticism of that argument in terms that I would embrace, see Ely, J., *The Wages of Crying Wolf: A Comment on Roe v. Wade*, YALE LAW JOURNAL 82:920 (1973). Dean Ely does not oppose abortion but does oppose the Court's anti-majoritarian imposition of its own abortion "statute" on the fifty state legislatures:

> Let us not underestimate what is at stake: Having an unwanted child can go a long way toward ruining a woman's life. And at the bottom *Roe* signals the Court's judgment that this result cannot be justified by any good that anti-abortion legislation accomplishes. This surely is an understandable conclusion—indeed it is one with which I agree—but ordinarily the Court claims no mandate to second-guess legislative balances, at least not when the Constitution has designated neither of the values in conflict as entitled to special protection. But even assuming it would be a good idea for the Court to assume this function, *Roe* seems a curious place to have begun. Laws prohibiting the use of "soft" drugs or, even more obviously, homosexual acts between consenting adults can stunt the "preferred life styles" of those against whom enforcement is threatened in very serious ways. It is clear such acts harm no one besides the participants, and indeed the case that the participants are harmed is a rather shaky one. Yet such laws survive, on the theory that there exists a societal consensus that the behavior involved is revolting or at any rate immoral. Of course the consensus is not universal but it is sufficient, and this is what is counted as crucial to get the laws passed and keep them on the books. Whether anti-abortion legislation cramps the life style of an unwilling mother more significantly than anti-homosexuality legislation cramps the life style of a homosexual is a close question. But even granting that it does, the *other* side of the balance looks very different. For there is more than simple societal revulsion to support legislation restricting abortion: Abortion ends (or if it makes a difference, prevents) the life of a human being other than the one making the choice.

Id. at 923-24. Other constitutional scholars have taken similar positions with respect to *Roe*. As one text has noted:

The Supreme Court abortion rulings provoked immediate criticism. Some of the most severe indictments of those decisions came from unexpected sources—pro-abortion writers. Criticism was aimed not only at what the Supreme Court had done (i.e., the substance of the new constitutional abortion doctrine), but also at how it had done it (by resort to the doctrine of substantive due process), and why (the legal arguments given in the official opinion to justify the result reached by the Court).

L. WARDLE & M. WOOD, A LAWYER LOOKS AT ABORTION (1982) at 4.

83. Henshaw, S., Martire, G., *Abortion and the Public Opinion Polls*, FAMILY PLANNING PERSPECTIVES 14(2):53 (March/April 1982).

84. *Id.* at 54.

85. *Id.* at 55-56; R. ADAMEK, ABORTION AND PUBLIC OPINION IN THE UNITED STATES (1982) at 3–5. The latter publication reports that a Gallup Poll in 1981 showed 52 percent of respondents thought that abortions should be legal only under "certain circumstances" and that a National Opinion Research Center poll in 1980 showed only 39 percent of respondents believed that a legal abortion should be available "[i]f the woman wants it for any reason." *Id.* at 4.

86. For creative suggestions as to ways in which courts could interact with legislatures over such issues, see G. CALABRESI, A COMMON LAW FOR THE AGE OF STATUTES (1982).

87. R. FISHER & W. URY, GETTING TO YES: NEGOTIATING AGREEMENT WITHOUT GIVING IN (1981).

88. *Id.* at 154.

Chapter 9

Personhood, Abortion, and the Right of Privacy

Harriet F. Pilpel

Somewhat to my surprise, I agree to a very substantial extent with Professor Baron's opinion in the preceding chapter,[1] although I take exception to his conclusion. While I agree that we should not become entangled over the concept of personhood in relation to the fetus, and that there are various entities which are persons for some purposes and not for others, I strongly disagree with his last suggestion that a widespread consensus cannot be reached on abortion. Senator Orrin Hatch (R-Utah), a proponent of the only anti-abortion amendment which has been favorably reported out of the Senate Judiciary Committee, said that there is no consensus in this country in favor of a so-called right to life, and I believe that to be true. However, there is a consensus that women should have a right to abortion in a wide variety of circumstances. Polls indicate that approximately 65 to 70 percent of the general public believe in such a right to abortion, as do more than 50 percent of Catholics.[2] This consensus accentuates the difference between Professor Baron's position and the opinion in *Roe v. Wade*.[3] Basically, the pro-life position is that no woman, no matter what her religious and ethical beliefs may be, should have a right to decide whether to have an abortion in any circumstances except, perhaps, when an abortion is necessary to save her life. The pro-choice groups ask that women, with the concurrence of their physicians, have the right to choose abortion in many circumstances in addition to life endangerment.

While this paper will address the terms listed in its title, I wish to consider them in reverse order. But before I address the right of privacy issue, a brief discussion of our constitutional system seems worthwhile and appropriate.

AN OVERVIEW OF OUR CONSTITUTIONAL SYSTEM
We have a federal system of government and under that system certain

activities, such as interstate and foreign commerce and the mails, are exclusively within the domain of the federal government. There are, however, two other ways in which the federal government reaches into our lives, and one of them has to do with the conditions that the government attaches to grants of money. For example, recipients of federal funds agree not to practice discrimination in their employment practices.

Second and more important is the fact that we have a federal Constitution which is supreme in this country. Insofar as our fundamental liberties are concerned, it governs what happens in every state. The genius of our federal Constitution lies in its protection of our fundamental rights which not even a majority of the people can take away from the minority or from individuals. The fundamental right of privacy in matters relating to marriage, family, and sex is the kind of right which is guaranteed by the federal Constitution,[4] and cannot be taken away from minorities or from individuals by any majority—federal, state or local.

Another important aspect of our legal system is that there are basically two sources for our laws—legislation and court decisions. Our constitutional framework charges the legislative branch of the government with enacting the various laws and statutes which the legislature deems necessary or desirable and places the responsibilty of interpreting those enactments on the judiciary. The early and landmark case of *Marbury v. Madison*,[5] decided by the United States Supreme Court, firmly established that the Constitution is the supreme law of the land and that "it is emphatically the province and duty of the judicial department to say what the law is."[6] No matter what the law or constitution of a particular state is as to rights protected by the federal Constitution, the United States Supreme Court's interpretation of those guarantees takes precedence.

One other fundamental feature of our constitutional system merits mention, and that is that those of us who are already born do not have any "right to life." The Fourteenth Amendment starts with the words: "All persons born or naturalized in the United States." The specific use of the word born indicates, almost surely, that the framers of that amendment did not have the unborn in mind. While it would be nice if we did develop a doctrine of entitlement which would provide all persons who are born with rights to education, health service, food, shelter, and the other necessities of life, unfortunately our constitutional system does not grant us those rights. It merely gives us the right not to have the government take away our lives, liberty or property without due process of law.[7] This is a very important distinction. Thus, for example, if you killed someone, you probably would not have violated the United States Constitution, but you would have violated the criminal law of the state where the killing took place. In other words, the so-called right-to-life amendments confer on unborn persons constitutional rights which born persons do not have.

Many people who have taken issue with the Supreme Court's abortion decision in *Roe v. Wade* act as though the Court suddenly created a basic constitutional right of privacy. However, a basic right of privacy was deemed to be inherent in our system of ordered liberty many years ago. As early as 1890 Justice Brandeis referred to it in a now famous law review article.[8] It was described as "the right most valued by civilized man" (and woman), the right as against the government to be left alone.[9] The Court invoked the basic right of privacy in a variety of contexts long before *Roe v. Wade*. For example, the right of privacy supported court decisions which invalidated miscegenation laws;[10] laws which told parents that they could not send their children to private schools;[11] and laws which stated that parents could not have their children learn German.[12] The right of privacy, though not mentioned specifically, underlay the Court decision invalidating an Oklahoma statute which attempted to force sterilization upon certain persons.[13] In 1965 the United States Supreme Court, in *Griswold v. Connecticut*, after 25 years of effort on the part of pro-choice forces, decided that the basic right of privacy included matters relating to marriage, family, and sex and that this right of privacy included the right to use a contraceptive.[14] In a subsequent decision, the United States Supreme Court made clear that the basic constitutional right of privacy to decide when and whether to have a child applied to unmarried persons as well as married persons.[15] A year later, in the landmark decision of *Roe v. Wade*, the Court held that a woman's right of privacy encompassed her right to have an abortion and that this right could be limited only in the presence of a compelling state interest—an interest that becomes more compelling as the pregnancy progresses.[16]

HISTORY OF ABORTION LAWS

A review of the history of abortion laws in the United States indicates that *Roe v. Wade* was the logical next step in the development of the right of privacy. The history of abortion laws in the United States is unusual. Although some laws prohibiting abortion were enacted early in the nineteenth century, early abortion was not a violation of any law when this country was founded. If one reviews the early years of this nation, one finds freedom of choice in regard to early abortion—a position taken even by the Catholic Church at the time.[17] It was not until the third decade of the nineteenth century that some states began to pass laws against abortion, and it was not until after the middle of the nineteenth century that a majority of states had passed laws severely limiting abortion.[18]

To the best of my knowledge, the early anti-abortion laws never mentioned the "fetus"; nor did they attribute personhood to it. The anti-abortion laws were passed because abortion until relatively recently was indeed a dangerous procedure. There were no antibiotics, and little knowledge about anesthesia or antiseptics. To have an abortion in the early nineteenth century, or even in the middle of the nineteenth century, was to have a dangerous operation. Today, of course, early abortion is far safer than childbirth. Concern for the fetus began much, much later, probably not until the twentieth century.

In a speech introducing his special brand of anti-abortion amendment, Senator Hatch claimed that the states had prohibited abortion during colonial times and during the Industrial Revolution.[19] Senator Hatch was mistaken. Abortion was *not* prohibited by the states in the early days of this country. When the states eventually did enact restrictive abortion laws, most of them in the mid-nineteenth century, it was for reasons of the health of the woman, not the protection of the conceptus. Moreover, after the Supreme Court in *Griswold* held that the basic right of privacy included the use of contraceptives, various states began passing laws permitting abortion for a wide variety of reasons in addition to saving the life of the pregnant woman.

The first state to do so was Colorado. In 1967, it enacted a statute based on a draft of a model law prepared some years before by the American Law Institute, an organization composed of leading lawyers, judges, and law professors.[20] The draft provided that abortion should be available when the life of the mother was at stake, when her mental or physical health was threatened, to avoid the birth of a defective offspring and in cases of rape and incest.[21] By the time of the *Roe v. Wade* decision in 1973, 14 states had adopted versions of this model law, and four states, including New York, passed laws which made early abortion available on request.[22] One of those four states—Washington—adopted its law by popular referendum. Thus, by 1973 when the Supreme Court decided *Roe v. Wade*, 18 states had changed their old abortion laws. Proposals to modify or change the laws were pending in virtually every other state in the union. Also, a number of important courts, including the Supreme Court of California and a prestigious federal district court in the District of Columbia, had held that laws prohibiting abortion except to save the life of the woman were unconstitutional.[23]

THE *ROE V. WADE* DECISION

The United States Supreme Court stated in *Roe v. Wade* that a statute which prohibited abortion except to save the life of the woman was an unconstitutional infringement of her basic right of privacy to decide when and whether to have a child.[24] The Court pointed out that whatever the status of a fetus, all agree that the life of the fetus can be terminated if the woman's life is threatened. Thus, at the very least, a fetus differs from a "born" human being. If a fetus were considered the equivalent of a "born" person, and the law permitting abortion when the mother's life is threatened were constitutional, then by the same reasoning a lover or husband who threatened the woman's life might have his life taken to save hers. Many battered women may think this is a good idea, but it has not yet been accepted in this country and I am sure — and hope — that it will never be. In other words, even in a strict anti-abortion state like Texas, there was a difference between a "fetus-person" and a "born" person.

In *Roe v. Wade*, the Court held that pregnancy falls into three distinct stages.[25] During the first trimester, i.e., for approximately 13 weeks after conception, the states may not regulate abortion except to require that a physician, rather than a nonphysician, perform an abortion. The Court, of course, has never stated that anyone had to have an abortion or that anyone could force another to have an abortion. It only held that a woman who wants an abortion is constitutionally entitled to have one during the first trimester of pregnancy if her doctor concurs.

The term "viability" is defined as the fetus' ability to survive outside the woman's body. From the end of the first trimester (13 weeks) until viability (generally 26 weeks), the Court said the states may legislate in the interests of the health of the woman but not in the interest of fetal life. Only from viability to birth can the government prohibit abortion, and even then the law must make an exception for the protection of the life and health of the mother. When it came to the question of personhood, the Supreme Court in *Roe v. Wade* declared that: "We need not resolve the difficult question of when life begins,"[26] noting that "when those trained in the respective disciplines of medicine, philosophy, and theology are unable to arrive at any consensus, the judiciary, at this point in the development of man's knowledge, is not in a position to speculate as to the answer."[27] The state of Texas did argue that the fetus was a person, but the Court held that "the fetus, at most, represents only the potentiality of life."[28] While it is true that unborn children have been recognized as acquiring rights by way of inheritance, those rights have generally been contingent upon live birth. In short, the unborn have never been recognized by the law as persons in the whole sense.

PENDING ABORTION LEGISLATION

Roe v. Wade stimulated violent reaction on behalf of an articulate minority in this country, and a variety of proposals are now pending in Congress that seek to undo it. Some proposals are for human life amendments; others are for human life statutes. Senator Hatch has introduced a bill that he has described as a human life federalism amendment. There is also much activity in connection with a proposed constitutional convention on the subject of abortion and a possible states' rights amendment. Some of the proposed human life amendments and statutes (several of which have been introduced by Senator Jesse Helms, R-N.C.) provide that a fetus is a human being from the moment of conception.[29] That is a very puzzling provision for many reasons, including the fact that it is not possible to identify the moment of conception. Consequently, if the law were to state that a fetus is a person from the moment of conception, a woman would not know if she had a "person" inside of her for some time after that "person" came into being. Some have suggested that a more sensible version of the proposed legislation would mandate that a fetus be considered a person from the moment of implantation because implantation can be ascertained scientifically. However, that is not what Senator Helms or his supporters want; they insist on personhood from conception. Bear in mind that recent research by a physician in Virginia has indicated that approximately 80 percent of fertilized eggs never implant, and that even when a fertilized egg has implanted, there is a wastage of 25 to 30 percent in the form of miscarriage.[30] One of the many dangers inherent in the type of proposal that would make the fetus a person is that any woman who had a miscarriage could be suspected of homicide. She would have the burden of proving that she did not do anything to cause the miscarriage—a virtually impossible burden on her right of privacy.

Another kind of "human life" proposal states that fetuses are to be entitled to the protection of the Fourteenth Amendment. Such a proposal would give fetuses the same rights that "born" people have, i.e., the government could not take away their lives without due process. Some of the human life amendments go much further and give fetuses rights that "born" people do not have. Some of these amendments prohibit any person from taking the life of a fetus. No person is prohibited by the Constitution from taking my life or the life of any born person — fetuses alone would have constitutional protection for their lives. Endless confusion and litigation would flow from any such constitutional provision.

The United States Constitution can be amended in two ways. Either two-thirds of each house of Congress can pass an amendment for ratification by three-quarters of the states, or two-thirds of the states can request Congress to call a constitutional convention for the purpose of proposing amendments to the Constitution which would also have to be ratified by three-quarters of the states. At the present time, the sponsors of human life amendments appear unable to obtain a two-thirds vote in either the

House or the Senate. Consequently, two alternatives have been proposed to get around this obstacle. One is a human life statute. Senator Helms has proposed a variety of different bills which call for Congress to make a finding that life begins at conception.[31] Since this would be a statutory enactment, it would not need two-thirds majority but could be passed by a simple majority vote. Although the human life statutes submitted to Congress contain endless variations, all are likely to be declared unconstitutional. This opinion is shared by 12 leading professors of constitutional law who signed a public statement to that effect[32] and six former Attorneys General of the United States who signed a similar statement. All of these scholars state that regardless of their position on abortion (and some of them are strongly against abortion), they consider an attempt to overrule the United States Supreme Court decision by a statute to be totally inconsistent with our system of checks and balances and clearly unconstitutional.

Another approach is the so-called human life federalism amendment proposed by Senator Hatch. He proposes a two-step process through which it will be established that fetuses are persons from the moment of conception. The first part of this strategy aims to deconstitutionalize abortion by a constitutional amendment stating that abortion is not protected by the federal Constitution, that both the state and federal governments shall have the right to restrict and prohibit abortions, and that in the case of conflict between the state and federal governments, the more restrictive law shall apply.[33] Senator Hatch relies on the Eighteenth Amendment as a precedent for this suggestion. If I were he, I would not do so. The Eighteenth Amendment is the only amendment to the Constitution which sought to take away a right—that is, of course, the right to drink intoxicating liquors, a right which most people would concede is not as important as the right to decide whether to have a child. The amendment was so dismally unsuccessful that it is the only one in our history to be repealed shortly after it was passed. In addition, it left us with a heritage of organized crime from which we still suffer.

Senator Hatch's human life federalism amendment was reported out of the Senate Judiciary Committee in March 1982 by a vote of 10 to 7. Some of those committee members voting for the bill reportedly did so only to get it out of the committee, not necessarily because they would vote for it on the Senate floor. It seems unlikely that the bill's supporters will amass the two-thirds necessary to pass the measure.

A constitutional convention and a possible states' rights amendment are other avenues open to anti-abortionists. At the moment it looks as if there will be insufficient consensus to pass any of the amendments or statutes discussed above, but support may exist for what Professor Baron really wants—a states' rights amendment. Such an amendment would simply say that every state can regulate abortion as it wishes. At present that proposal does not have the support of either the pro-choice or the so-called pro-life groups. The pro-life groups dislike it because they want a fetus to be a constitutionally protected person in every state from the moment of conception and they fear that there would be some states where abortion would remain available on a variety of grounds. The pro-choice people dislike it because they believe it would create the situation which existed before *Roe v. Wade*, and which exists today, for example, in the divorce field. They fear that there will be abortion "meccas"—perhaps New York, California, Illinois, or Michigan—to which people who have money could travel for abortions. Thus, abortion would become an option available only to those who can afford to travel to states with liberal abortion laws or to foreign countries.

In my opinion, the states' rights amendment should not be passed because it will hopelessly confuse the law of abortion and create an unjustifiable imbalance of individual rights from state to state. Such an amendment might pass if two-thirds of Congress want to avoid the problems concerning abortion that have constantly come before them. A states' rights amendment might provide Congress with an easy buck-passing solution. In some ways, the worst of the pending proposals is the call for a constitutional convention—an alternative to the congressional method of proposing an amendment. We have not had a national constitutional convention in this country since the first one in 1787, which was called for the purpose of amending the Articles of Confederation. Instead the convention threw out the Articles and drafted the Constitution, for which we can all be grateful. However, I would not like a convention today to throw out the Constitution and substitute something else.

No one, no matter how he or she feels about the abortion issue, knows whether a convention called for the purpose of passing an anti-abortion amendment could be restricted to that amendment. Congress has legislation before it now which would restrict a convention to the subject matter for which it was called, but since it is a statute, it could be changed by a subsequent Congress or be invalidated by the courts. Currently, nineteen states have requested Congress to call a constitutional convention on the subject of abortion; 34 are needed to do so. (Thirty-one states have asked Congress to call a convention to pass a balanced federal budget amendment.) The founding fathers inserted the provision for a constitutional convention in the amendment section of the federal Constitution for a very specific reason which is not applicable here. In 1787, the states were jealous of their power, having all too recently emerged from the dictates of George III. Therefore, they wanted some method whereby they could call a constitutional convention if the federal government seemed to be stomping all over them. Hence it was provided that two-thirds of the states could request and force Congress to call such a convention. Clearly, the abortion question was not the kind of problem that the framers of the Constitution had in mind when they provided this alternative method of amending it. Virtually every constitutional lawyer and every constitutional law professor with whom I have spoken believes that calling a constitutional convention at this time might seriously imperil the entire Constitution, including the Bill of Rights, and everything else that has worked so well for us for almost 200 years. Our Constitution, of course, has served as a model for constitutions of many nations, including the Philippines and India. Is it wise to open the door to wholesale tampering with something which has worked so well in so many ways, including the protection of individuals against arbitrary governmental invasion of their fundamental rights?

PERSONHOOD

If the fetus were considered a person from the moment of conception, countless legal and social questions would arise. What consequences would follow if a laboratory assistant inadvertently dropped a test tube or a petri dish, and thus destroyed the fertilized egg contained in it? Has he or she committed a homicide, or perhaps even a murder if it could be shown that he or she intended to drop the test tube or dish and thereby end the "life" that it contained?

The kind of consequences which would affect women if the fetus were a person from the moment of conception have been alluded to elsewhere in this text.[34] Fertile women of child-bearing age would, in effect, have no right of privacy at all. If the fetus is a person from the moment of conception, would we celebrate our conception days instead of our birthdays? In fact, birth would cease to have any real legal significance. The Fourteenth Amendment speaks of all persons born or naturalized in the United States and would have to be expanded to cover all persons born or naturalized or unborn. In addition, could a fetus sue its mother if she did not take proper care of herself during the pregnancy? This concept is not as farfetched as it might sound. A Royal Commission in Great Britain recently studied the question of whether a child born defective by reason of action taken or not taken by its mother during pregnancy should be able to sue its mother. The Royal Commission finally recommended that the fetus, when born, should not be able to sue its mother because such action would be destructive of family harmony.[35]

Professor Baron alludes to the question of whether the "fetus-person" can inherit property, and he also mentions the problems we would face with fertilized eggs in test tubes. It does not help to use labels; as Professor Baron has said, we should not get "hung up" on the concept of "personhood." I agree that we should not use personhood as a battleground, and that there are various entities which are persons for some purposes and not for others. A recent case in Illinois involved a woman who was transfused with the wrong blood at age 13 and who, eight years later, gave birth to a defective child because she had received the wrong blood years earlier. The court held that the child was entitled to damages;[36] yet, no person existed eight years before conception. This case illustrates why invoking the concept of personhood in regard to the fetus does not answer any questions and raises many.

Professor Roger Fisher of the Harvard Law School has suggested that the way to approach major problems is by fragmenting them.[37] For example, if you ask people if they are in favor of war or peace, their answers could only be generalities; if you ask the same people if they want to be involved in a war in El Salvador, the chances are they will be far more specific. One way to face up to the problems of personhood, right of privacy, and abortion is to define exactly what consequences will flow in connection with the unborn (or whatever one decides to label them). Should they be able to inherit property? Should women be under suspicion of murder if they have miscarriages? If the unborn fetus is a person, then should every fertile woman of childbearing age be required to have a monthly pregnancy test? Do we want that? Many other difficult questions must be faced very specifically. I believe that if they are, we will get to the heart of *Roe v. Wade*—that with reference to abortion and personhood, we should not tell anyone what to do or think, and we should not allow anyone else to tell us what to do or think. Individual autonomy and the right to privacy must be scrupulously protected in any country that deserves to be called a democracy.

NOTES

1. *See* Baron, C.H., *The Concept of Person in the Law,* Chapter 8.
2. Henshaw, S., Martine, G., *Abortion and the Public Opinion Polls,* FAMILY PLANNING PERSPECTIVES 14(2):53 (March/April 1982).
3. Roe v. Wade, 410 U.S. 113 (1973).
4. *See id.* at 152-53. "The Constitution does not explicitly mention any right to privacy. In a line of decisions, however, . . . the [Supreme] Court has recognized that a right of personal privacy, or a guarantee of certain areas or zones of privacy, does exist under the Constitution."
5. Marbury v. Madison, 5 (1 Cranch) U.S. 137(1803).
6. *Id.* at 177.
7. U.S. Const. amend. XIV, §1 states that "nor shall any State deprive any person of life, liberty or property, without due process of law . . ."

8. Brandeis, L.D., Warren, J.D., *Right to Privacy*, HARVARD LAW REVIEW 4:193 (1890).

9. Olmstead v. United States, 277 U.S. 438, 477 (1928) (Brandeis, J., dissenting).

10. Loving v. Virginia, 388 U.S. 1, 8-13 (1967).

11. Pierce v. Society of Sisters, 268 U.S. 510, 534-35 (1925).

12. Meyer v. Nebraska, 262 U.S. 390, 399-400 (1923).

13. Skinner v. Oklahoma, 316 U.S. 390, 399-400 (1923).

14. Griswold v. Connecticut, 381 U.S. 479 (1965).

15. Eisenstadt v. Baird, 405 U.S. 438, 453 (1972).

16. 410 U.S. at 163.

17. *See id.* at 133 n. 22.

18. *See id.* at 129, 138.

19. 127 Cong. Rec. S10197 (daily ed. September 21, 1981).

20. COLO. REV. STAT. §§18-6-101, 104 (Cumm. Supp. 1981).

21. ALI MODEL PENAL CODE §230.3; *reprinted in* Doe v. Bolton, 410 U.S. 179, 205 (1973) (Appendix B).

22. 410 U.S. at 140 n. 37.

23. People v. Barksdale, 105 Cal. Rptr. 1 (1972); United States v. Vuitch, 305 F. Supp. 1032 (D.D.C. 1969), *reversed*, 402 U.S. 62 (1971).

24. 410 U.S. at 164.

25. *Id.* at 164–65.

26. *Id.* at 159.

27. *Id.*

28. *Id.* at 162.

29. *See e.g.*, S.J. 19, 97th Cong., 1st Sess. (1981).

30. *See* Towers, B., *Ethical and Legal Responsibilities of Physicians Toward the Dying Newborn*, in LEGAL AND ETHICAL ASPECTS OF TREATING CRITICALLY AND TER-MINALLY ILL PATIENTS (A.E. Doudera, J.D. Peters, eds.) (AUPHA Press, Ann Arbor, Mich.) (1982) at 228, 229.

31. S. 158, 97th Cong., 1st Sess. §1 states: "Congress finds that present day scientific evidence indicates a significant likelihood that actual human life exists from conception. . ."

32. *Human Life Bill: Hearings on S. 158 Before the Subcommittee on Separation of Powers of the Senate Comm. on the Judiciary*, 97th Cong., 1st Sess. 1092 (1981) (letter from panel of constitutional law professors, June 18, 1981).

33. S.J. 110, 97th Cong., 1st Sess. (1981).

34. *See* Golbus, M.S., *Advances in Fetal Diagnosis and Therapy*, Chapter 5; and Ryan, G.M., *Medical Implications of Bestowing Personhood Status on the Unborn*, Chapter 6.

35. Report on Injuries to Unborn Children (Prepared by British Law Commission No. 60 for the Lord High Chancellor and presented by him to Parliament, August 1974). See also a California statute enacted in 1981 that prohibited parent-child litigation:

> No cause of action arises against a parent of a child based upon the claim that the child should not have been conceived or if conceived, should not have been allowed to have been born alive.

1981 Cal. Stats., Ch. 331(a) (to be codified at CAL. CIV. CODE 43.6).

36. Renslow v. Mennonite Hosp., 367 N.E.2d 1250 (Ill. 1977).
37. *See* Fisher, R., *Fractionating Conflict*, in INTERNATIONAL CONFLICT AND BEHAVIORAL SCIENCE (R. Fisher, ed.) (Basic Books, New York) (1964) at 91.

Chapter 10

Medicolegal Implications of a Human Life Amendment

John A. Robertson

Groups opposed to abortion have proposed several kinds of constitutional amendments to undo the effect of *Roe v. Wade*, the 1973 Supreme Court decision which held that "the right of privacy . . . is broad enough to encompass a woman's decision whether or not to terminate her pregnancy."[1] One kind of amendment speaks directly to abortion, and explicitly grants Congress or the states the power to prohibit it. Another set of proposals, known as human life amendments (HLAs) tries to achieve the same end by stating that "person" within the Fifth and Fourteenth Amendments includes "unborn offspring at every stage of biological development including fertilization." While the "human life" or HLA approach has taken many forms, a version endorsed by the National Right To Life Committee is representative:

> Section 1. The right to life is the paramount and most fundamental right of a person.
>
> Section 2. With respect to the right to life guaranteed to persons by the fifth and fourteenth articles of amendment to the Constitution, the word "person" applies to all human beings, irrespective of age, health, function, or condition of dependency, including their unborn offspring at every stage of biological development including fertilization.
>
> Section 3. No unborn person shall be deprived of life by any person; provided, however, that nothing in this article shall prohibit a law permitting only those medical procedures required to prevent the death of a pregnant woman; but this law must require every reasonable effort be made to preserve the life and health of the unborn child.
>
> Section 4. Congress and the several States shall have power to enforce this article by appropriate legislation.[2]

The legal impact of any of these anti-abortion amendments will depend on their wording and on the subsequent legislation passed under their authority. There are, however, significant differences in the scope of the impact of the proposed amendments. Amendments dealing directly with abortion will impact only on abortion. Human life amendments, however, because they attempt to reach their anti-abortion goal by defining person-hood, have potential impacts in many areas of law. Specifically, the HLA approach appears to have an impact on medical practice in many areas beyond abortion. This paper discusses the medicolegal implications of a human life amendment for abortion, contraception, prenatal diagnosis, fetal therapy, novel means of reproduction, and medical care of the pregnant woman.

LEGAL EFFECT OF THE HLA: NO IMPLEMENTING LEGISLATION

There has been much speculation about the legal effect of the HLA, but little analysis. Discussion of it often seems to proceed on the assumption that the HLA would be self-executing—that its passage would without further legislation ban abortion and any other activity endangering the fetus. The American Civil Liberties Union, for example, asserts:

> If the fertilized egg becomes, constitutionally, a "person," any action that carries even a risk of causing fetal damage could be construed as a crime. . . .[3]
> Enforcement of the HLA would be a nightmare. Because a fetus would have an affirmative "right-to-life" under the Constitution, it would be the government's obligation to seek out and protect all fetuses. . . .[4]

The mere fact that people think that passage of the HLA will have such effects could, if such an amendment passes, deter women and doctors from performing abortions and undertaking other medical activities that might endanger the fetus. But while passage alone will have a chilling effect on medical activities, further legislation would be necessary to legally ban abortion and other activities endangering the fetus. Consider the matter first at the state and then the federal level.

STATE LAW

Would the HLA by its mere passage bring fetuses within the ambit of all state laws protecting persons, including the criminal code's laws against homicide and other bodily harms? A good argument could be made that it would not. The meaning of "person" in the Constitution is not necessarily equivalent to "person" in the criminal code. Suppose a prosecutor charged a doctor and woman who had participated in an abortion the day after the HLA was passed with first degree murder (or some other homicide charge). I think a good defense would be that the state legislature, in making homicide a crime, did not intend to include "fetus" within the meaning of person.

Passage of the HLA would, however, authorize states to protect fetuses in a variety of ways not now possible under current law. Nonetheless (as the discussion of this topic below shows), the state's power under such an amendment would not be nearly as broad as some have imagined. Whatever its limits, it is a power which the individual states have to exercise by enacting legislation. The passage of the HLA defines the value that must be accorded fetuses. It does not inform as to how the variety of conflicts that can arise between fetuses and other persons is to be resolved.

At the same time that the HLA authorizes the states to pursue fetal over maternal interests, it also places limits on state action infringing the rights of fetuses. Since the HLA makes fetuses "persons" within the meaning of the Fourteenth Amendment, states could not deny them equal protection or due process of law. It is, however, not clear what that obligation means in practical terms. Even if the right to life is in some sense paramount, it would not impose a duty on the state to protect fetuses at the expense of the rights of other persons. Since constitutional rights are negative and not positive (e.g., they are rights against state interference and not claims on the state to act positively on behalf of someone), it would protect fetuses from state deprivations of life, but would not require that the state take steps to protect fetuses, particularly at the expense of other persons. A state that did not prohibit abortion after passage of an HLA would not necessarily deny fetuses equal protection, since there would only be state inaction and not state action. In any event, even if state action were found, it is far from clear that fetuses subject to abortion would be found by the courts to be denied equal protection. Even under the strict scrutiny analysis, a state's interest in preserving the reproductive and bodily autonomy of the pregnant woman could be sufficient to justify exclusion of fetuses from protection from harm.

FEDERAL LEVEL

A similar analysis would apply to federal laws. Congress may not pass legislation that impinges on fetuses in a way that would violate a person's rights under the Fifth Amendment, but the inclusion of "fetus" within the Fifth Amendment would not automatically change every federal statute using the term person. The HLA amends the Constitution, and not every statute passed by Congress. Such laws could not reasonably be interpreted to protect fetuses since their language and their legislative history clearly show otherwise. Nor is the argument persuasive that Congress intended to protect "persons" as defined under the Constitution at the time the question arises, because "person" has been subject to both progressively broad and narrow interpretations. Furthermore, such a result would assume that Congress would make the same trade-offs between the fetuses and other interests that it would make between "persons" and those interests. Yet it is likely that Congress would not want to protect fetuses to the same extent as other persons in every case. Thus, passage of the HLA would not make every abortion or activity endangering a fetus a civil or criminal violation of the federal civil rights acts.

Nor would passage of an HLA obligate Congress to amend the laws to protect fetuses to the same extent as other persons, since (1) state inaction does not equal state action, and (2) different treatment of fetus-persons from children and adults can still be justified under the equal protection clause because of dissimilarity in situation. Protecting the woman's interest in procreative autonomy and bodily integrity would be a sufficiently substantial reason to withstand even strict scrutiny under the equal protection component of the Fifth Amendment.

In sum, the widespread belief that the HLA would, by its very passage, bring fetuses within the protection of any federal and state statute using the term "person" or "human being" is open to serious question. Doctors and pregnant women need not fear that prosecution under the federal civil rights acts or state criminal codes must occur for any action that harms a fetus. Despite the chilling effect of the confusion over its direct impact, the main legal effect of the HLA is the authority it gives the federal and state legislatures to protect fetuses.

LEGAL EFFECT: IMPLEMENTING LEGISLATION

It is also widely thought that the HLA would empower the states to enact a wide variety of legislation restricting procreative choices, including limits on abortion, contraception, novel means of reproduction, prenatal diagnosis, and medical treatment of pregnant women. The assumption is that if the fertilized egg, embryo, and fetus have all the rights of persons, and the right to life is paramount, then the state must be able to override the rights of the pregnant woman to protect that interest. But making the fetus a person does not necessarily mean its right to life automatically takes precedence over that of the mother. Rather, there would be a conflict between the fetus' interest in life and the mother's interest in bodily integrity and procreative privacy. Mere passage of the HLA does not tell us how this conflict would be resolved. Indeed, favoring the fetus over the mother could violate the mother's rights to bodily integrity, procreative privacy, and equal treatment—rights which the HLA does not abolish.

To understand this possibility, it is essential to clarify a central confusion or ambiguity in the meaning of abortion. Induced abortion involves an interruption of the pregnancy, leading to expulsion of the fetus from the mother's body. It may or may not cause the death of the fetus—a fact that depends on the method and timing of the abortion, the stage of the pregnancy, and the efforts taken after delivery to protect the newborn.

Abortion, then, at least in some circumstances, may be thought of as the removal of the fetus-person from the mother's body (ejection from lodging or life-support system). Viewed in this context, banning abortion means that a woman must lend her body to support another. But imposing such a duty on the mother implicates rights of equal protection and bodily integrity that need further discussion in the context of a particular ban.

RESTRICTIONS ON ABORTION

Ban on First Trimester Abortions

Suppose, after passage of the HLA, a state banned all abortions including those in the first trimester. Such a ban would infringe a woman's rights of privacy or bodily integrity, as set forth in *Roe v. Wade* and other Supreme Court decisions. But since those rights can be infringed to promote a compelling state interest, the fetus' interest in life would now be a sufficient basis to sustain the legislation. But it could be argued, as Donald Regan has done in a stimulating article,[5] that forcing women to lend their bodies to aid another person when the law does not mandate similar burdens on other people, would violate the woman's right to equal protection. An evaluation of that argument is beyond the scope of this paper. However, it is worth noting that it does provide a legal handle to enjoin prosecution of abortion laws until the Supreme Court—which might just strike down abortion laws on equal protection grounds—hears the case.

Ban on Abortions after Viability

States prohibiting abortions after passage of the HLA would no doubt also ban abortions after the fetus had reached viability. In *Roe v. Wade* the Supreme Court made viability the point at which the state could, in order to protect the potential personhood of the fetus, ban abortion. Viability was defined as the potential "[t]o live outside the mother's womb, albeit with artificial aid."[6] It was the compelling point for protecting "the State's important legitimate interest in potential life . . . because the fetus then presumably has the capability of meaningful life outside the mother's womb."[7]

If the fetus is defined as a person, however, it would appear that at viability abortion (understood in the narrow sense of terminating the pregnancy and removing the fetus from the mother without directly destroying it) should be permitted. At this stage, the fetus can survive and the mother can regain control of her body. As improvements in perinatology and the development of artificial uteruses push the point of viability back earlier and earlier in the pregnancy, the ability to terminate a pregnancy at viability by removal without destruction of the fetus will be even more important. While it will not prevent a woman from knowing that her genes exist in a child, with its attendant psychosocial harm, this technological development will relieve her of the physical burdens of several months of pregnancy.

Suppose, however, that the state prohibits post-viability abortions despite the possibility of reconciling the mother's interest in her body and the fetus' interest in life. Such a statute would be subject to constitutional attack and could conceivably be struck down. Protecting the life of the fetus-person would not justify the burden imposed on the mother's rights of privacy, bodily integrity, and reproductive choice because abortion— termination and removal from the mother—will not always cause the death of the fetus. A viable fetus by definition can survive outside the mother. Furthermore, forcing a woman to lend her body to someone who does not really need it, while other persons are not obligated to lend their bodies, could be found to violate equal protection rights. The state could regulate the abortion method to improve the chance of fetal survival, but banning abortions after viability would not be justified.

Prohibitions on Abortions Necessary to Save Mother's Life or Health

Suppose state laws passed after the HLA banned abortions deemed medically necessary to save the mother's life or health. Again, such a law would pose a conflict between the fetus' interest in occupying the mother's body and the mother's interest in bodily autonomy, and in this case, her interest in her own life and health. This conflict should be considered only in the pre-viable situation, since banning post-viable abortions (as we have just seen) would be invalid, whatever the effect of the pregnancy on the mother's life or health. In the pre-viable context, the choice then is between the mother's life or health and the fetus' life (since by definition pre-viable termination, however done, will lead to its death).

Looking first at pregnancy that threatens the mother's health, the question is whether the state could prefer the fetus-person's life over that of the mother. One can only speculate about the answer, particularly since such an extreme law is unlikely to be passed. If it were passed, a woman or doctor prosecuted under it could argue that it was unconstitutional in that it deprived her of life without sufficient justification. In addition, she could argue that it denied her a right of self-defense that other persons had. While her complicity or role in bringing about the life-threatening situation might distinguish her case, the innocence of the fetus would not. The law of self-defense allows a person to kill another who threatens his or her life, even if the other is totally innocent.

A law prohibiting abortions necessary to protect the mother's health would also be subject to an equal protection challenge. The law of self-defense allows one person to kill another to prevent serious bodily harm, even when an innocent person threatens that harm. Prohibiting pregnant women from removing a threat of serious bodily harm, but not others, could violate their right to equal treatment. However, when the threat to health is less serious the preference for the fetus over the mother's health may be constitutional, since the woman would then be treated the same as other persons faced with nonserious threats to health.

Prohibitions on Abortions of Fetuses with Severe Congenital Defects

Suppose the state law passed after the HLA banned abortions on pre-viable fetuses who had been diagnosed as having serious congenital defects, such as Down syndrome, meningomyelocele, or sickle cell anemia. Many persons choose to abort such fetuses. Could the state, after passage of the HLA, prevent that option? If a ban on pre-viable abortions is otherwise constitutional, then a ban on such abortions when the fetus is congenitally defective would also be constitutional. If the state may prefer the pre-viable fetus' life over the mother's interest in privacy and bodily integrity, it may do so even if the life protected will be handicapped in significant ways. As long as life is a good for the handicapped fetus, the state could impose burdens on the mother for its benefit, just as it could to benefit a normal fetus. Of course, such a policy would be rational only if the state also prohibited nontreatment of defective children once they had been born.

Prohibitions on Abortion Methods

One thing seems clear: after passage of the HLA the state may regulate the methods used to terminate a pregnancy. Since it may choose to regard fetuses as persons and to protect them accordingly, the state could protect fetuses by restricting termination of pregnancy to methods that will maximize fetal survival. Indeed, as we have seen, the state may not be able to prevent a woman from terminating pregnancy either before or after viability, because to do so would burden a woman with a duty that is not imposed on other persons. The state could, however, require techniques such as prostaglandin induction which will not directly kill the fetus. It could also mandate the presence of doctors and equipment at such abortions to assure fetal survival. It should be noted, however, that these restrictions would apply only to abortions where the fetus might survive. If pre-viable abortions could not be banned, then neither could the methods employed be restricted to those which seek to protect the fetus since its expulsion from the mother by any method will lead to its death.

RESTRICTIONS ON CONTRACEPTION AND STERILIZATION

Would the HLA authorize state laws restricting contraception and sterilization? To answer this question it is necessary to distinguish contraceptive techniques that prevent fertilization, and those that prevent implantation of the fertilized egg in the uterine wall.

Prevention of Fertilization

It is doubtful that state laws restricting contraceptive techniques which prevent fertilization from occurring would be constitutional even after passage of the HLA. Passage of the HLA does not change the fundamental right status of the decision not to procreate.[8] It merely authorizes the state to prefer the life of the fertilized egg, embryo, and fetus (once it exists) over the mother's interest in privacy and procreative autonomy. The question would be whether a state's interest in bringing into existence fertilized eggs and fetuses would override the potential parents' interest in preventing conception altogether. I think it would not, for the state's interest in bringing more beings into existence would not (absent severe underpopulation) be compelling. The state's interest in protecting a person in existence—the fetus—would be more compelling than bringing such persons into existence by prohibiting contraception.

Prevention of Implantation

Would the outcome change if the contraceptive technique worked by preventing further development or implantation of the fertilized egg rather than prevention of conception in the first place, as intrauterine devices, the morning-after pill, and menstrual extraction techniques appear to do? Here the state's justification for limiting the right not to procreate would, after the HLA, be protection of another person—the fertilized egg or embryo. The answer would depend on the answer to the validity of bans on first trimester, pre-viable abortions. Preventing use of post-conception, pre-implantation contraceptive techniques would, in effect, force a woman to aid or rescue an embryo in need. If the embryo existed in a petri dish outside her body and needed to be "housed" in her uterus to survive, it is doubtful whether a law mandating insertion into her and implantation would stand. Imposing a duty of rescue on her would be to impose a much greater duty than is imposed on other persons. The question, thus, would be whether the presence of the embryo inside her should be treated differently. This will depend on whether her participation in bringing the embryo into existence justifies imposing a duty to lend her body that is not generally imposed on others. The answer to that question will determine the constitutionality of state bans on contraceptive techniques that operate after fertilization but before implantation.

Restrictions on Prenatal Diagnosis

Questions have also been raised about the effect of the HLA on prenatal diagnosis. Could a state after passage of the HLA ban amniocentesis, sonography, fetoscopy, or other prenatal diagnostic techniques (either directly, by criminalizing their use, or indirectly, by imposing civil liability)? The state might justify such a law on the grounds that it would prevent abortions of defective fetuses or that it would prevent harm to the fetus from the diagnostic procedure itself.

Neither of these reasons, however, would justify the burden on the mother's right to have the diagnostic procedures done. A court could find that the mother's decision to have prenatal diagnosis is an exercise of her fundamental right of privacy, in that it involves intimate bodily matters, involves medical decisions, and is relevant to procreative decision making. Yet the state's asserted interest in protecting the fetus by preventing maneuvers that might harm it directly or indirectly by providing information that could lead to abortion would not constitute the compelling justification necessary to infringe a fundamental right, and indeed, might not even satisfy a rational basis test.

If abortion is otherwise prohibited, the added incentive to have one resulting from a prenatal diagnosis would not be so great as to justify the restriction. After all, identifying a congenital anomaly in utero would probably benefit more than harm the fetus. Identification may allow in utero therapies to be applied to correct the anomaly, improve management of the birth and immediate postnatal care, or influence the method and timing of birth to protect the child. In addition, prenatal diagnosis could also reassure the mother and perhaps prevent an abortion that she would otherwise have. Given these benefits, it is unlikely that the minimal risks to the fetus of the procedure or the incentive to seek an abortion (illegally, or legally in another jurisdiction) would justify such a ban. In sum, even after passage of the HLA, the benefits to unborn children of restrictions on prenatal diagnosis are too small to be constitutional, in light of the harm they can cause those same children and the mother.

Effect on Relief of Infertility

It is also supposed that passage of the HLA might interfere with developing techniques of relieving infertility through artificial insemination donors (AID) or in vitro fertilization and implantation. Would state laws preventing relief of infertility by these means be constitutional? It seems unlikely, for these techniques allow conception to occur and children to be born in cases where this would ordinarily be impossible. Perhaps the strongest case for the state would be that in vitro fertilization creates "persons"—fertilized eggs and embryos—that will frequently be destroyed. While prohibition of experimentation or manipulation of fertilized eggs and their destruction could be prohibited, the aim of in vitro fertilization is to allow birth to occur. The interference with the mother's interest in procreating could not be justified by preventing the destruction or miscarriage of some of the fertilized eggs that result from the procedures. Otherwise, women prone to miscarriage could be prohibited from conceiving on the theory that this will prevent the same destruction of embryos and fetuses. In any event, it is not clear how a "person" is harmed if he or she is brought into being by the only method possible, and then dies because there is no way to continue that life.

Effect on State Efforts to Protect Unborn Children

It is also widely thought that passage of the HLA would empower the state to enact a variety of measures designed to protect the unborn child. For example, the ACLU lists the following interventions into the body or freedom of a woman that would be possible for the state to enact to protect unborn children:

> A woman with cancer could be prohibited from continuing radiation therapy; women of childbearing age could be excluded from heavy work or toxic environments; the physical activities, travel, and other normal routines of pregnant women could be regulated. To reduce the possibility of miscarriage, the state might be permitted to prescribe dangerous experimental drugs, notwithstanding their impact on a woman's health. Under an HLA,

women would become machines bearing "human life," and the machines would be expendable, while fertilized eggs would acquire unprecedented legal protection.[9]

Although the list of steps the state might take to protect a fetus is speculative, it is true that passage of the HLA could lead to state restrictions on women to benefit fetuses beyond prohibition of abortion and other reproductive-related decisions. As long as these restrictions did not otherwise violate equal protection, due process, or other constitutional guarantees, they would be lawful. However, it is unclear whether the HLA would increase the state's power in this regard in a significant way. Under *Roe v. Wade*, the state has considerable power to intrude on the freedom and even body of a pregnant woman to protect the unborn child. First, activities during any stage of pregnancy that would cause the death of or serious harm to a child that would otherwise be born can be punished criminally or civilly. Second, after viability (and possibly before, if no abortion is planned) the state may mandate or even directly coerce medical or surgical treatments for the sake of the unborn child. In utero transfusions for Rh factor, confinement of a mother during the last trimester of pregnancy, and even an undesired caesarean section can be imposed on the mother for the benefit of the unborn child.[10]

Given the state's existing power to protect unborn children, the main effect of the HLA on the health of fetuses would be to prohibit abortion. If an abortion is not planned, the state already has authority to intervene and regulate the activities of pregnant women to protect the unborn child.

Effect on Medical Treatment of Pregnant Women

It is also thought that the HLA would interfere with the proper medical care of pregnant women, because such treatment could harm the fetus or even cause abortion. Dr. George Ryan, writing in this volume, identifies several situations in which conflicts between maternal and fetal health might arise, and assumes that the HLA would prevent proper treatment of the mother.[11] These include removal of a tubal or ectopic pregnancy before it ruptures and becomes life-threatening to the woman; dilation and curettage when miscarriage is inevitable but has not yet occurred; inducing labor or early delivery to protect the mother; appendectomy during pregnancy which could induce miscarriage; and radiation treatment of a pregnant woman with cancer that could harm the fetus.

In evaluating this claim, however, it is essential to recall that the HLA will not by its passage alone criminalize any preference in treatment for the mother over the fetus. Until some specific law is passed, a doctor treating a woman in a way that harms or causes the death of the fetus (say by radiation of her cancer or a surgical procedure that precipitates a miscarriage) would not be committing a crime.

The important question about the legal effect of the HLA on the medical treatment of pregnant women concerns the limitations which state laws designed to protect the pre-viable fetus and enacted pursuant to the HLA would place on such cases. One limitation would arise from laws banning pre-viable abortions even when necessary to protect the mother's health. If a ban on pre-viable abortions is constitutional, then two questions arise which would determine the restrictions, if any, on medical treatment of a pregnant woman.

The first is whether a maternal treatment that harms the fetus is an "abortion" within the statutory prohibition. If the purpose of the procedure is to help the pregnant woman while making every attempt not to injure the fetus, the fact that the fetus is harmed does not mean that treatment is an abortion. Similarly, the abortion statute would not necessarily cover removal of ectopic pregnancies or dilation and curettage where miscarriage is inevitable since death of the fetus would naturally occur in those cases anyway.

The second question would arise only if a medical treatment of the mother that harmed or removed the fetus were considered an abortion within the meaning of a statute forbidding it, or were otherwise prohibited. Here the question, discussed above, would be whether denying the mother a means of self-defense available to others would deny to her equal protection and thus be invalid. As we have seen, there is a strong legal argument, at least where the threat to her health is significant, that her rights would be violated.

This reasoning would also apply to state laws passed after the HLA that directly regulated the health care that could be given to pregnant women. If the law preferred fetal over maternal health, it would have to meet equal protection standards to be valid.

Conclusion

Analyzing the medicolegal effects of the HLA shows that they are not nearly so drastic or far-reaching as some people have asserted. This is because the HLA is not self-executing and will require further legislation to achieve the desired protection of fertilized eggs, embryos, and fetuses. It is unclear how far a congress or a state legislature would then be willing to go to protect fetuses by restricting abortions and other medical activities harmful to the fetus. In addition, the HLA may have a more limited impact than thought because granting the fetus constitutional rights as a person will not guarantee that its rights will always trump the rights of other persons. Indeed, the HLA might not even be sufficient to authorize prohibitions on abortion before viability, and most likely would not support a ban on post-viability abortions.

But my claim that the HLA will not be as far-reaching as intended or feared and, indeed, might not even ban abortion, is not intended as a defense of the proposal. In fact the confusion that would be generated by its passage, and the chilling effect on doctor and patient activity while implementing legislation is passed and these questions are sorted out by the courts, are sufficient reasons to oppose it. If a constitutional amendment reversing *Roe v. Wade* is intended, it should be done directly and not through the circuitous route of making fertilized eggs, embryos, and fetuses "persons" within the meaning of the Constitution.

NOTES

1. 410 U.S. 113, 153 (1973).
2. *The So-Called "Human Life" Amendment*, American Civil Liberties Union Foundation, 2-3 (undated).
3. *Id.* at 8.
4. *Id.* at 12.
5. Regan, D.H., *Rewriting* Roe v. Wade, MICHIGAN LAW REVIEW 77 (7): 1569 (1979).
6. *Supra* note 1, at 160.
7. *Id.* at 163.
8. *See* Carey v. Population Services International, 431 U.S. 678 (1977); Eisenstadt v. Baird, 405 U.S. 438 (1972); Griswold v. Connecticut, 381 U.S. 479 (1964).
9. *Supra* note 2.
10. Robertson, J., *The Right to Procreate and In Utero Fetal Therapy*, JOURNAL OF LEGAL MEDICINE 333 (September 1982).
11. Ryan, G.M., *Medical Implications of Bestowing Personhood on the Unborn*, Chapter 6.

Chapter 11

Beyond Abortion: The Potential Reach of a Human Life Amendment

David Westfall

INTRODUCTION

Just as it is axiomatic that hard cases make bad law, so it is also true that difficult social issues often provoke ill considered and unsound legislative proposals. The question of whether a woman may choose to terminate a pregnancy by abortion provokes a greater intensity of feeling and involves a more complex amalgam of powerful and contradictory values than any other contemporary social issue. These include fundamental ethical and religious views on the value of human life, society's high regard for individual privacy and autonomy, and public concerns over teenage pregnancies and the population explosion.

It is no surprise that the Supreme Court's decision in *Roe v. Wade* [1] (which held that the constitutionally protected right of privacy includes the right of women to terminate pregnancies free of state interference until the fetus is viable) did not set the matter to rest. The inevitable sequel was a tidal wave of litigation, legislative activity, and heated public discussion. As subsequent decisions struck down various forms of state interference with women's constitutionally protected freedom to abort,[2] the anti-abortion forces naturally sought legislative redress.[3]

The most significant result of this effort, the Hyde amendment,[4] has virtually cut off direct federal funding for abortions.[5] The federal legislative triumph for the anti-abortion forces has received the imprimatur of constitutionality from the Supreme Court[6] and is a major roadblock for poor women who want abortions but lack financing. But similar efforts to

This article is an expanded version of the paper presented by Professor Westfall at the conference in Houston; it was originally published in the AMERICAN JOURNAL OF LAW & MEDICINE 8(2):97 (Summer 1982).

secure state legislation to ban or restrict abortions, making them unavailable even for those able to pay, generally have been held unconstitutional.[7]

Thus the stage was set for a direct attack on the decisions which accord women the right (although not the means) to have an abortion. Like other disappointed litigants in constitutional cases,[8] the anti-abortion forces propose to remove the source of that right by constitutional amendment.

The most straightforward of these efforts would prohibit abortion outright. A prohibition of abortion per se would bear heavily on women who are too poor to finance travel to a jurisdiction permitting abortion. But an amendment explicitly prohibiting abortion and nothing else is not subject to the criticism that it would have unintended effects in other areas of law. [9]

A second group of proposed amendments would not undertake to deal directly with abortion as a matter of federal law, but rather would authorize the states to allow, regulate, or prohibit abortion.[10] Again, state legislation authorized by the amendment would bear more heavily on poor women than on those who have the resources to travel elsewhere. The impact of the amendment would be limited to abortion itself and would not extend to other matters.

This article focuses on a third, less direct approach: amendments which seek to accomplish the desired end of banning or limiting the availability of abortions by broadening the definition of "person" to include unborn individuals.[11] A variant of the "right to life" theme, the Helms-Hyde human life bill,[12] purports to achieve a similar result without a constitutional amendment by legislation pursuant to the Congressional power under section 5 of the Fourteenth Amendment.

This article does not deal with the soundness of *Roe v. Wade* and its progeny or with the desirability of constitutional amendments which seek to overturn the decisions directly. Instead, it addresses the implications of the less direct approach embodied in the proposed "human life" statute and amendments—which will be collectively referred to as an "HLA"—in areas unrelated to abortion.

Seventeen separate HLAs were introduced during the 97th Congress, but they reflect only a limited number of differences with a single, basic approach. This article focuses on the following three proposed constitutional amendments and the Helms-Hyde bill:

(1) The Ashbrook proposal:

> Section 1. With respect to the right to life guaranteed in this Constitution, every human being, subject to the jurisdiction of the United States, or of any state, shall be deemed, from the moment of fertilization, to be a person and entitled to the right to life.

Section 2. Congress and the several States shall have concurrent power to enforce this article by appropriate legislation.[13]

(2) The Garn-Rhodes proposal:

Section 1. With respect to the right to life the word "person," as used in this article and in the fifth and fourteenth articles of amendment to the Constitution of the United States, applies to all human beings, irrespective of age, health, function, or condition of dependency, including their unborn offspring at every stage of their biological development.

Section 2. No unborn person shall be deprived of life by any person: Provided, however, that nothing in this article shall prohibit a law permitting only those medical procedures required to prevent the death of the mother.

Section 3. Congress and the several States shall have the power to enforce this article by appropriate legislation within their respective jurisdictions.[14]

(3) The Helms-Dornan proposal:

The paramount right to life is vested in each human being from the moment of fertilization without regard to age, health or condition of dependency. [15]

(4) The Helms-Hyde human life bill:

Section 1. The Congress finds that present day scientific evidence indicates a significant likelihood that actual human life exists from conception. The Congress further finds that the Fourteenth Amendment to the Constitution of the United States was intended to protect all human beings. Upon the basis of these findings, and in the exercise of the powers of the Congress, including its power under section 5 of the Fourteenth Amendment to the Constitution of the United States, the Congress hereby declares that for the purposes of enforcing the obligation of the states under the Fourteenth Amendment not to deprive persons of life without due process of law, human life shall be deemed to exist from conception, without regard to race, sex, age, health, defect, or condition of dependency; and for this purpose "person" shall include all human life as defined herein.[16]

The Ashbrook and Garn-Rhodes versions are similar in their reliance on redefinition of "person" as used in the Constitution as the vehicle for overturning *Roe v. Wade*. Both were evidently inspired by dicta in the Court's opinion indicating that if fetuses were held to be persons within the language and meaning of the Fourteenth Amendment, their "right to life would . . . be guaranteed specifically by the Amendment."[17] Both also are alike in conferring concurrent enforcement power on both Congress and the states.

There are two major differences between the two versions. Garn-Rhodes expressly applies to life-depriving acts of individuals and excludes from its ban laws permitting "medical procedures required to prevent the death of the mother."[18] The Ashbrook version does not expressly deal with either of these matters.

The Helms-Dornan version differs from both Ashbrook and Garn-Rhodes in referring to the "paramount right to life" rather than to any right presently protected by the Constitution, raising the question of whether it would supersede existing law with respect to capital punishment.[19] It omits any express authorization to Congress or the states to enact legislation to enforce the amendment.

The Helms-Hyde bill is essentially an attempt to achieve by statute the result sought by the Helms-Dornan proposed Constitutional amendment, based on a congressional finding that "actual human life exists from conception." It raises constitutional issues not present in the other proposals. [20]

The proposed constitutional amendments would likely receive a broader construction than the proposed statute, under the doctrine favoring statutory construction in a manner which avoids constitutional issues.[21] This article will examine the potential consequences of the use of an HLA to ban or restrict abortions, rather than anticipate the precise course judicial construction of any given form would be likely to follow. To avoid value-laden terminology[22] this article will use the term "conceptus" to refer to the unborn.[23]

POSSIBLE JUDICIAL APPROACHES

This section will address two threshold issues. First it will discuss applications of an HLA to private persons, and whether state action must be present in order to invoke an HLA. Then it will consider the various approaches courts may take in determining the nature and extent of the rights conferred on conceptuses by an HLA.

APPLICATION TO PRIVATE PERSONS AND
THE REQUIREMENT OF STATE ACTION

Only the Garn-Rhodes version expressly applies to private persons. The other three HLAs discussed here leave unsettled whether they have any application in the absence of "state action." The Fourteenth Amendment refers to actions of states, rather than conduct of private persons. What constitutes state action, however, is not always clear.[24] For example, the Supreme Court has recently indicated that a state's failure to provide a civil remedy for the private taking of life is not "state action" constituting a denial of due process.[25] One commentator has suggested that in other situations, however, "inaction may carry a greater aura of State action . . .

than the mere denial of a civil action. . . ."[26] Thus the latter three versions of an HLA might require courts to confront the state action issue in a variety of contexts.

DETERMINING THE RIGHTS OF A CONCEPTUS

If a conceptus is to be considered a "person" for purposes of the Four-teenth Amendment, courts will have to determine the extent of its rights. At least three alternative approaches could be followed: (1) the only right of the conceptus is protection from destruction by abortion; (2) the concep-tus enjoys protection from any form of bodily injury to the same extent as other persons, but no protection of property rights or other nonbodily interests; and (3) the conceptus enjoys the same rights as other persons, subject to legislative authority to adopt reasonable classifications of per-sons. There are major problems with all three approaches.

Protection from Abortion Alone

A *tour de force* of judicial construction could limit the rights of the concep-tus to protection from destruction by abortion. This approach, however, requires the courts to treat an HLA's references to "human life" or "right to life" as mere code words without substantive effect[27] designed to enlist public support.[28] The redefinition of "person" effected by such an HLA would be merely a stratagem to overturn *Roe v. Wade.* The "abortion only" approach is a cynical interpretation that ignores the language of an HLA actually enacted.

Protection from Bodily Injury Alone

Support for limiting protection of the conceptus to freedom from bodily injury in any form comes from the explicit reference in many versions of HLAs to the "right to life," and the absence of references to "liberty" and "property" interests.[29]

Serious problems with this approach arise from the special physical relationship between the conceptus and its mother. Because of this rela-tionship, absolute protection of the conceptus would make paramount the role of actual or potential mothers for all pre-menopausal women who had not been sterilized.[30] In an era of increasing concern for equal treatment of men and women, this absolutist approach would encounter determined opposition.

If absolute protection of the conceptus is viewed judicially as an unwarranted limitation on a woman's right to privacy, a balancing test could be employed. It would be possible to weigh the potential detriment to the conceptus from given forms of conduct by the woman against the potential interference with her privacy and autonomy interests. Any such judicial balancing inevitably has a strongly subjective flavor. Application of a balancing test to possible governmental restrictions on a woman's activity could lead to years of litigation and uncertainty.

Equal Protection with Other Persons

A third possible judicial approach is "equal protection": conceptuses are "persons" within the meaning of the Fourteenth Amendment and other provisions of the Constitution, entitled as such to full protection of their rights, subject only to legislative authority to adopt reasonable classifications.[31] This interpretation assumes that human life begins at the moment of conception to its logical conclusion and extends to the conceptus the full panoply of rights accorded those already born.

This last approach is most consistent with the underlying premise of an HLA: that conceptuses are indistinguishable, for purposes of constitutional law, from newborn infants. The Fourteenth Amendment appears to define "persons" in the same manner for both the due process and equal protection clauses as it uses the same word twice in proximity.[32] Elsewhere in the Constitution, distinctions have been drawn between different classes of "persons." For example, only "citizens," and not all "persons," are protected under the Fourteenth Amendment from abridgment of their "privileges and immunities"[33] and are entitled to vote under the Twenty-sixth Amendment.[34] Furthermore, *Roe v.Wade* seems to treat "person" in the same manner for due process and equal protection purposes.[35]

One of the strongest proponents of an HLA has stated "[t]he amendment would merely apply the existing principles of due process of law and the equal protection of the laws to all human beings, including the child in the womb."[36] If this view receives judicial acceptance, a critical question will be the level of justification required to support legislative classifications which treat some or all conceptuses differently from other persons.

It would unduly prolong this article to explore the full range of possible judicial approaches in applying constitutional guarantees to challenged state or federal statutes. At one extreme is the rational relationship test, under which such legislation survives if a reasonable connection between a permissible legislative goal and the challenged enactment can be supplied by an exercise of judicial ingenuity, without regard to whether the connection actually had been contemplated by any legislator.[37] At the other pole is strict scrutiny, usually applied in a manner which invalidates the challenged enactment.[38] There are also intermediate positions variously characterized as intermediate scrutiny, balancing of interests, and less restrictive alternatives.[39]

It is impossible to predict exactly where on this spectrum of constitutional scrutiny any given legislative classification affecting conceptuses differently from other persons might fall. However, substantial support is readily apparent for strict scrutiny of such legislation. Conceptuses bear some of the traditional indicia of a suspect class or a discrete and insular minority.[40] First, they are politically helpless.[41] Second, conceptuses have endured a history of discrimination matched by that of few, if any, other minorities. As one commentator argued: "[i]t is not unreasonable to conclude that unborn children are subject to a badge of servitude when they as a class, unlike all other human beings, are made subject to death at the convenience of others.[42] Classifications affecting the rights of conceptuses in areas other than abortion could be subject to strict scrutiny and may require justification by a compelling state interest.[43] Strict scrutiny would be appropriate if, in the words of a proponent of an HLA, "the right to live is superior to these other [fundamental constitutional] rights."[44]

No one can predict with confidence which, if any, version of an HLA will be adopted, or what judicial approach would predominate in determining its consequences in areas other than abortion. Indeed, there is no reason to assume that any single approach will be adopted and consistently applied; no court is likely to paint with such a broad brush. But whatever approaches are followed in applying an HLA, the technique which it embodies in redefining the point at which human life begins ensures that it will impose three kinds of major social costs: (1) litigation to determine the effect of an HLA in areas other than abortion, with attendant expense for litigants and burdens on the judicial system; (2) legislative and administrative responses to an HLA and to decisions determining its consequences, with resulting diversion of available legislative and administrative resources from other tasks; and (3) planning and transaction costs for individuals and firms which may flow from uncertainty as to the consequences of an HLA and its impact on business and social arrangements. These burdens on society will be examined in more detail later in this chapter.

The fundamental reason to anticipate such wide-ranging costs to society from using an HLA as the means to prohibit abortion is that so much existing law in widely divergent subject areas is construed and applied in light of three assumptions: (1) rights accrue only on a live birth; (2) many duties are owed to individuals only after birth; and (3) age is measured from birth rather than from conception. In a wide range of situations, interested parties will have powerful incentives to test the validity of these assumptions in light of an HLA. Existing law already recognizes that some duties are owed to conceptuses,[45] and it is reasonable to anticipate that an HLA would lead to a substantial expansion of both rights and duties in this area. Although the extent of the expansion will turn on the predominant judicial approach to an HLA, any significant growth will add to judicial, legislative, and administrative dockets, as well as to individual planning and transaction costs.

These costs are wholly unnecessary if the sole objective of an HLA is to ban abortion. Such costs could be substantially reduced even if the sponsors' goals extend beyond abortion and include, for example, prohibiting the use of other methods of birth control.[46] All that is required to reduce the scope of judicial, legislative, and administrative inquiry that could be compelled by an HLA is specifying what is to be accomplished, beyond banning abortion, rather than leaving the problem for later resolution. Chief Justice Burger has argued persuasively that both excessive judicial caseloads and judicial "legislating" are at least partly attributable to sloppy drafting by members of Congress who "just drop the controversial element of the legislation and say 'let the courts work it out.'"[47]

POTENTIAL SUBSTANTIVE EFFECTS OF AN HLA

An HLA may have substantive effects in areas other than abortion. In each of these areas, an HLA could create chaos, confusion, and uncertainty for years after its enactment.

LEGISLATIVE APPORTIONMENT

The impact of an HLA could be greater for federal election purposes than for state and local elections, because the constitutional requirement that each person's vote carry equal weight is more rigorously applied to the former.[48] But an HLA may have major effects on state and local elections as well.

Congressional Elections

The Constitution provides that representatives in Congress shall be allocated according to "the whole number of person's in each State"[49] and that the people of the several States will choose these representatives.[50] As judicially construed, each person's vote must carry equal weight in electing representatives.[51] Thus, the critical question is whether a conceptus is a "person" for these purposes.

An affirmative answer can be justified; the fact that a conceptus cannot vote is immaterial. "Persons" include many groups that are not entitled to vote, including children, aliens, and persons convicted of crimes.[52] Like members of such groups, conceptuses have an interest in how voting rights are allocated because that allocation determines the weight to be given the votes of their parents and others directly concerned with their welfare. When the Fourteenth Amendment was being debated in Congress, Representative Blaine pointed out that "the nonvoting classes have a vital interest in the conduct of the Government."[53]

If conceptuses are "persons," an HLA would require that they be counted for purposes of congressional elections and apportionment of representatives.[54] This follows from the fact that application of the "one person, one vote" standard in federal elections has been rigorous and pregnancies are not necessarily distributed geographically in the same proportion as persons who have been born.

The Supreme Court has held that article I, section 2 of the United States Constitution requires congressional districts to be equal in size so that each person's vote has the same value, leaving no room for any classification of people in a way that unnecessarily abridges their voting rights.[55] Even an average variation between districts as small as 1.6 percent has been held an impermissible deviation from the required mathematical equality of population.[56]

A required inclusion of conceptuses for electoral purposes could control the allocation of congressional representation among states. One court has pointed out that "small shifts in population can make a significant difference in apportionment, especially at the state level. . . . The present 435th seat in Congress was awarded to Oklahoma rather than Oregon. If Oregon had had 250 more persons in its apportionment population, it would have been the other way around."[57] In 1973, the first year in which abortions generally were permissible under *Roe v. Wade* and *Doe v. Bolton* without regard to state restrictions, Oregon reported approximately 10,800 more abortions than Oklahoma.[58] Consequently, had an HLA been in effect in 1970 and conceptuses included in the census, there is a substantial likelihood that Oregon would have been entitled to the seat.

State and Local Elections

The potential effect of an HLA in state and local elections is less clear, as the standard for equality of representation[59] is less rigorous than in federal elections. Minor deviations from mathematical equality between districts do not make out a prima facie case of invidious discrimination.[60] Larger deviations may be permissible because of the acceptance of nonpopulation criteria, such as the integrity of political subdivisions.[61]

This conclusion assumes that a state could not explicitly exclude conceptuses for apportionment purposes. Although there is authority that states must use the same apportionment base as the federal government, at least in drawing up congressional districts,[62] for state political purposes they are not required to use total population figures derived from the federal census. Thus they need not count "aliens, transients, short-term or temporary residents, or persons denied the vote for conviction of crime."[63] But whether the states would be free under an HLA to exclude conceptuses is another matter.

The Constitution expressly forbids use of certain factors, such as military service,[64] for excluding persons from apportionment computation. No case has been found which considered whether minors or conceptuses are similarly protected from exclusion. If they are protected, or if a state chooses to count them as part of its legislative implementation of an HLA, the results under the more relaxed constitutional standard for state legislative apportionment are likely to be far less dramatic than in apportioning congressional representation.[65]

DISTRIBUTION OF GOVERNMENTAL FISCAL BENEFITS

A recent survey found 107 federal benefit programs which use census data as a factor in allocating funds.[66] Whether an HLA would require including conceptuses in the census figures for this purpose is uncertain. However, it is generally accepted that "Congress has far greater flexibility in allocating federal funds than is allowed in the distribution of political power."[67] Thus it is less likely that the effects of an HLA would be felt in this area.

In *Burns v. Alcala*,[68] the term "dependent child" as used in § 406 (a) of the Social Security Act[69] was held, as a matter of congressional intent, not to include the unborn. Whether this holding would survive an HLA is uncertain. If an HLA took the form of a statute, it would constitute a later expression of congressional intent than that which is embodied in the statutory provision construed in *Burns*. If an HLA were a constitutional amendment, it probably would be more important as evidence of congressional intent than as a limitation on congressional power.

CIVIL LIBERTIES

In addition to limiting or abolishing their constitutionally protected right to terminate pregnancies, an HLA might deprive women of other civil liberties they now enjoy. They might be required to lead less active lifestyles in order to preserve the life of a conceptus (or possible conceptus). The interests of the conceptus will often diverge from those of the woman in such matters. From the standpoint of the conceptus, a passive carrier who exposes it to the minimum risk of miscarriage or prenatal injury is preferred. She should not smoke, drink, or use any drugs with possible adverse effects on the conceptus. Coffee may be interdicted. Skiing, working in hazardous environments, flying, and riding in automobiles might be prohibited for such women in order to minimize possible adverse effects on the conceptus. Indeed, the Victorian regimen for upper-class pregnant women that minimizes activities either inside or outside the home might be ideal. Restricting the activities of potentially pregnant women might similarly be justified on the ground that such classification is necessary to protect the conceptus during the period between conception and proof of pregnancy.[70]

How far an HLA would lead the Court to go in requiring, or in allowing federal or state legislatures to require, such emphasis by pregnant or fertile women on their childbearing role is difficult to predict. Prior to *Roe v. Wade* the New Jersey Supreme Court had held that a pregnant woman could be compelled to undergo blood transfusions against her will in order to protect her life and that of the conceptus within her.[71] The potential sweep of an HLA goes much further. The worst, and least likely, scenario would include a full-scale state bureaucratic apparatus charged with regulating and monitoring the lifestyles of all pregnant or fertile women, seeking to maximize the safety of the conceptus regardless of costs to maternal privacy.[72] A far more plausible possibility would be class actions on behalf of conceptuses to enjoin various forms of behavior by pregnant or fertile women. Such suits might be authorized by an HLA itself, if it created an equitable liability for potential injury to conceptuses.[73]

At a minimum, an HLA could be expected to prohibit "abuse and neglect" of a conceptus by its carrier under existing statutes previously applied to children.[74] A harbinger of the possible scope of such prohibitions is *Hoener v. Bertinato*,[75] in which a New Jersey court ordered that blood transfusions be given the infant after delivery on the ground that the parents' refusal to authorize such transfusions constituted neglect.

FEDERAL INCOME TAX

The Internal Revenue Code is a somewhat unique domain in that deductions allowed in computing taxable income are often viewed by the courts as a matter of legislative grace,[76] seldom hindered by constitutional limitations. Because of such judicial deference, it is possible that an HLA would have no significant income tax consequences. But if this hurdle is overcome, the possible consequences surely would shock the proponents of an

HLA. In its most expansive potential application, an HLA could result in a tax expenditure in excess of $1 billion per year.

Section 151 (e)(l) of the Internal Revenue Code[77] allows an exemption (currently $1000)[78] for each dependent of the taxpayer, defined in § 152 (a) to include children as well as "[a]n individual . . . who . . . has as his principal place of abode the home of the taxpayer and is a member of the taxpayer's household."[79] To date, exemptions have not been allowed for conceptuses either as children or under the language just quoted,[80] and an HLA might not change this result.

If such exemptions are allowed, the consequences could be startling. The $1,000 exemption would be available for a woman during her pregnancy, which might include portions of two taxable years, whether or not the conceptus was born alive. Treasury Regulation § 1.152-1(b) provides: "(t)he fact that the dependent dies during the year shall not deprive the taxpayer of the deduction if the dependent lived in the household for the entire part of the year preceding his death."[81]

Assuming an average marginal tax rate of 25 percent, the cost of a $1,000 exemption for each of the reported 1,320,300 abortions in 1977[82] would have been $330 million. This does not take account of miscarriages, nor the possibility that two taxable years might be included in the period of pregnancy. A total revenue loss in excess of $1 billion per year is possible.

Ironically, an HLA could turn the dependency exemption into a mechanism for financing travel to procure abortions in other countries where the operation remains legal. Many abortions are legal under Canadian law,[83] and the round trip bus fare from Detroit to Toronto is currently about $50—far less than the value of a $1,000 exemption for a great many taxpayers.

In addition to the dependency exemption for the conceptus, the cost of a foreign abortion itself might be deductible as a medical expense. The Internal Revenue Service has ruled that the cost of an abortion "not illegal under state law" is deductible within the limits provided by § 213 [84] of the Internal Revenue Code.[85] If the availability of the deduction is determined by the law of the place where the operation is performed, rather than the taxpayer's state of residence,[86] the cost of Canadian abortions could be deducted by American taxpayers.

The variety of arguments that may be grounded on a determination that life begins at conception or fertilization is suggested by *Greer v. United States*,[87] in which a taxpayer contended that insurance proceeds received upon the death of a five-day-old racing horse are taxable as a long-term capital gain, on the ground that the taxpayer's holding period began with conception rather than birth. Although the Court of Appeals said that to so hold would not be to read the tax statute in its "ordinary and natural sense,"[88] the case illustrates the kind of suits with which courts could be required to deal.

Internal Revenue agents are trained to use delicacy and tact in dealing with the taxpaying public. But the audit of claimed exemptions for aborted or miscarried conceptuses, as well as for a pregnancy preceding a live birth, would place unusual strains on the often fragile taxpayer-agent relationship.

CRIMINAL LAW

The differences between the various versions of an HLA may have important consequences in relation to capital punishment and state-created criminal liabilities for abortions.

Capital Punishment

Although the various HLAs discussed in this article all refer to a "right to life," they do so in strikingly different terms which may affect the impact of a given HLA on capital punishment. The Ashbrook version refers to "the right to life guaranteed in this Constitution"[89] and arguably would have no effect on capital punishment, which is not unconstitutional per se.[90] Similarly, the Garn-Rhodes version would forbid depriving any unborn person of life but contains no comparable provision limiting post-birth deprivation.[91] Conversely, the Helms-Dornan[92] and Helms-Hyde[93] proposals refer to the right to life as "paramount," without qualification, and thus raise the question of whether such a paramount right can be reconciled with capital punishment under any circumstance.

State-created Liabilities for Abortion

Under *Roe v. Wade,* a woman may abort without fear of state-created criminal liability up to the point of viability.[94] Beyond that point, states are constitutionally free to impose criminal liability for abortion. However, as of 1980, 28 states and the District of Columbia had failed to do so.[95]

Similarly, destruction of the conceptus as a result of a third party's violent or reckless conduct, without the consent of the woman, generally is not considered homicide. Homicide prosecutions under statutes like Model Penal Code § 210[96] have typically failed because courts consider the statute inapplicable until the conceptus has been born alive, which is usually indicated by separate breathing.[97] Although California has amended its homicide statute to include viable conceptuses,[98] there is a virtually unbroken line of decisions elsewhere dating from 1797 which hold that the state must show actual physical independence of a conceptus to sustain a conviction for homicide.[99]

A number of states do make it a lesser criminal offense to cause the destruction of a "quick" conceptus.[100] However, many courts have concluded that the legislative concern was for the woman's life and health rather than for protection of the conceptus, and have required, as an essential element of the offense, that the injuries be inflicted with a malicious intent to kill the woman.[101]

The effect of an HLA on this aspect of criminal law would depend both on the particular version adopted and the extent to which a given state has exercised authority given by an HLA to criminalize conduct adversely affecting the conceptus. All versions presumably would *permit* the states to criminalize abortion. Some states would not choose to do so; several had decriminalized a large number of categories of abortions even before *Roe v. Wade* was decided.[102] Whether an HLA would permit Congress to criminalize abortions not involving interstate movement in some way may be affected by the language of the particular version adopted. [103]

TORTS

Tort law is an area in which an HLA would be unlikely to do more than accelerate a trend, already well established in many states, toward full recognition of conceptuses as "persons." The major result of an HLA might be to impose more uniform standards in this area.

Wrongful Death Actions

Until 1949, no state permitted a wrongful death action on behalf of *any* stillborn. In *Dietrich v. Northampton*,[104] the Supreme Judicial Court of Massachusetts, speaking through Justice Holmes, held that a child in the womb has no action for injuries leading to its premature birth and death. Erosion of the *Dietrich* rule began in *Bombrest v. Kotz*,[105] which allowed recovery for direct injury to a viable conceptus subsequently born alive. Today, a conceptus born alive generally is allowed to sue for prenatal injuries.[106]

Verkennes v. Corniea[107] extended the *Bombrest* rule to allow an action for the wrongful death of a stillborn conceptus. At least 25 states now permit such actions,[108] but most still require viability at the time of injury.[109] Only Rhode Island[110] and Georgia [111] permit actions for wrongful death of a conceptus from an injury occurring prior to viability.

Most jurisdictions now construe "person" as used in wrongful death statutes to include viable conceptuses. In *Roe v. Wade,* however, the Supreme Court explained that states which permit such suits do so "to vindicate the parents' interest and do not confer legal recognition of fetuses as 'persons' in the whole sense."[112]

Actions for Prenatal Injuries

Suits for prenatal injuries brought by a conceptus who is born alive generally are permitted.[113] The significant difference among states is that some require the injuries to have occurred after viability while others permit recovery for pre-viability injuries.[114] In effect, the latter group defines "person" for this purpose as including *any* conceptus that is later born alive, while the former group restricts the definition to *viable* conceptuses later born alive.

　　Thus, the major issue an HLA would raise is whether all states would be required to allow recovery for pre-viability as well as post-viability injuries. This in turn would depend on the reasonableness of a legislative classification based on the distinction between the two classes.[115]

HEALTH CARE AND MEDICAL MALPRACTICE

In *Roe v. Wade*, the Supreme Court expressed substantial concern for doctors' ability to exercise professional judgment free from state interference. The impact of an HLA on health care and in medical malpractice actions likely would be felt in the areas of medical treatment of pregnant women, birth control, physicians' reporting responsibilities, and the so-called "right to die."

Medical Treatment of Pregnant Women

Under *Roe v. Wade*, state regulation of medical procedures in the interest of the conceptus cannot commence until viability;[116] under an HLA, such regulation could commence with conception. If it does, medical procedures which may be harmful to a conceptus could become difficult to obtain. For example, dilation and curettage is a standard procedure for certain gynecological disorders. It consists of surgically scraping the lining of the uterus and therefore has the incidental effect of destroying any conceptus.[117] Physicians might be barred from using this procedure on pregnant women. Because of uncertainty as to whether a female patient is pregnant, doctors might be required to conduct a pregnancy test before using the procedure on any woman of child-bearing age.

Birth Control

The effects of an HLA on the utilization of birth control devices depend upon the precise moment identified as the starting point of "human life." The Ashbrook and Helms-Dornan versions refer to "fertilization;"[118] the Garn-Rhodes version leaves the matter unsettled by referring to "each stage of biological development."[119] Under all three versions, intrauterine devices, minipills, and "morning after" pills could be banned because they prevent pregnancy after fertilization or conception has occurred. The meaning of the Garn-Rhodes reference to "each stage of biological development" would remain for judicial interpretation. Thus the present freedom of contraceptive devices from state regulation[120] would be sharply curtailed.

Physician's Reporting Responsibilities

Many states require physicians to report injuries to or abuses of children to state agencies.[121] If an HLA leads to judicial construction of these statutes as including conceptuses in the class for which reporting is required, doctors would be required to report suspected injuries to or abuses of conceptuses as well. Depending on the scope of the physician's reporting requirement, pregnant women may be forced to curtail activities that may be detrimental to conceptuses.[122]

The So-called "Right to Die"

One of the most controversial areas which could be greatly affected by an HLA is the qualified right individuals now enjoy to refuse life-saving medical treatment.[123] Courts derive this "right to die"[124] from several sources. The earliest cases, which usually involved Jehovah's Witnesses who refused blood transfusions because of their religious beliefs, were concerned with the patient's religious freedom[125] and the common law right to be free from unconsented-to touching.[126] Later cases have focused on the individual's right to privacy, which includes the right to determine what will be done with one's body.[127] *In re Quinlan*[128] recognized this right to privacy and held that incompetent persons have the same right as competent persons to refuse treatment, even though someone else actually makes the choice on behalf of the incompetent. Currently, statutes in at least ten states provide for a "right to die," generally allowing individuals to direct a physician to withhold medical treatment at some later date.[129] The directive usually becomes effective when the patient is unable to exercise his right to refuse medical treatment and is not expected to recover.

Courts have identified four state interests[130] to be balanced against the interest of an individual in refusing treatment: (1) the preservation of life; (2) the maintenance of the ethical integrity of medical treatment; (3) the protection of the interests of innocent third parties; and (4) the prevention of suicide. Of these four, the first two have generally been considered the most important.[131] In balancing the individual and state interests, courts have considered whether the individual is an adult or a minor, whether competent or incompetent, whether the treatment is likely to cure the disease or merely prolong life, and whether the treatment involves an extensive invasion of the individual's person.[132]

Courts have split over whether competent adults in nonemergency situations can refuse treatment, though they are more likely to permit refusal when the physical invasion is great or the prognosis with further treatment unfavorable.[133] There seems to be a greater tendency now for courts to uphold the individual's right to refuse treatment.[134]

When the patient is incompetent, the court assumes a different role. Since incompetent adults have the same right as competent adults to refuse treatment,[135] and because they are unable to exercise that right themselves, courts,[136] parents, or guardians ad litem[137] use "substituted judgment" and make the decision based on what the patient would choose if competent. If the choice is to refuse treatment, the patient's interest in refusing is balanced against the state's interests in the same way as a competent adult's interest is so balanced. The value or quality of a handicapped or retarded individual's life does not enter the analysis.[138]

The process in a case involving a minor is similar to that for an incompetent adult. Courts, in their role as *parens patriae,* will use "substituted judgment," rejecting the parents' refusal and ordering treatment if it is in the best interest of the child.[139]

By making the right to life "paramount," the Helms-Dornan version[140] could supersede an individual's right to die. Alternatively, it could be viewed as merely requiring that greater weight be given the state's interest in the preservation of life. That interest and the individual's privacy interest in this area have been compared to their counterparts in the abortion cases,[141] where the woman's privacy interest conflicts with the state's interest. If a balancing of interests is required in the right to die area, it is difficult to predict the extent to which an HLA would affect the balance.

LABORATORY RESEARCH AND IN VITRO FERTILIZATION

At present there is extensive federal[142] and state[143] regulation of laboratory work involving conceptuses. Generally such work is permitted, but with strict controls on the permissible level of risk. Under an HLA, it would be no more permissible to experiment on conceptuses than on individuals after birth. Statutes permitting research on conceptuses outside of the uterus would probably be unconstitutional violations of equal protection, leading to what one commentator has described as the "anomalous result of requiring physicians to let fetuses die, only to be studied and experimented upon after death."[144]

In vitro fertilization, which now offers hope otherwise denied to childless women, might likewise be curbed because of serious doubt as to whether a physician would be permitted to discard ova which are fertilized outside the womb and not implanted. Without an affirmative answer to this issue, in vitro fertilization could be effectively blocked.

GENDER-BASED EMPLOYMENT DISCRIMINATION

The struggle to secure equal employment opportunities for women was painfully slow until the enactment of Title VII of the Civil Rights Act of 1964.[145] As a result of Title VII, many women have entered a wide-ranging variety of occupations previously reserved for men. In recent years, however, many companies have adopted a policy of excluding fertile women from jobs in which they might come in contact with certain chemicals known as teratogens. These chemicals destroy more cells in the conceptus than can be replaced by later proliferation.[146] Some women, faced with the alternative of losing a high-paying job, have chosen to be sterilized.[147] Others have sued their employers, asserting that such a policy violated Title VII of the Act.[148]

As yet, no reported case appears to deal with this issue.[149] An HLA could have a large impact in such litigation, and may require or encourage governmental action to exclude fertile or pregnant women from jobs involving possible hazards to the conceptus. Such exclusion could severely restrict women's job opportunities. The Equal Employment Opportunity Commission (EEOC) estimates that as many as 20 million jobs may involve exposure to alleged reproductive hazards.[150]

Present Law

Bona Fide Occupational Qualification Requirement Under Title VII, explicit exclusionary employment practices based on sex are permissible only if sex is a "bona fide occupational qualification (BFOQ) reasonably necessary to the normal operation of (an employer's) particular business or enterprise."[151] Additionally, facially neutral employment policies that have discriminatory impact[152] will violate Title VII unless they arise from business necessity. Although often confused by the courts,[153] these two forms of discrimination are distinct, having separate defenses.

Both the courts[154] and the EEOC[155] have interpreted the BFOQ defense very narrowly, using varying expressions of the standard which employers seeking to invoke the defense must satisfy. In *Weeks v. Southern Bell Telephone & Telegraph*,[156] the Fifth Circuit Court of Appeals demanded that the employer have "reasonable cause to believe, that is, a factual basis for believing, that all or substantially all women would be unable to perform safely or efficiently the duties of the job involved." In *Diaz v. Pan American World Airways*[157] the same court required that the essence of the business operation be undermined by hiring members of both sexes. The Supreme Court quoted these formulations in *Dothard v. Rawlinson*.[158] A somewhat different view was applied by the Ninth Circuit Court of Appeals in *Rosenfeld v. Southern Pacific Co.*,[159] which required that the job call for specific physical characteristics necessarily possessed by one sex.

Permissible explicit sex-based discrimination in employment was further curtailed by the 1978 Pregnancy Amendment[160] to Title VII. This amendment was enacted in response to the Supreme Court's decision in *General Electric Co. v. Gilbert*,[161] which held nondiscriminatory an employer's health insurance plan that covered almost everything except pregnancy. The amendment includes the following definition:

> The terms "because of sex" or "on the basis of sex" include, but are not limited to, because of or on the basis of pregnancy, childbirth, or related medical conditions; and women affected by pregnancy, childbirth, or related medical conditions, shall be treated the same for all employment related purposes . . . as are other persons not so affected but similar in their ability to work.[162]

Although fertility is not expressly included in the Pregnancy Amendment, the House Report states that the bill's "protection extends to the whole range of matters concerning the childbearing process."[163] The amendment should be interpreted to include fertility as well as pregnancy; otherwise, women could be excluded from certain jobs before, but not after, becoming pregnant—an anomalous result.

Present law probably would not allow employers to rely on the BFOQ defense as a basis for excluding fertile women from toxic workplaces.[164] The EEOC issued (but later withdrew) guidelines which stated that the defense would not apply to such an exclusion as no question concerning the woman's ability to perform a job is raised by the fact that she is fertile.[165]

Employers are more likely to assert a duty to protect the conceptus rather than the woman herself as a reason for excluding fertile women from a given job.[166] Safety has indeed been a factor in the courts' determination of the validity of BFOQ defenses, but it has been the safety of other employees or customers,[167] not of either the employee alleging discrimination[168] or the conceptus.[169] Cases dealing with a BFOQ defense based in part on safety of the conceptus have dealt with airlines' mandatory leaves for pregnant flight attendants.[170] Although the decisions are divided,[171] the courts were concerned in each instance with whether a flight attendant's pregnancy would reduce the safety of air travel, not whether it would reduce the safety of the attendant herself or of the conceptus.[172] One judge noted: "Eastern does not have a sufficiently compelling interest in the health of its flight attendants to override the discriminatory impact of its policy. Eastern's business is transportation by air, not maternity care."[173] Possible dangers to the conceptus were likewise dismissed because they did not "give rise to a significant operational concern."[174]

An employer's assertion of a duty to protect conceptuses as a justification for explicit discrimination against women presents a problem of underinclusiveness: both maternal and paternal exposure to toxic workplaces can injure conceptuses. Given the nature of the toxic substances that affect conceptuses, it is unlikely that fertile women are sufficiently more vulnerable than fertile men to justify increased protection of women.

There are three varieties of toxic substances that affect conceptuses: mutagens, teratogens, and transplacental carcinogens.[175] Mutagens damage the genetic material of the parent prior to conception.[176] Teratogens pass through the placenta[177] destroying more cells in the conceptus than can be replaced by later proliferation.[178] Although the woman must be exposed to the teratogen before it can affect the conceptus, this exposure can result from exposure to another person, who functions as a carrier, introducing the teratogen into the environment.[179] Transplacental carcinogens act on the cells in the conceptus to cause cancer.[180] Currently, the only known agent that works this way is diethylstilbesterol (DES), which causes vaginal adenosis in young women prenatally exposed to it.[181] Consequently, only if the workplace hazard is either a transplacental carcinogen or a teratogen without carry-home effects could an employer's duty to protect conceptuses support a BFOQ defense against charges of explicit discrimination against pregnant or fertile women.

Discriminatory Effect, Business Necessity and Concern for Possible Tort Liability The business necessity defense, available in Title VII actions alleging that facially neutral employment policies have a discriminatory impact, has been narrowly applied.[182] Nevertheless, employers might attempt to rely on a duty to protect conceptuses as giving rise to a defense of business necessity. In such a case, the relevant analysis would be essentially similar to that for the BFOQ defense discussed above.

Some employers may regard the Occupational Safety and Health Act of 1970[183] as partially superseding Title VII's requirements of non-discrimination in employment. The Act was passed "to assure so far as possible every working man and woman in the Nation safe and healthful working conditions and to preserve our human resources."[184] It is administered by the Occupational Safety and Health Agency (OSHA), which is authorized to "provide medical criteria which will assure insofar as practicable that no employee will suffer diminished health, functional capacity, or life expectancy as a result of his work experience."[185] Industries for which OSHA has not established a standard are governed by the Act's general duty clause, which requires that every employer "shall furnish to each of his employees employment and a place of employment which are free from recognized hazards that are causing or are likely to cause death or serious physical harm to his employees."[186]

The focus of the Act is on the worker's health and safety.[187] Although the inability to bear a healthy child would be included in the phrase "diminished . . . functional capacity," it would be ironic if OSHA chose to protect fertile females by requiring or permitting employers to exclude them from the workplace while leaving fertile males unprotected.[188] OSHA's lead exposure standards do seek to protect conceptuses as well as employees, but OSHA does not pursue this goal by barring fertile females from particular jobs.[189]

Possible Effects of an HLA

The adoption of an HLA could cut off access to jobs for women by strengthening both the BFOQ defense to charges of explicit discrimination and the business necessity defense to charges of discriminatory effect. In addition, it could validate state legislation which seeks to protect women and their potential offspring from the hazards of the workplace by excluding them from employment opportunities.[190]

Explicit Discrimination and BFOQ Defense An HLA could be construed to make the protection of the life and well-being of the conceptus the duty of the employer and part of the essence of the business enterprise. Such a duty could justify explicit discrimination against pregnant or fertile women by providing the employer with a BFOQ defense. Exclusion of women who are fertile but not pregnant might be justified because of the problem of determining pregnancy in its early stages. If only pregnant women were excluded, employers would be permitted, or even required, to administer regular pregnancy tests to fertile female employees.[191] How a duty to protect conceptuses against teratogens with carry-home effects could be carried out is unclear: the employer might not know who might be contaminated by male employees carrying home teratogens.

In view of these difficulties in finding a BFOQ defense for employers based on a duty to protect conceptuses, courts may be inclined to avoid the problems by finding no such duty. But before either conclusion is reached, extensive litigation could be required to deal with employers' real or feigned concerns in this area.

Discriminatory Effect, Business Necessity and Possible Concern for Tort Liability An HLA could strengthen the business necessity defense by increasing employers' exposure to tort liability.[192] This threat could then be seen as sufficiently compelling to justify the exclusion of fertile men and women from certain jobs. Excluding fertile women, but not fertile men, could more readily be justified if changes occurred in tort liability for wrongful termination of and prenatal injuries to conceptuses.[193] If the workplace hazard was teratogenic with a carry-home effect, exclusion of women but not men would be difficult to justify.

State "Protective" Legislation Restricting Employment of Women A mass of state legislation and administrative regulations formerly sought to protect women and their potential offspring from the hazards of the workplace.[194] Such legislation severely hampered women in the quest for equal employment opportunities. Because "such laws and regulations do not take into account the capacities,[195] preferences, and abilities of individual females,"[196] the EEOC has regarded them as invalid discriminations on the basis of sex. Many have been struck down as violating Title VII.[197]

An HLA could breath new life into this body of legislation. An explicit grant of legislative authority to the states could provide a basis for broadly defined exclusions of pregnant or fertile women from a variety of allegedly hazardous occupations.

ESTATES, PROPERTY, AND TRUSTS

The key to the property rights of a conceptus has always been the requirement of live birth. No case has been found in which a share of a decedent's estate vested in a conceptus that was never born alive. The common understanding that birth alive is necessary for a property interest to vest in a claimant is reflected in § 2-1.3(a) of the New York Estates, Powers and Trust Law (NYEPTL): "Unless the creator expresses a contrary intention, a disposition of property to persons described in any instrument as the issue . . . children, descendants, heirs . . . of the creator or another, includes: . . . children conceived before, but *born alive* after such disposition becomes effective."[198] This is a statutory embodiment of *Marsellis v. Thalhimer*,[199] the first American case to consider whether one could inherit through a stillborn child. The live birth requirement has been adhered to ever since.[200]

Were the live birth requirement superseded by an HLA, there would be chaos in the law of estates, property, and trusts. The illustrations in this section are from the NYEPTL but could be duplicated under the laws of many jurisdictions.

Lapse Statutes

NYEPTL § 3-3.3(a) provides: "Whenever a testamentary disposition is made to the issue or to a brother or sister of the testator, and such beneficiary dies during the lifetime of the testator leaving issue surviving such testator, such disposition does not lapse but vests in such surviving issue, per stirpes."[201] If the testator's brother predeceases the testator, leaving a wife who is pregnant, but who later miscarries, did the brother leave "issue surviving"? If he did, the estate of the conceptus would take a share which would then pass to his mother by intestacy.

Intestacy Statutes

NYEPTL § 4-1.1(a) provides for distribution of shares of the estates of intestate decendents to "children" or "issue."[202] If these terms include a conceptus which was never born alive, its share would in turn pass by intestacy to its parents under § 4-1.1(1)(3), not to its siblings.[203] The result would be anomalous. For example, assume an intestate male decendent is survived by a wife, a child, and a conceptus that was later miscarried. Under § 4-1.1,[204] the wife would receive $4,000 and one-third of the residue, the child would receive one-third, and the estate of the conceptus one-third. If the wife were the mother of the conceptus, she would be the sole heir of its estate and would thus receive two one-third shares of the residue of her husband's estate, instead of the one-half share mandated by the legislature for men who die intestate leaving a wife and one child. If the mother of the conceptus were another woman, she would similarly be entitled to the estate of the conceptus. Thus an incentive would be created for women to assert that they were pregnant with the conceptus of an intestate decedent when he died, and that the conceptus did not miscarry until after his death.

Miscellaneous Provisions

Under NYEPTL § 5-1.1,[205] the size of the share of a surviving spouse who elects against a decedent's will depends on whether the decedent is survived by issue. Is a conceptus, later stillborn, issue for this purpose?

Under NYEPTL § 5-3.1, if there is no surviving spouse, an exemption of specified property from disposition as part of a decedent's estate is provided for the benefit of "children under the age of 21 years. . . ."[206]

NYEPTL § 5-3.2 provides,[207] under specified circumstances, a share of a decendent's estate for a child born after the execution of the will. Would this include a conceptus, later stillborn?

NYEPTL § 6-5.6[208] provides for construction of certain remainders as referring to "persons living at the death of the person named as ancestor," which might be held to include a conceptus later stillborn. Section 6-5.7(b)[209] raises a different issue by referring specifically to the effect on certain dispositions of "the birth of a child conceived before but born *alive* after the death of such person" (emphasis added). It could be contended that this is an unconstitutional discrimination against a conceptus who was not born alive.

POTENTIAL SOCIAL COSTS AND UNCERTAINTIES CREATED BY AN HLA

> *Afflictions sorted, anguish of all sizes,*
> *Fine nets and stratagems to catch us in,*
> *Bibles laid open, millions of surprises.*
> —George Herbert, The Temple, "Sin," Stanza 2 (1633)

The substantive effects of an HLA in areas other than abortion could be severely limited by judicial decisions. If that happens, the problems posed earlier will be resolved in due course. But the years required to complete this process may stretch into a decade or more. The social costs of chaos and confusion in the legal system while this process is taking place would be very high. There is *no* justification for incurring these costs merely to achieve a more favorable charisma for a constitutional amendment to limit or ban abortion.[210] The potentially heavy cost of finding out what an HLA means will be felt by the courts, Congress, state legislatures, administrative agencies, and the private sector.

COURTS

The initial impact of an HLA undoubtedly would be greatest in the courts, as litigants seek to determine its impact in areas other than abortion. Chief

Justice Burger has suggested that congressional committees prepare "court impact statements" for legislation creating new rights, which would include estimates of the number of new judges and support personnel required to handle the new cases generated by the legislation. These statements would insure "that Congress consider the needs of the courts along with the need for the new legislation."[211] If such a statement were to be prepared for an HLA, the estimated cost figures would be very high.

Whether an HLA is to be construed broadly or narrowly can only be determined by litigation in many different areas. Until the Supreme Court has clearly defined the scope of an HLA, lawyers are likely to bring test cases in all of the areas described earlier. Where deeply held opinions are involved or significant sums are at stake, novel arguments will be advanced by resourceful plaintiffs. For instance, class actions seeking to regulate the conduct of pregnant (or potentially pregnant) women may be expected.[212] Would-be heirs of a stillborn's estate are certain to litigate,[213] and the Internal Revenue Service will be forced to respond to conceptus-related exemptions and deductions.[214] Government operations may be impeded by census litigation to determine whether conceptuses were properly counted or even needed to be counted.[215]

In the area of property and estates, New York's experience with the impact of constitutional uncertainties of probate practice is instructive. In *In re del Drago's Estate*[216] the Court of Appeals held that the predecessor to §2-1.8 of the NYEPTL, dealing with the manner in which persons interested in an estate share the burden of federal estate taxes, violated the supremacy clause.[217] Almost a year followed before the United States Supreme Court reversed the decision.[218] During that year, the administration of many New York estates was severely impeded because of uncertainty as to the size of the shares of the legatees. In *del Drago*, moreover, the facts were undisputed. In many cases dealing with the effects of an HLA, major evidentiary problems are sure to arise. In the words of the Commission on Civil Rights:

> [S]uch litigation would probably be characterized by disputes over whether the woman was pregnant, when the moment of conception occurred, what the potential value of the fetus was, based on its stage of development, and such other matters which are not easily determined. . . . [S]uits will, more than ever before, proceed with crowds of medical witnesses.[219]

Finally, an HLA may authorize the states to pass implementing legislation. If experience under the Twenty-first Amendment, prohibiting transportation of liquor into a state in violation of its laws, is any guide, litigation over the scope of state legislative authority under an HLA is likely to be substantial.[220]

CONGRESS AND STATE LEGISLATION

Just as an HLA could be expected to spur litigants to test its effect in various fields, so it will prompt legislative bodies to rewrite or attempt to clarify numerous laws in light of the new status accorded to conceptuses. Legislative revision may be required to indicate the circumstances under which a conceptus will be treated as a person. If differences in treatment for any given statutory purpose are believed (or held) unconstitutional, further revisions would be required to meet constitutional standards.

One danger inherent in any such process of legislative revision is that consensus may prove to be a fragile creature in the context of controversial legislation. If an HLA creates a need for revision of a large number of statutory laws, it may be difficult to secure agreement on the form such revision shall take.

ADMINISTRATIVE AGENCIES

Three types of practical administrative problems can be anticipated: (1) obtaining a correct count of conceptuses in the population, broken down by states and political subdivisions; (2) determining the age of individuals; and (3) revising administrative regulations to conform to judicially determined requirements stemming from the HLA. The last is similar to the tasks for legislatures and courts described above. The first two merit further analysis.

Counting Conceptuses

Population counts are critical in legislative apportionment[221] and distribution of governmental fiscal benefits.[222] If income tax consequences are to follow from recognition of "life" as existing from the moment of conception,[223] the Internal Revenue Service as well as the Census Bureau will be involved. Counting conceptuses as part of the population, or as dependents, requires that the census taker recognize the moment of conception, something that medical science is unable to do: pregnancy cannot be identified at the moment of conception, fertilization, or even implantation.[224] As a result, some miscarriages will go undetected and, conversely, some fraudulent claims based on nonexistent conceptuses will be difficult to unmask. Further, it is administratively impossible to count conceptuses at a single point in time; this problem cannot be avoided by counting them retroactively after birth. According to one estimate, as many as 60 percent of all pregnancies terminate from natural causes, often before the woman knows she is pregnant.[225]

Proponents of an HLA have asserted without explanation that an HLA's requirements would apply "only when the existence of the child [sic] is knowable"[226] or after positive proof of pregnancy.[227] However, as two commentators have responded: "[t]his may be one solution to the dilemma created by these amendments, but it is not what the amendments themselves say."[228] The most practical solutions are a set of arbitrary count-back lines, comparable to the 300-day presumptions used by some states in paternity suits,[229] or a statutory requirement that all positive pregnancy tests be reported to a registrar in same way live births are reported. As a conceptus can be identified, before birth, only by the name of the mother, this would require a governmental index of the names of pregnant women.

Determining the Age of Individuals

The Constitution sets minimum ages for eligibility for public offices[230] and for exercise of the right to vote.[231] A host of legislative provisions use age to measure either the time for receipt of benefits or the imposition of obligations, such as military service and school attendance. Property interests often vest upon attainment of designated ages. Up to now, age has been measured from birth. If a conceptus is a "person" from the moment of conception, should age be measured from the moment of conception? Possibly the answer would depend upon the purpose for which age was being determined. Even if an HLA ultimately requires no change in current practice, the issue provides another basis for litigation.

THE PRIVATE SECTOR

Until an HLA has been extensively tested in the courts, no one will know what its actual effects will be. This uncertainty may impede business transactions and estate planning and will add to legal fees. For some companies, the cost of doing business may increase, as is illustrated above in the context of employment discrimination.[232] Furthermore, businesses may be inhibited from making commitments which depend on either the validity or invalidity of a given statute or rule in light of an HLA.

For individuals, there will be a premium on all-inclusive estate planning to foresee every contingency under an HLA, including its anomalous effects on rules of inheritance.[233] But the most serious surprises are, by definition, the unpredictable ones. The best illustrations of unanticipated results which can attend constitutional amendments come from our national experience with prohibition[234] and repeal,[235] the only post-Reconstruction constitutional amendments to address a broad social question and to authorize implementing state legislation. Both provided their share of surprising judicial decisions. In *Lambert v. Yellowly*,[236] for example, the Supreme Court held that the Eighteenth Amendment gave Congress the power to prohibit even medical uses of alcohol. In *United States v. Mack*,[237] the Court held that the Twenty-first Amendment did not render unenforceable existing contractual liabilities premised on prohibition. The biggest surprise to stem from the Twenty-first Amendment was a decision almost 40 years after its adoption that it limited liberties previously protected by the Bill of Rights. In *California v. Larue*,[238] the Supreme Court sustained an ordinance forbidding live entertainment in establishments licensed to sell liquor, holding that the ordinance was authorized by the power granted states under the amendment. Then, in *New York State Liquor Authority v. Bellanca*,[239] the Court held that the amendment conferred "broad powers"[240] on a state to prohibit topless dancing in establishments where liquor is served even though such activity would normally be protected by the First Amendment. Justice Stevens, dissenting, complained that "a state may [now] ban any protected activity" on premises where liquor is sold "no matter how innocuous, or, more importantly, how clearly protected."[241]

This surprising result arose because, as one commentator has noted, the Twenty-first Amendment is the "only presently operative portion of the Constitution which the Supreme Court has construed as granting power to the states."[242] An HLA would similarly create concurrent state and federal enforcement authority and may likewise usher in surprising new exercises of state legislative power, but on far broader fronts than the Twenty-first Amendment.

CONCLUSION

All versions of an HLA share two fundamental flaws: (1) they could create chaos throughout our legal system in areas having no direct connection with abortion; and (2) they could create needless uncertainty until the courts determined their implications. If abortions are to be banned or restricted, the appropriate way to do so is through a constitutional amendment dealing directly with abortions, and not by defining "persons" to include conceptuses.

NOTES

1. 410 U.S. 113 (1973). For reviews of the constitutional issues involved in Roe v. Wade, see L. TRIBE, AMERICAN CONSTITUTIONAL LAW § 15-10 (1978): Ely, *The Wages of Crying Wolf: A Comment on* Roe v. Wade, 82 Yale L.J. 920 (1973); Epstein, *Substantive Due Process by Any Other Name: The Abortion Cases*, 1973 SUP. CT. REV. 159; Henkin, *Privacy and Autonomy*, 74 COLUM. L. REV. 1410

(1974); Heymann & Barzelay, *The Forest and the Trees: Roe v. Wade and its Critics*, 53 B.U.L. REV. 765 (1973); Perry, *Abortion, the Public Morals, and the Police Power: The Ethical Function of Substantive Due Process*, 23 U.C.L.A. L. REV. 689 (1976); Regan, *Rewriting* Roe v. Wade, 77 MICH. L. REV. 1569 (1979); Tribe, *Foreword: Toward a Model of Roles in the Due Process of Life and Law*, 87 HARV. L. REV. 1 (1973).

2. *See, e.g.*, Doe v. Bolton, 410 U.S. 179 (1973) (invalidating state requirements that abortions take place in an accredited hospital with committee approval and written concurrences by two doctors other than the performing physician that an abortion was justified); Planned Parenthood v. Danforth, 428 U.S. at 75-79 (state cannot restrict abortions by requiring a virtually unavailable medical procedure); Colautti v. Franklin, 439 U.S. 379 (1979) (state cannot chill the exercise of a woman's right to choose by creating vague definitions of viability for the purpose of determining physicians' criminal liability). Requirements of spousal or parental consent have also been invalidated. *See* Planned Parenthhood v. Danforth, 428 U.S. 52, 67-75 (1976) (spousal consent or parental consent in the case of an unmarried minor); Bellotti v. Baird, 443 U.S. 662 (1979) (parental consent in the case of a minor). *But see* H.L. v. Matheson, 450 U.S. 398 (1981) (upholding state statute requiring physicians to notify unmarried minor's parents before performing abortion).

3. *See generally* A. MERTON, ENEMIES OF CHOICE—THE RIGHT TO LIFE MOVEMENT AND ITS THREAT TO ABORTION (1981).

4. The amendment, a rider to an appropriations bill for the Department of Health, Education and Welfare, was enacted in 1976. Pub. L. No. 94-439, § 209, 90 Stat. 1418, 1434 (reenacted in Pub. L. No. 96-123, § 109, 93 Stat. 923, 926 (1979)). For its background see Harris v. McRae, 448 U.S. 297, 302-03 (1980).

5. Indirect support continues through the allowance of an income tax deduction for medical expenses. *See infra* notes 84-85 and accompanying text.

6. *See* Harris v. McRae, 448 U.S. 297 (1980). *See also* Maher v. Roe, 432 U.S. 464 (1977) (upholding state welfare department regulation limiting Medicaid benefits to first trimester abortions that were medically necessary).

7. *See supra* note 2.

8. Similar responses greeted the Supreme Court's decision barring public school prayer; *see Senate Fails to Amend School Prayer Ruling*, 22 CONG. Q. ALMANAC 512 (1966); requiring equal weight for each person's vote, *see* Monroe, *To Preserve the United States: A Brief for the Negative on Three Current Plans to Amend the Constitution*, 8 ST. LOUIS U.L.J. 533, 539 (1963); and approving forced busing to remedy racial discrimination, *see* 118 CONG. REC. 4625 (1972) (comments of several constitutional law scholars).

9. *See, e.g.*, Rice, *Overriding* Roe v. Wade: *An Analysis of the Proposed Constitutional Amendments*, 15 B.C. INDUS & COM. L. REV. 307, 341 (1973).

10. *E.g.*, H.R.J. Res. 96, 94th Cong., 1st Sess. (1975): "Section 1. Nothing in this Constitution shall bar any State or Territory or the District of Columbia, with

regard to any area over which it has jurisdiction, from allowing, regulating, or prohibiting the practice of abortion."

11. *See infra* notes 13-14 and accompanying text.

12. *See infra* note 16 and accompanying text.

13. H.R.J. Res. 13, 97th Cong., 1st Sess. (1981). Identical versions have been introduced by Representatives Guyer and Hyde; *see* H.R.J. Res 32, 97th Cong., 1st Sess. (1981).

14. S.J. Res. 17, 97th Cong., 1st Sess. (1981); H.R.J. Res. 62, 97th Cong., 1st Sess. (1981). Identical versions have been introduced by Senator Grassley and by Representatives Emerson, Luken, Mazzoli, Oberstar and Fish. S.J. Res. 18, 97th Cong., 1st Sess. (1981); H.R.J. Res. 27, 97th Cong., 1st Sess. (1981); H.R.J. Res. 99, 97th Cong., 1st Sess. (1981); H.R.J. Res. 122, 97th Cong., 1st Sess. (1981); H.R.J. Res. 125, 97th Cong., 1st Sess. (1981); H.R.J. Res. 133, 97th Cong., 1st Sess. (1981). In addition, four variations of the Garn-Rhodes proposal have been introduced by Representatives Hansen, Volkmer, Zablocki, and Russo. Representative Hansen's proposal differs as follows:

> Section 2. This article shall not apply in an emergency when a reasonable medical certainty exists that continuation of the pregnancy will cause the death of the mother.

H.R.J. Res. 39, 97th Cong., 1st Sess. (1981). Representative Volkmer's proposal differs as follows:

> Section 4. This article shall be inoperative unless it shall have been ratified as an amendment to the Constitution by the legislatures of three-fourths of the several States, within ten years of the date of its submission to the States by the Congress.

H.R.J. Res. 92, 97th Cong., 1st Sess. (1981). Representative Zablocki's proposal differs as follows:

> Section 2. No unborn person shall be deprived of life by any person: Provided, however, that nothing in this article shall prohibit a law permitting those medical procedures required to save the life of the mother when a reasonable medical certainty exists that continuation of pregnancy will cause the death of the mother, and requiring that person to make every reasonable effort, in keeping with good medical practice, to preserve the life of her unborn offspring.

H.R.J. Res. 127, 97th Cong., 1st Sess. (1981). Representative Russo's proposal differs as follows:

> Section 2. No abortion shall be performed by any person except under and in conformance with a law which (1) authorizes the performance of an abortion only when a reasonable medical certainty exists that continuation of the pregnancy would result in the death of the mother, and (2) requires that the person performing the abortions make every reasonable effort, in keeping with good medical practice, to preserve the life of any person who is the subject of the abortion.

H.R.J. Res. 198, 97th Cong., 1st Sess. (1981).

15. S.J. Res. 19, 97th Cong., 1st Sess. (1981): H.R.J. Res. 104, 97th Cong., 1st Sess. (1981). Identical versions have been introduced by Representative Gaydos, H.R.J. Res. 106, 97th Cong., 1st Sess. (1981), and Representative Paul, H.R. 392, 97th Cong., 1st Sess. (1981).

16. S. 158, 97th Cong., 1st Sess. (1981); H.R. 900, 97th Cong., 1st Sess. (1981).

17. 410 U.S. at 156-57.

18. *See supra* note 14 and accompanying text.

19. *See infra* notes 89-92 and accompanying text.

20. For a discussion of these issues, see L. TRIBE, AMERICAN CONSTITUTIONAL LAW § 5-14 (1978).

21. *Id.* § 3-8.

22. *See* Nat'l Right to Life News, June 15, 1981, at 5, col. 4. ("[I]f you can repeat 'kill babies' in proper context and often enough, you will win more minds and hearts than your anti-life opponents.")

23. Conceptus is defined as "the sum of derivatives of a fertilized ovum at any stage of development from fertilization until birth, including extraembryonic membranes as well as the embryo or fetus." DORLAND'S ILLUSTRATED MEDICAL DICTIONARY 296 (26th ed. 1981).

24. *See generally* L. TRIBE, AMERICAN CONSTITUTIONAL LAW § 18 (1978).

25. Martinez v. California, 444 U.S. 277 (1980).

26. Dale, Potential Implications of S. 158 for the Legal Rights of the Unborn in Traditional Areas of Tort, Property, and Criminal Law 33 (Apr. 21, 1981) (unpublished manuscript available from Congressional Research Service).

27. *See Hearing on S.J. Res. 199 and S.J. Res. 139 Before Subcomm. on Constitutional Amendments of the Senate Comm. on the Judiciary*, 93d Cong., 2nd Sess., 78 (1974) (testimony of Senator Buckley stating that idea of fetuses acquiring substantial rights is "silliness").

28. *See, e.g.*, Boston Sunday Globe, Apr. 12, 1981, at 11, col. 1. ("[Senator] East indicated that, by focusing on the definition of life, he hoped to avoid a general debate on the abortion issue itself, and thus get quicker Congressional approval.")

29. *See supra* notes 13-16 and accompanying text.

30. *See infra* notes 70-75 and accompanying text.

31. *See generally* L. TRIBE, AMERICAN CONSTITUTIONAL LAW § 16 (1978).

32. "[N]or shall any state deprive any person of life, liberty, or property, without due process of law; nor deny to any person within its jurisdiction the equal protection of the laws." U.S. CONST. amend. XIV, § 1.

33. *Id.*

34. U.S. CONST. amend. XXVI, § 1.

35. *See* Roe v. Wade, 410 U.S. 113, 156-62 (1973).

36. *See* Rice, *supra* note 9, at 326. Professor Tribe appears to concur in the equal protection approach. *See* Tribe, *Foreword: Toward a Model of Roles in the Due Process of Life and Law*, 87 HARV. L. REV. 1, 32-33 n.144 (1973).

37. *See* L. TRIBE, AMERICAN CONSTITUTIONAL LAW § 16-3 (1978).

38. *See id.* § 16-6.

39. *See id.* § 16-30.

40. *See* United States v. Carolene Prods. Co., 304 U.S. 144, 152-53 n.4 (1938) (dictum). Justice Stone defined such minorities in terms of political powerlessness.

41. Byrn, *The Abortion Amendments: Policy in the Light of Precedent*, 18 St. Louis U.L.J. 380, 405 (1974).

42. Rice, *supra* note 9, at 340.

43. *See, e.g.,* Korematsu v. United States, 323 U.S. 214, 216 (1944). *See generally* J. Nowak, R. Rotunda & J. Young, Handbook on Constitutional Law 524 (1978).

44. *See* Byrn, *supra* note 41, at 394.

45. *See infra* notes 88-99 and accompanying text.

46. *See infra* notes 99-101 and accompanying text.

47. *Burger is Critical of Writing of Laws,* N.Y. Times, June 2, 1981, at B9, col. 6 (quoting Chief Justice Burger).

48. *Compare* White v. Weiser, 412 U.S. 783 (1973) (small deviation in population among congressional districts not permitted) *with* cases cited *infra* at note 63.

49. U.S. Const., amend. XIV, § 2.

50. U.S. Const., art. I, §§ 2,3.

51. *See* Wesberry v. Sanders, 376 U.S. 1 (1964).

52. Federation for Am. Immigration Reform v. Klutznick, 486 F. Supp. 564 (D.D.C.), *appeal dismissed,* 447 U.S. 995 (1980) (illegal aliens must be included).

53. Cong. Globe, 39th Cong., 1st Sess. 141 (1866).

54. *See* U.S. Const., art. I., § 2, cl.3.

55. Wesberry v. Sanders, 376 U.S. 1 (1964).

56. White v. Weiser, 412 U.S. 783 (1973).

57. Federation for Am. Immigration Reform v. Klutznick, 486 F. Supp. at 570 n.10.

58. U.S. Bureau of the Census, Statistical Abstract of the United States: 1980 at 70 (1981).

59. *See* Reynolds v. Sims, 377 U.S. 533, 568 (1964) (equal protection clause requires that the seats in a state legislature be apportioned on a population basis).

60. *See* Swann v. Adams, 385 U.S. 440, 444 (1967) ("De minimus deviations are unavoidable, but . . . none of our cases suggest that differences of this magnitude (30-40 percent) will be approved without a satisfactory explanation grounded on acceptable state policy."); Mahan v. Howell, 410 U.S. 315, 322 (1973) (approving 16.4 percent deviation because "broader latitude has been afforded the states"); Gaffney v. Cummings, 412 U.S. 735, 745 (1973) ("[m]inor deviations from mathematical equality among state legislative districts are insufficient to make out a prima facie case of invidious discrimination under the Fourteenth Amendment so as to require justification by the State").

61. Abate v. Mundt, 403 U.S. 182, 185 (1971).

62. *See* Young v. Klutznick, 497 F. Supp. 1318, 1325 (E.D. Mich. 1980), *rev'd on other grounds,* 652 F.2d 617 (6th Cir. 1981), *cert. denied,* 102 S. Ct. 1430 (1982) (Constitution requires that decennial census govern apportionment within states); Borough of Bethel Park v. Stans, 319 F. Supp. 971, 979 (W.D. Pa. 1970), *aff'd,* 449 F.2d 575 (3d Cir. 1971) ("under the Constitution, total population is a proper basis for the apportionment of both congressional and State legislative districts").

63. Burns v. Richardson, 384 U.S. 73, 91-92 (1966).

64. Carrington v. Rash, 380 U.S. 89 (1965), *discussed in* L. Tribe, American Constitutional Law § 13-14 (1978).

65. A court's remedial power may be more limited in state apportionment cases. *See* Minnesota State Senate v. Beens, 406 U.S. 187 (1972) (per curiam) (invalidating court's reduction of number of legislative districts from 67 to 35).

66. Staff of House Subcomm. on Census and Population of the Comm. on Post Office and Civil Service, 95th Cong., 2d Sess., Report on the Use of Population Data in Federal Assistance Programs 11 (Comm. Print 1978).

67. Note, *Demography and Distrust: Constitutional Issues of the Federal Census,* 94 Harv. L. Rev. 811, 863 (1981).

68. 420 U.S. 575 (1975).

69. Social Security Act § 406(a), 42 U.S.C. § 606(a) (1974).

70. *See* Williams, *Firing the Woman to Protect the Fetus: The Reconciliation of Fetal Protection with Employment Opportunity Goals under Title VII,* 69 Geo. L.J. 641, 697 n.318. Pregnancy can now be detected 8 to 10 days after conception. *See* J. Greenhill & E. Friedman, Biological Principles and the Practice of Obstetrics 57 (1974); R. Hatcher, Contraceptive Technology 134-35 (10th ed. 1980).

71. Raleigh Fitkin-Paul Morgan Memorial Hosp. v. Anderson, 42 N.J. 421, 201 A.2d 537, *cert. denied,* 377 U.S. 985 (1964).

72. The obvious candidate for this responsibility would be OSHA. *See infra* notes 190-95 and accompanying text.

73. At least one class action has already been brought on behalf of conceptuses. *See* Byrn v. New York City Health & Hosps. Corp., 38 A.D.2d 316, 329 N.Y.S.2d 722, *aff'd,* 31 N.Y.2d 194, 286 N.E.2d 887, 335 N.Y.S.2d 390 (1972), *appeal dismissed,* 410 U.S. 949 (1973) (class action seeking to enjoin municipal hospitals from performing abortions except to save the woman's life). *See also* Rice, *supra* note 9, at 337.

74. *See, e.g.,* N.Y. Penal Law § 260.10 (1977).

75. 67 N.J. Super, 517, 171 A.2d 140 (Juv. Ct. 1961).

76. *See, e.g.,* Deputy v. du Pont, 308 U.S. 488 (1940). *But see* Griswold, *An Argument Against the Doctrine That Deductions Should be Narrowly Construed as a Matter of Legislative Grace,* 5 Tax Couns. Q. 419 (1961).

77. I.R.C. § 151(e) (1) (West Supp. 1981).

78. Economic Recovery Tax Act of 1981, § 104(c)(2); *Id.* § 151(f) (provides for cost-of-living adjustment of exemption amount, beginning 1985).

79. *Id.* § 152(a).
80. *See* Rev. Rul. 73-156, 1973-1 C.B. 58 (dependency exemption for child who lived only momentarily depends on whether State or local law recognizes child as live born and there is official documentation thereof).
81. Treas. Reg. § 1.152-1(b) (1957).
82. U.S. BUREAU OF THE CENSUS, STATISTICAL ABSTRACT OF THE UNITED STATES: 1980 at 56 (1981).
83. The Canadian Criminal Code provides that abortion is legal if it is approved by a therapeutic committee and continuation of the pregnancy would, or would be likely to, endanger the woman's life. *See* CAN. REV. STAT. ch. C-34, § 251(4) (1970).
84. I.R.C. § 213 (West Supp. 1981).
85. *See* Rev. Rul. 73-201, 1973-1 C.B. 140.
86. This issue has not yet been addressed by the Internal Revenue Service.
87. 408 F.2d 631 (6th Cir. 1969).
88. *Id.* at 636, *quoting* Helvering v. San Joaquin Fruit & Investment Co., 297 U.S. 496, 499 (1936).
89. *See supra* note 13 and accompanying text.
90. *See* Gregg v. Georgia, 428 U.S. 153, 168-69 (1976).
91. *See supra* note 14 and accompanying text.
92. *See supra* note 15 and accompanying text.
93. *See supra* note 16 and accompanying text.
94. 410 U.S. at 163.
95. Wood & Hawkins, *State Regulation of Late Abortion and the Physician's Duty to the Viable Fetus,* 45 MO. L. REV. 394, 410-11 (1980).
96. MODEL PENAL CODE § 210 (1974).
97. SEE KING, *The Juridical Status of the Fetus: A Proposal for Legal Protection of the Unborn,* 77 MICH. L. REV. 1647, 1658-59 (1979); Dale, *supra* note 26, at 28.
98. CAL. PENAL CODE § 187 (West 1980); *see* People v. Apodaca, 76 Cal. App. 3d 479, 142 Cal. Rptr. 830 (1978).
99. *See* State v. McKee, 1 Add. 1 (Pa. 1797); State v. Winthrop, 43 Iowa 519 (1876); Wallace v. State, 10 Tex. App. 255 (1881); Morgan v. State, 148 Tenn. 417, 456 S.W. 433 (1923); Montgomery v. State, 202 Ga. 678, 44 S.E.2d 242 (1947); Keeler v. Superior Ct. of Amados County, 2 Cal. 3d 619, 87 Cal. Rptr. 481 (1970); State v. Dickinson, 23 Ohio App. 2d 259, 263 N.E.2d 253 (1970); State v. Gyles, 313 So. 2d 799 (La. 1975); State v. Brown, 381 So. 2d 916 (La. 1979). *But see* People v. Chavez, 77 Cal. App. 2d 621, 176 P.2d 92 (1947).
100. *See* FLA. STAT. ANN. § 782.09 (West 1976); LA. REV. STAT ANN. § 14.87.1 (West 1974); MICH. COMP. LAWS ANN. § 750.322 (1968); MISS. CODE ANN. § 97-3-37 (1972); MO. ANN. STAT. § 565.026 (Vernon 1979); NEV. REV. STAT. § 200.210 (1979); N.Y. PENAL LAW § 125.00 (Consol. 1977); OKLA. STAT. ANN. tit.21, § 613-14 (West 1958).
101. Annot., 40 A.L.R.3d 445, 450 (1971); *see* Note, *Live Birth: A Condition Precedent to Recognition of Rights.* 4 HOFSTRA L. REV. 805, 817 (1976).
102. *See, e.g.,* N.Y. PENAL LAW § 125.05(3) (Consol. 1977).

103. For example, both the Ashbrook and Garn-Rhodes versions would explicitly authorize the enactment of enforcement legislation by both Congress and the states. *See supra* notes 13-14 and accompanying text.

104. 138 Mass. 14 (1884).

105. 65 F. Supp. 138 (D.D.C. 1946).

106. There is disagreement among jurisdictions as to whether the conceptus must be viable at the time of the injury in order to recover. *See* W. PROSSER, HAND-BOOK OF THE LAW OF TORTS § 55 (4th ed. 1971); Comment, *Negligence and the Unborn Child: A Time for Change,* 18 S.D.L. REV. 204, 213 n.74 (1973).

107. 229 Minn. 365, 38 N.W.2d 838 (1949).

108. *See* King, *supra* note 97, at 1662 n.74.

109. *Id.*

110. *See* Presley v. Newport Hosp., 117 R.I. 177, 365 A.2d 748 (1976) (dictum).

111. Porter v. Lassiter, 91 Ga. App. 712, 87 S.E.2d 100 (1955).

112. 410 U.S. at 162. One commentator has argued that this limited recognition "should be seen as a desire . . . to fulfill the purpose of tort law by providing compensation for the parents' loss of a 'potential child.'" Note, *supra* note 101, at 824.

113. *See* King, *supra* note 97, at 1660.

114. *See* Dale, *supra* note 26, at 5 n.18.

115. *See supra* notes 41-44 and accompanying text.

116. 410 U.S. at 163.

117. *See* STEDMAN'S MEDICAL DICTIONARY 343, 395 (4th ed. 1976).

118. *See supra* notes 13, 16 and accompanying text.

119. *See supra* note 14 and accompanying text.

120. *See* Carey v. Population Servs. Int'l., 431 U.S. 678 (1977); Eisenstadt v. Baird, 405 U.S. 438 (1972); Griswold v. Connecticut, 381 U.S. 479 (1965).

121. *See, e.g.,* MASS. GEN. LAWS ANN. ch. 119, § 51A (West 1981).

122. *See supra* notes 70-75 and accompanying text.

123. *See generally* Horan, *Termination of Medical Treatment,* 16 FORUM 470 (1981); Walfoort, *The Proper Guardian: Medical Care Decisions for Fatally Ill Children,* 16 FORUM 131 (1980); Comment, *The Right to Refuse Medical Treatment: Under What Circumstances Does it Exist?* 18 DUQ. L. REV.607 (1980); Note, *The Right of Privacy and the Terminally Ill Patient: Establishing the "Right-to-Die,"* 31 MERCER L. REV. 603 (1980); Note, *The Refusal of Life Saving Medical Treatment v. The State's Interest in the Preservation of Life: A Clarification of the Interests at Stake,* 58 WASH. U.L.Q. 85 (1980).

124. One court has said there is no constitutional right to choose to die. John F. Kennedy Memorial Hosp. v. Heston, 58 N.J. 576, 580, 279 A.2d 670, 672 (1971).

125. *See* John F. Kennedy Memorial Hosp. v. Heston, 58 N.J. 576, 279 A.2d 670 (1971); United States v. George, 239 F. Supp. 752 (D. Conn. 1965); *In re* President of Georgetown College, Inc., 331 F.2d 1000 (D.C. Cir.), *cert. denied,* 377 U.S. 978 (1964).

126. *See, e.g.,* Long Island Jewish-Hillside Medical Center v. Levitt, 73 Misc. 2d 395, 342 N.Y.S.2d 356 (Sup. Ct. 1972).
127. *See* Satz v. Perlmutter, 362 So. 2d 160 (Fla. Dist. Ct. App.1978), *aff'd* 379 So. 2d 359 (Fla. 1980); *In re* Spring, 1980 Mass Adv. Sh. 1209, 405 N.E.2d 115; *In re* Quackenbush, 156 N.J. Super. 282, 383 A.2d 785 (1978); Superintendent of Belchertown State School v. Saikewicz, 373 Mass. 728, 370 N.E.2d 417 (1977).
128. 70 N.J. 10,355 A.2d 647 (1975), *cert. denied,* 429 U.S.922(1976).
129. *See, e.g.,* CAL. HEALTH AND SAFETY CODE §§ 7185-7195 (West 1977). These statutes are collected in Horan, *supra* note 126, at 470-71 nn.1-2(1981).
130. These interests are referred to in Superintendent of Belchertown State School v. Saikewicz, 373 Mass. at 739, 370 N.E.2d at 425, and have been cited in subsequent cases. *See, e.g.,* Satz v. Perlmutter, 362 So. 2d 160, 162-64 (Fla. Dist. Ct. App. 1978); *In re* Spring, 1979 Mass. App. Ct. Adv. Sh. 2469, 399 N.E.2d 493, 497 (1979).
131. *In re* Quackenbush, 156 N.J. Super. 282, 290, 383 A.2d 785, 790 (1978); Superintendent of Belchertown State School v. Saikewicz, 373 Mass. at 739-40, 370 N.E.2d at 425-26; *In re* Quinlan, 70 N.J. 10, 41, 355 A.2d 647, 663 (1975), *cert. denied,* 429 U.S. 922 (1976); John F. Kennedy Memorial Hosp. v. Heston, 58 N.J. at 584, 279 A.2d at 674.
132. *See* Comment, *The Right to Refuse Medical Treatment: Under What Circumstances Does it Exist?* 18 DUQ. L. REV. 607 (1980).
133. *Compare* United States v. George, 239 F. Supp. 752 (D. Conn. 1965) (interests of hospital and staff in providing proper medical care a factor that may overcome patient's religious objection to blood transfusion) *and* John F. Kennedy Memorial Hosp. v. Heston, 58 N.J. 576, 279 A.2d 670 (1971) (same as to religious objections of patient's mother) *with In re* Osborne, 294 A.2d 372 (D.C. 1972) (patient's religious objections to blood transfusion override state interests involved), *In re* Quackenbush, 156 N.J. Super. 282, 383 A.2d 785 (1978) (competent adult's right of privacy stronger than state interest in life where extensive bodily invasion required despite absence of dim prognosis), *and* Satz v. Perlmutter, 362 So. 2d 160 (Fla. Dist. Ct. App. 1978), *aff'd,* 379 So. 2d 359 (Fla. 1980) (competent adult has right of privacy to refuse or discontinue treatment that would temporarily and artificially prolong life).
134. *See, e.g.,* Satz v. Perlmutter, 362 So. 2d at 163 (characterizing earlier cases where blood transfusions were ordered as involving incompetent patients, equivocal refusals, or refusals of treatment by family members but not actually the patient).
135. *See, e.g., In re* Quinlan, 70 N.J. at 41, 355 A.2d at 663; Superintendent of Belchertown State School v. Saikewicz, 373 Mass. 728, 738, 370 N.E.2d 417, 424 (1977).
136. The highest court in Massachusetts required that the "ultimate decision making responsibility" be in the courts. Superintendent of Belchertown State School v. Saikewicz, 373 Mass. 728, 370 N.E.2d 417 (1977).

137. The New Jersey Supreme Court entrusted the decision to the patient's guardian, family, doctors, and hospital ethics committee, *In re* Quinlan, 70 N.J. at 54, 355 A.2d at 671.

138. Superintendent of Belchertown State School v. Saikewicz, 373 Mass. 728, 370 N.E.2d 417 (1977).

139. Custody of a Minor, 378 Mass. 732, 393 N.E.2d 836 (1979); Walfoort, *The Proper Guardian: Medical Care Decisions for Fatally Ill Children*, 16 FORUM 131 (1980).

140. *See supra* note 16 and accompanying text.

141. *See In re* Quinlan, 70 N.J. at 41, 355 A.2d at 663.

142. *See* NATIONAL RESEARCH ACT, PUB. L. NO 93-348, § 213, 88 STAT. 342, 353 (1974); DEPARTMENT OF HEALTH AND HUMAN SERVICES, ADDITIONAL PROTECTIONS PERTAINING TO RESEARCH, DEVELOPMENT, AND RELATED ACTIVITIES INVOLVING FETUSES, PREGNANT WOMEN, AND HUMAN IN VITRO FERTILIZATION, 45 C.F.R. §§ 46.201-211 (1978).

143. *See, e.g.*, CAL. HEALTH & SAFETY CODE § 25956 (West Supp. 1981); PA. STAT. ANN. tit. 35, §6605 (Purdon 1979). The statutes are collected in King, *supra* note 97, at 1647 n.6.

144. Comment, *Fetal Experimentation: Moral Legal and Medical Implications*, 26 STAN. L. REV. 1191, 1201 (1974).

145. 42 U.S.C. §§ 2000e to 2000e-17 (1976 & Supp. 1980).

146. *See* Bronson, *Issue of Fetal Damage Stirs Women Workers at Chemical Plant*, Wall St. J., Feb. 9, 1979, at 1, col. 1 (American Cynamid Co., Allied Chemical, Olin Corp.); Richards, *Face Off on Hazardous Jobs: Women's Right: Fetus Safety*, Wash. Post, Nov. 3, 1979, at A6, col. 5 (Hercules Co., Gulf Resources and Chemical Corp., General Motors); Shabecoff, *Job Threats to Workers' Fertility Emerging as Civil Liberties Issue*, N.Y. Times, Jan. 15, 1979, at Al, col. 2 (Dow Chemical, Monsanto, Du Pont, Bunker Hill Smelting, Eastman Kodak, Firestone Tire & Rubber). Many companies force fertile women from higher paying to lower paying jobs. *See* Bronson, *supra*. Some transfer only pregnant women and allow them to keep both their seniority and original pay. *See* Shabecoff, *supra*.

147. Bronson, *supra* note 146; Richards, *supra* note 146; Shabecoff, *supra* note 146.

148. At least six cases have been filed. *See* Williams, *supra* note 70, at 641-42 nn.2, 11.

149. *See id.* Other articles on the topic include: Andrade, *The Toxic Workplace: Title VII Protection for the Potentially Pregnant Person*, 4 HARV. WOMEN'S L.J. 71 (1981); Furnish, *Prenatal Exposure to Fetally Toxic Work Environments: The Dilemma of the 1978 Pregnancy Amendment to Title VII of the Civil Rights Act of 1964*, 66 IOWA L. REV. 63 (1980); Nothstein & Aryes, *Sex-Based Considerations of Differentiation in the Workplace: Exploring the Biomedical Interface Between OSHA and Title VII*, 26 VILL. L. REV. 239 (1981); Sloan, *Employer's Tort Liability When a Female Employee Is Exposed to Harmful Substances*, 3 EMPLOYEE REL. L.J. 506 (1978); Trebilcock, *OSHA and Equal Employment Opportunity Laws for Women*, 7 PREVENTIVE MED. 372 (1978); Zener, *Women in the Workplace: Toxic Substances*

and *Sex Discrimination,* 1 Toxic Substances J. 226 (1979); Comment, *Employment Rights of Women in the Toxic Workplace,* 65 Calif. L. Rev. 1113 (1977); Note, *Exclusionary Employment Practices in Hazardous Industries: Protection or Discrimination,* 5 Colum. J. Envtl. L. 97 (1978) [hereinafter cited as *Exclusionary Employment*].

150. EEOC Interpretive Guidelines on Employment Discrimination and Reproductive Hazards, 45 Fed. Reg.7514 (Feb. 1, 1980) (corrected in 45 Reg. 16,501 (1980)).

151. 42 U.S.C. § 2000e-2(e) (1976).

152. The Supreme Court extended Title VII's prohibition of discriminatory employment practices to include such policies in Griggs v. Duke Power Co., 401 U.S. 424 (1971). The Court said, "The Act proscribes not only overt discrimination but also practices that are fair in form, but discriminatory in operation. The touchstone is business necessity. If an employment practice which operates to exclude Negroes cannot be shown to be related to job performance, the practice is prohibited." *Id.* at 431. The Court struck down the company's educational and testing requirements because it found them irrelevant to job performance. The prohibition of practices having a disparate impact on women was first recognized in Nashville Gas Co. v. Satty, 434 U.S. 136 (1977).

153. *See* cases cited in *Exclusionary Employment, supra* note 149, at 149 n.204.

154. *See, e.g.,* Dothard v. Rawlinson, 433 U.S. 321, 333-34 (1976).

155. 29 C.F.R. § 1604.2 (1980). The only BFOQ the EEOC guidelines recognize is for "authenticity or genuineness" (e.g. actor or actress). *Id.*

156. 408 F.2d 228, 235 (5th Cir. 1969) (exclusion of women from being switchmen because of required heavy lifting violates Title VII).

157. 422 F.2d 385, 388, (5th Cir. 1971), *cert.denied,* 404 U.S. 950 (1971) (exclusion of men as flight attendants because women are more soothing to passengers violates Title VII).

158. 433 U.S. 321 (1976). The case involved both disproportionate impact and explicit exclusion attacks. Alabama's height and weight requirements for prison guards were struck down as not sufficiently related to the job requirement of strength. However, the exclusion of women from contact positions with male prisoners, 20 percent of whom had been convicted of sex offenses, was upheld as a BFOQ defense because "[t]he employee's very womanhood would thus directly undermine her capacity to provide the security that is the essence of a correctional counselor's responsibility." *Id.* at 336. The decision was limited to the facts before it—a male, maximum-security, unclassified penetentiary with "rampant violence" and a "jungle atmosphere." *Id.* at 344.

159. 444 F.2d 1219, 1224-25 (9th Cir. 1971).

160. 42 U.S.C. § 2000e-(k) (Supp. 1980).

161. 429 U.S. 125 (1976).

162. 42 U.S.C. § 2000e-(k) (Supp. 1980).

163. H.R. Rep. No. 948, 95th Cong., 2d Sess. 5, *reprinted in* 1978 U.S. Code Cong. & Ad. News 4749, 4753.

164. *See* Andrade, *supra* note 149; Furnish, *supra* note 149; Williams, *supra* note 70; *Exclusionary Employment, supra* note 149. *But see* Sloan, *supra* note 149; Zener, *supra* note 149; Nothstein & Ayres, *supra* note 149.

165. *See* Interpretive Guidelines on Employment Discrimination and Reproductive Hazards, 45 Fed. Reg. 7514 (1980) (withdrawn at 46 Fed. Reg. 3916 (1981)): "The BFOQ exception does not apply to the situations covered by these guidelines. That narrow exception pertains only to situations where all or substantially all of a protected class is unable to perform the duties of the job in question. Such cannot be the case in the reproductive hazards setting, where exclusions are based on the premise of danger to the employee or fetus and not on the ability to perform." *Id.* at 7516.

166. Zener, *supra* note 149, at 227-29.

167. *See* Dothard v. Rawlinson, 433 U.S. 321 (1977) (safety of prison guards and prisoners considered in determining whether women could be excluded from security guard jobs in maximum-security, all-male prisons); Burwell v. Eastern Airlines, Inc., 458 F. Supp. 474 (E.D. Va. 1978) (court considered safety of passengers in determining validity of mandatory leave for pregnant flight attendants), *aff'd in part, rev'd in part, and remanded,* 633 F.2d 361 (4th Cir. 1980) (per curiam); Harriss v. Pan Am. World Airways, Inc., 437 F. Supp. 413, 434 (N.D. Cal. 1977) (same); Usery v. Tamiami Trail Tours, Inc., 531 F.2d 224 (5th Cir. 1976) (passenger safety considered in upholding exclusion of older persons from bus-driver jobs).

168. *See, e.g.,* Weeks v. Southern Bell Tel. & Tel. Co., 408 F.2d 228, 236 (5th Cir. 1969). "Men have always had the right to decide whether the incremental increase in remuneration for strenuous, obnoxious, boring, or unromantic tasks is worth the candle. The promise of Title VII is that women are now on an equal footing."

169. *See, e.g.,* Burwell v. Eastern Airlines, Inc., 458 F. Supp. at 496-97; Harriss v. Pan Am. World Airways, Inc., 437 F. Supp. at 422 n.13; *In re* Nat'l Airlines, 434 F. Supp. 254, 261 n.15 (S.D. Fla. 1977). *But see* Zener, *supra* note 149, at 229 (comparing the safety of fetuses to the safety of other third parties).

170. These cases have used both the BFOQ and business necessity defenses. *See, e.g.,* Burwell v. Eastern Airlines, Inc., 458 F. Supp. 474 (E.D. Va. 1978), *aff'd in part, rev'd in part, and remanded,* 633 F.2d 361 (4th Cir. 1980) (per curiam); Harriss v. Pan Am. World Airways, Inc., 437 F. Supp. 413 (N.D. Cal. 1977).

171. *Compare* Burwell v. Eastern Airlines, Inc., 633 F.2d 361 (4th Cir. 1980) (per curiam) *and In re* Nat'l Airlines, 434 F. Supp. 254 (S.D. Fla. 1977) (mandatory leave for pregnant flight attendants during first trimester violates Title VII) *with* Harriss v. Pan Am. World Airways, Inc., 437 F. Supp. 413 (N.D. Cal. 1977) (mandatory leave valid BFOQ).

172. Burwell v. Eastern Airlines, Inc., 458 F. Supp. at 496-97; Harriss v. Pan Am. World Airways, Inc., 437 F. Supp. at 422 n.13, 423; *In re* Nat'l Airlines, 434 F. Supp. at 259.

173. Burwell v. Eastern Airlines, Inc., 458 F. Supp. at 496.

174. Harriss v. Pan Am. World Airways, Inc., 437 F. Supp. at 422 n.13.

175. Furnish, *supra* note 149, at 121-22; Manson, *Human and Laboratory Animal Test Systems Available for Detection of Reproductive Failure,* 7 PREVENTIVE MED. 322,

326 (1978); Williams, *supra* note 70, at 655-57; *Exclusionary Employment, supra* note 149, at 99-100.

176. Furnish, *supra* note 149, at 121-22; Manson, *supra* note 175, at 326; Williams, *supra* note 70, at 656; *Exclusionary Employment, supra* note 149, at 100.

177. Warshaw, *Employee Health Services for Women*, 7 PREVENTIVE MED. 385, 391 (1978).

178. Manson, *supra* note 175, at 325.

179. *Id.* at 327-28; Williams, *supra* note 70, at 657 nn.102-03; Comment, *Employment Rights of Women in the Toxic Workplace*, 65 CALIF. L. REV. 1113, 1117 nn.16-17.

180. Manson, *supra* note 175, at 326-27.

181. *Id.* at 327.

182. *See supra* note 152 and accompanying text.

183. 29 U.S.C. §§ 651-678(1976).

184. *Id.* § 651(b).

185. *Id.* § 651(b)(7).

186. *Id.* § 654(a)(1).

187. *See id.* §§ 651-678 (1976).

188. *See* Andrade, *supra* note 149, at 90-91; Williams, *supra* note 70, at 663.

189. *See* Andrade, *supra* note 149, at 90.

190. *See generally* J. BAER, THE CHAINS OF PROTECTION: THE JUDICIAL RESPONSE TO WOMEN'S PROTECTIVE LABOR LEGISLATION (1978). Protective labor legislation for women only was first upheld by the Supreme Court in Muller v. Oregon, 208 U.S. 412 (1908). The Court upheld state limitations on hours women could work in factories, mechanical establishments and laundries, after striking down similar limitations for bakers in Lochner v. New York, 198 U.S. 45 (1905). The court reasoned:

> That woman's physical structure and the performance of maternal functions place her at a disadvantage in the struggle for subsistence is obvious. This is especially true when the burdens of motherhood are upon her. Even when they are not, by abundant testimony of the medical fraternity continuance for a long time on her feet at work, repeating this from day to day, tends to injurious effects upon the body, and as healthy mothers are essential to vigorous offspring, the physical well-being of woman becomes an object of public interest and care in order to preserve the strength and vigor of the race.

Muller v. Oregon, 208 U.S. 412, 421 (1908).

191. Under guidelines proposed and later withdrawn by the EEOC, "if the hazard is shown, by reputable scientific evidence, to affect the fetus through women only, the class excluded must be limited to pregnant women and not all women of childbearing capacity." 45 Fed. Reg. 7514, 7515 (1980) (withdrawn in 46 Fed. Reg. 3916 (1981)). *See also* Cheatwood v. South Cent. Bell Tel. & Tel. Co., 303 F. Supp. 754 (M.D. Ala. 1969) ("Title VII surely means that all women cannot be excluded from consideration because some of them become pregnant.").

192. *See* Sloan, *supra* note 149, at 510-14.

193. *See supra* note 114 and accompanying text.

194. *See supra* note 190 and accompanying text.
195. *Id.*
196. 29 C.F.R. § 1604.2(b)(1)(1981).
197. *See, e.g.,* Rosenfeld v. Southern Pac. Co., 444 F.2d 1219 (9th Cir. 1971); Kober v. Westinghouse Electric Corp., 480 F.2d 240 (3d Cir. 1973); Manning v. General Motors Corp., 466 F.2d 812 (6th Cir. 1972), *cert. denied,* 410 U.S. 946 (1973). "[B]y mid-1973, the [courts] had found state hours, weight, and job prohibition laws invalid under Title VII." B. BABCOCK, A. FREEDMAN, E. NORTON & S. ROSS, SEX DISCRIMINATION AND THE LAW: CAUSES AND REMEDIES at 270 (1975).
198. N.Y. EST. POWERS & TRUSTS LAW § 2-1.3(a) (Consol. 1977) (emphasis supplied).
199. 2 Paige Ch. 35 (N.Y.Ch. 1830).
200. *See, e.g., In re* Peabody, 5 N.Y.2d 541, 158 N.E.2d 841, 186 N.Y.S.2d 265 (1959).
201. N.Y. EST. POWERS & TRUSTS LAW § 3-3.3(a) (Consol. 1977).
202. *Id.* § 4-1.1(a).
203. *Id.* § 4-1.1(a)(3).
204. *Id.* § 4-1.1.
205. *Id.* § 5-1.1.
206. *Id.* § 5-3.1.
207. *Id.* § 5-3.2.
208. *Id.* § 6-5.6.
209. *Id.* § 6-5.7(b).
210. *See supra* note 28 and accompanying text.
211. W. Burger, Report on the Problems of the Judiciary, Remarks at the Meeting of the American Bar Association (Aug. 14, 1972), 92 S.Ct. 2923, 2925 (1972).
212. *See supra* note 73 and accompanying text.
213. *See supra* notes 199-200 and accompanying text.
214. *See supra* notes 82-85 and accompanying text.
215. *See supra* notes 48-68 and accompanying text. After the 1980 census, approximately 50 lawsuits were brought by state and local governments. *See, e.g.,* Carey v. Klutznick, 653 F.2d 732 (2d Cir. 1981).
216. 287 N.Y. 61, 38 N.E.2d 131 (1941), *rev'd sub nom.* Riggs v. del Drago, 317 U.S. 95 (1942).
217. *See id.* at 79, 38 N.E.2d at 140.
218. 317 U.S. 95 (1942).
219. U.S. COMMISSION ON CIVIL RIGHTS, CONSTITUTIONAL ASPECTS OF THE RIGHT TO LIMIT CHILDBEARING 90-91 (Apr. 1975).
220. At least 146 cases dealing with the scope of state power over liquor have been reported since 1933, the year the Twenty-first Amendment was adopted. Over 30 have been decided since 1979.
221. *See supra* notes 48-65 and accompanying text.
222. *See supra* notes 69-71 and accompanying text.
223. *See supra* notes 76-88 and accompanying text.
224. *See* J. GREENHILL & E. FRIEDMAN, BIOLOGICAL PRINCIPLES AND THE PRACTICE OF OBSTETRICS (1974).

225. *See* Manson, *supra* note 175, at 326. Another study estimates that fewer than 60 percent of all conceptions survive the first month. J. LANGMAN, MEDICAL EMBRYOLOGY, HUMAN DEVELOPMENT—NORMAL AND ABNORMAL 47-48 (1975).

226. *Hearings on S.J. Res. 119 and S.J. Res. 130 Before the Subcomm. on Constitutional Amendments of the Senate Comm. on the Judiciary,* 93d Cong., 2d Sess. 79 (1974) (testimony of Sen. James Buckley).

227. *See* Bopp, *Effect of NRLC Human Life Amendment on Birth Control Drugs and Devices,* NAT'L RIGHT TO LIFE NEWS, June 1, 1981, at 10, col.1.

228. *See* Goodman & Price, *Abortion and the Constitution: An Examination of the Proposed Anti-Abortion Amendments,* 7 RUT.-CAM. L. REV. 671, 692-93 (1976).

229. *See, e.g.,* CAL. CIV. CODE § 7004 (West 1980). This kind of presumption deals with the timing problem arbitrarily.

230. U.S. CONST., art. I, § 3, art. II, § I.

231. U.S. CONST., amend. XXVI, § 1.

232. *See supra* notes 145-97 and accompanying text.

233. *See supra* notes 199-200 and accompanying text.

234. U.S. CONST., amend. XVIII.

235. U.S. CONST., amend. XXI.

236. 272 U.S. 581 (1926).

237. 295 U.S. 480 (1935).

238. 409 U.S. 109 (1972). For a discussion of this decision see Kamenshine, California v. LaRue: *The Twenty-First Amendment as a Preferred Power,* 26 VAND. L. REV. 1035 (1973). *See also* Note, *The Effect of the Twenty-First Amendment on State Authority to Control Intoxicating Liquors,* 75 COLUM. L. REV. 1578 (1975).

239. 452 U.S. 714 (1981).

240. *Id.* at 718.

241. *Id.* at 719.

242. *See* Kamenshine, *supra* note 238, at 1038-39. *But see* National League of Cities v. Usery, 426 U.S. 833 (1976) (the tenth amendment creates a sphere of state autonomy into which the federal government may not intrude).

Audience Discussion

Leonard Riskin, Moderator

WARREN M. HERN, M.D., M.P.H. (Boulder Abortion Clinic, Boulder, Colorado): My question is for Professor Robertson. In your presentation, you seemed to be saying that those who provide abortion services would be able to continue unimpeded by the Human Life Amendment. I thought that the purpose of the Human Life Amendment was to prevent abortions. Will it, or won't it, and if not, why not?

Also, at the beginning of your presentation, in relation to abortion if not fetal surgery, you talked about one person's rights conflicting with another's, and yet, in the Human Life Amendment or the Human Life Bill, the woman is referred to as a "mother." A woman who is pregnant with an unwanted fetus, unborn child, or baby, or whatever you'd like to say, clearly does not wish to be a mother even though the law may say she is a mother. If she does not wish to be a mother, I presume, she must go through some process by which she severs her parental responsibility. If there are parental rights and responsibilities, and if the fetus' rights are protected by a Human Life Amendment or Statute, what is the process by which a woman who is unwillingly pregnant may terminate her parental rights and responsibilities? If she succeeds in doing this, and by some miracle the fetus survives the event, who, then, has the responsibility for that medical procedure including liability for injury to the infant, who has the financial responsibility for maintenance of that individual, and who provides parental care for that individual in an emotional sense? If the individual is institutionalized from birth, what are the emotional and social consequences for millions of such individuals?

JOHN ROBERTSON (Conference Faculty): If I understand your question, you're asking if a human rights amendment passed, who would have the responsibility for an unwanted fetus? Well, it depends on how the woman severs her parental responsibility. If under such an amendment, she were able to do it simply by expelling the fetus–person from her body, and the fetus-person then died as a result, there'd be no problem with that. If the fetus-person lived, if she has legally terminated her responsibility, then she would have no further financial or other duties, and the duty there, I think, would devolve upon the state to take care of that person. This would be similar to the situation that exists in many states which have parental termination statutes. Under such laws you can terminate your rights and duties as a parent, and you have no further obligations to take care of that child. It's then up to the agency that assumes responsibility for the child.

REV. THOMAS O'DONNELL (St. Francis Hospital, Tulsa, Oklahoma): I just wish to state that whatever the Supreme Court, or Ms. Pilpel, or others think, neither the Catholic Church nor Thomas Aquinas has ever, under any circumstances, taught that early abortion was permissible.

JOSEPH M. GRAHAM (Texas Right to Life, Houston, Texas): First, in regard to a remark made by Professor Westfall, which I found extraordinarily interesting, concerning the fact that unborn horses are given legal recognition under the United States tax laws, but that unborn children are not, I'm not sure whether he wants to remove the legal status of the unborn horse or whether he wants to extend it to unborn persons. That's a point I'd like to hear a comment on.

I also sense a certain air of unreality among the gathering which is, as I understand, an information gathering and dispensing meeting, and one which I think is extraordinarily valuable. However, as you recall, when Senator East held hearings on the human life bill in the spring of 1981, there was a tremendous outcry when it was discovered that the vast majority of the people invited to speak and give authoritative testimony were, in fact, pro-lifers. Eventually, that balance was rectified and pro-choice individuals were asked to provide testimony. But the fact is that the hearings were held to provide information on a very valuable and important subject. Professor Westfall made the observation that the *Harvard Law Review* did not think anybody was even interested in this subject. Well, I believe a great number of people are interested, but Professor Westfall classified people such as myself and others as "enemies of choice" (which is surely not a term of endearment), as if we were, somehow, idiots for even thinking that maybe there is something to the other side.

This meeting does not indicate any awareness of the pro-life side. This morning over and over again we have been talking about the implications of a human life amendment and not one member of the faculty has admitted that they would be in favor of such an amendment. In fact, when two were accused of so being, they very righteously insisted that they were not. Now, whether you're in favor or against a human life amendment radically modifies how you would interpret the possible consequences of the passage of such an amendment. The same was the case when in *Brown v. Board of Education*[1] the United States Supreme Court tossed out *Plessy v. Ferguson*[2] and we heard all sorts of horrendous calculations about what was going to happen as a result of according equal rights and equal status to blacks in our society. Well, people have found out that most blacks weren't interested in marrying their daughters after all, but it was still a horrible and "real" threat in the beginning. Likewise, many of the issues that you're pointing to are in fact pseudo-issues which are extremities meant to frighten people out of their wits about the possibility of according legal status to the unborn. In fact, if unborn children were given status entitling their parents to a tax exemption, I'm all for it. The more of those, the better. So, it would seem that a truly significant discussion of the issue should have brought into the discussion somebody who believes that two million abortions annually performed in the United States is something very bad, who thinks that the unborn child is a person, and that abortion should be stopped whether by passage of an amendment or a statute or whatever. The conference fails in that we have not heard this position in this meeting.

LEONARD RISKIN, J.D. (University of Houston, College of Law, Houston, Texas): I think we've just heard the position, and I should add there are a great number of others in the audience who have enunciated that position.

DAVID WESTFALL (Conference Faculty): I would like to comment on one or two points that were made. In the first place, I'm afraid that my illustration of the horse was misunderstood. It was not mentioned to argue that unborn horses have rights, but rather as an illustration of the kinds of arguments that lawyers frequently make on behalf of their clients. In this case, it was with respect to the tax treatment of the compensation received for the horse which died after its birth, and it had nothing to do with the "rights" of unborn horses. Secondly, my reference to "enemies of choice" was in the context of a book by Andrew H. Merton entitled *Enemies of Choice*.[3] While one may regard that title as being somewhat one-sided, the book contains a great deal of relevant discussion of the background of the right-to-life movement. Moreover, I would be the last to describe anyone associated with the right-to-life movement as an idiot, for it's obvious that people in the right-to-life movement are highly intelligent, and it is for that reason that there is such a serious possibility that their views will be made persuasive and may prevail.

CHARLES BARON (Conference Faculty): I would like to make an observation that seems appropriate here. I think I hear, in the tone of voice of the two members of the Catholic clergy and the gentleman who just spoke from the Texas Right-to-Life organization, some quality of defensiveness, and I can readily believe they feel that way. In the abortion debate, people like you have taken a great deal of abuse for their position—a position, it seems obvious to me, which has been taken most often for reasons of conscience. One of the things that we all have to realize is that the chickens are now coming home to roost. I think those in the right-to-life movement have been abused in the past, and I for one feel bad about that. I think also people on the other side have been abused. There has been a lot of shouting back and forth, but we are all sensitive human beings and I think it's time for us to apologize to each other and to realize that getting along together is our challenge. In a way it's like marriage counseling: you've got spouses who are living in a relationship where an awful lot of bad words have been said in the past, and, if you want to save the marriage, people are going to have to relax a little bit and admit that right and wrong are not the bases of everything, that compromise and getting along together are really the important things. I may be opposed to the Human Life Amendment, and opposed to *Roe v. Wade*,[4] but I am very pro-society, and I think it's time we tried to make this societal marriage we are all a part of work a little better.

JOHN ROBERTSON: I'd also like to make a brief comment. My presentation on the medical-legal ramifications was not meant as a list of horribles. Indeed, the message for the right-to-lifers who want to ban abortion is that if you go the Human Life Amendment route, you may not end up banning abortion. If you want to ban abortion, do it directly. Otherwise, you're going to have to deal with some long traditions of law including one that says that one person does not have to lend her body to another.

MARGARET M. WHELTLE, S.T.M., J.D. (Mount de Sales Academy, Baltimore, Maryland): I'm a former practicing attorney with a later degree in theology, who is now an instructor and lecturer in law and theology. I'd like to reiterate the prior comment, that is, that a question must have some basis in reality. Too frequently, I think it is proposed for reasons of fear, duress, or confusion, and while I'm not accusing the speakers of that today, I think that may be the ultimate result. For example, consider Professor Westfall's remarks concerning the IRS: I have no fear that the IRS is capable of taking care of themselves, and I think with the stroke of a pen they will probably rule that a conceptus is not considered a person for provisions hereunder.

I also have a question for Professor Robertson, but before I get to it I would like to voice a criticism. It is my understanding that the proposed Human Life Amendment does not seek to give precedence to the fetus or conceptus, whatever you want to call it, over the mother. Rather, it seeks to provide equal rights to the fetus and then to have both sets of rights considered. If there is a weighing of evidence for the mother, the mother's rights would take precedence. If there is a weighing of evidence for the fetus, the fetus' rights would take precedence. If it's 50-50, there would be an equal dialogue on the rights, which is the purpose of the law. I'm a little disturbed that in this symposium the Human Life Amendment is being attacked and no speaker has been brought in to give us the perspective of why they have put the amendment up, and I think that's a very deep imbalance for a symposium of this sort. I do not mind pros and cons, but I'd like to hear both sides and there's nobody here to defend the amendment.

I have two questions. You can answer any or all as you like. I would like to know what your legal basis is for declaring a voluntarily conceived fetus as an unjust aggressor or, in your words, "an attacker." I do not think that has a basis in law. Also, what basis do you have for saying that a voluntarily conceived fetus cannot expect a duty to be cared for by its mother since its origin is not an intervening, free-choosing agent, but, in a sense, an invitee. An invitee, I should add, has a right to be protected from dangerous elements on another's property. Would not such an argument—a right to be protected if invited into another's being—apply to the fetus?

JOHN ROBERTSON: In order to give other people a chance to ask questions, let me just answer the last point. If you invite someone onto your property you have a duty not to expel them in an injured way, in a way that hurts them. If there's a storm outside and they could be injured, you have a duty to keep them in your house a while longer. But that duty does not extend to nine months keeping them there, and if they need your blood and kidneys, and body as well, the duty doesn't require that you lend it. So the mere fact that the fetus was considered to be a person while inside the mother's womb would not give that fetus-person a right to nine-month use of her body. To impose that burden on a woman would be to impose burdens that we impose on no one else in society, and I think would raise real equal protection problems.

NORMA RINGLER, PH.D. (University Hospital, Cleveland, Ohio): I would like to address my questions on another level, that is, addressing the legal implications of defining human life. Because of new technology and research, I wonder if the panel would address the issues of cloning and embryonic freezing that are being researched nationally and internationally.

JOHN ROBERTSON: They are important issues, but I'm afraid I cannot address them now because we are already doing a lot of speculation, and cloning and embryonic freezing and transfer are even further into the future. Perhaps we should be thinking about such issues now, but I'm not sure that that would change a lot of the analysis concerning the rights of the mother.

HARRIET PILPEL (Conference Faculty): Well, I can only say that one thing is clear and that is if a woman cannot control her reproductive life, she cannot control her life at all. The things that you're talking about apparently would not necessarily involve a woman's reproductive life and, therefore, perhaps different considerations might apply which I hope will be discussed tomorrow. But for a woman, her reproductive life, and control of it, is her destiny.

CAROLINE WHITBECK, PH.D. (Institute for the Medical Humanities, Galveston, Texas): I would like to ask a question of both the general audience and of the participants. Suppose you were able to do so, how many of you would like to have an abortion? As I suspected, none. I suggest that one of the things that goes out of sight in these discussions is that no one would really like to have an abortion, in the straightforward sense that people would like equal pay for equal work. There are many of us who would like safe abortions to be available, just as we would like safe mastectomies to be available, but that does not mean that we want mastectomies or abortions per se. This is something that frequently is forgotten. It was forgotten by Dr. Baron when he discussed the possibility of a woman in the third trimester deciding to have an abortion because the baby did not have blue eyes. To have a third trimester abortion for trivial reasons would be an act of major self-mutilation, as anyone who understands the experience of pregnancy will realize. Of course there are a few people whose self-hatred is so great that they do engage in self-mutilation, but their acts are bizarre and call for something other than moral or legal censure.

If we pay a little attention to the experience of a woman in pregnancy, then we will not perpetuate the fantasy that we need laws to keep women from doing things like having abortions in the third trimester because they do not like the fetus' eye color.

AUDRA C. GIER, M.S. (Cleveland Chiropractic College, Kansas City, Missouri): I am really excited by a lot of the things that are being said at this symposium because basically it gives me additional arguments to support the stands which I have already made. However, one of the things which I see as missing is the opportunity for the right-to-life people to present their position. This would have helped me to "disambiguate" how they can support this kind of legislation, and the restrictiveness that it entails, in a way which does not infringe upon my rights. One of the things I really appreciate about Professor Baron's remarks was his plea for an acceptance of the plurality upon which our society is based. I appreciate the defensiveness of some of the right-to-life people that are here; but I also know how defensive I feel when I'm being accused of supporting murder. I would really like to hear from some of those people concerning how they seek to protect fetal rights without destroying our pluralistic society, without imposing upon a lot of people who do not agree with them, things about which I feel as strongly morally as they do.

NOTES

1. 347 U.S. 483 (1954).
2. 163 U.S. 537 (1896).
3. A.H. MERTON, ENEMIES OF CHOICE: THE RIGHT-TO-LIFE MOVEMENT AND ITS THREAT TO ABORTION (Beacon Press, Boston) (1981).
4. 410 U.S. 113 (1973).

Part Four

Ethical, Cultural and Religious Perspectives

Chapter 12

When Human Rights Conflict: Two Persons, One Body

Ruth Macklin

Conflicts of rights are among the most intractable problems confronting moral philosophers and others who work in theoretical or applied ethics. This is partly because the framework of rights, at least in the moral domain, gives no clear guidance about priorities among various rights, and also because there remains a good deal of uncertainty about just which rights claims are valid and what sorts of entities are properly the bearers of rights. The topic addressed in this paper is further complicated by the ambiguity and vagueness surrounding the concept of a person, and the sharp disagreements among contributors to the bioethics literature on personhood. Since a motivating force behind this volume is the proposal (by politicians and other opponents of abortion) that the fetus be considered a person, and given the biological fact of pregnancy that the fetus and pregnant woman are indissolubly joined (at least for a while) in one body, the title of this paper reflects the problem that arises out of these features taken together. If we grant that persons are bearers of rights, and accept the assumption that the fetus is a person, how can we resolve the conflict of rights that occurs when two persons are joined in one body?

Since the task of addressing the issues requires an acceptance of the assumption that the fetus is a person, this discussion will grant that assumption for the sake of argument.

RIGHTS, PERSONS, AND CONFLICTS OF RIGHTS

The concept of rights exists in both the legal and moral domains. But while the existence of a particular legal right has some objective basis and can be defended by consulting statutory or common law, there is no corresponding objective source for moral rights. One major school of thought in philosophical ethics focuses on rights as the central moral concept (usually along with the correlative notion of duties),[1] while other approaches either eschew the language of rights altogether[2] or treat the concept of rights as a derivative notion, the central moral concepts being utility, happiness,[3] or some other candidate for "the good."[4] But even among those who put forward ethical theories couched in the language of rights and duties, there is no overall agreement about the source of human rights or about precisely which potential candidates for rights actually deserve that status. In short, when there is disagreement about the existence or nature of rights in particular cases, it is generally easier to put forward relevant and cogent reasons or evidence in support of the claim that something is a legal right than it is to justify claims about moral rights.

Among the problems that arise in assessing rights claims in ethics are two categories directly relevant to the present topic: the adjudication of conflicts of rights, and the determination of the moral status of entities to which rights are attributed. If we grant the assumption that the fetus is a person and therefore enjoys the same moral status as that of full-fledged members of the moral community, the problem at once reverts to the first category, that of conflicts of rights. The chief right that concerns us among several candidates for fetal rights is the obvious one: the right to life (other rights claimed on behalf of the fetus are the right to be born well and the right to genetic health). But here is where an asymmetry begins, since it is only in very rare cases that the pregnant woman's own right to life conflicts with the fetus's right to life. The right that pro-abortionists typically claim on behalf of pregnant women is "the right to control one's own body."[5] Even in the absence of a fully worked out hierarchy of moral rights, it is evident that if any right stands at or near the top of the list, it is the right to life. Hence, the difficulty of balancing the rights of the fetus against the rights of the pregnant woman: the right to life would seem to override virtually all others, so how can destruction of a fetus be morally permissible when the right served by that act falls lower on a hierarchy of human rights? Put succinctly by one foe of abortion:

> [H]uman beings with equal rights often come in conflict with each other, and some decision must be made as to whose claims are to prevail. Cases of conflict involving the fetus are different only in two respects: the total inability of the fetus to speak for itself and the fact that the right of the fetus regularly at stake is the right to life itself.[6]

Yet it is possible to make some further distinctions among rights, and to raise additional questions about balancing and weighing one set of rights against another. The lack of any authoritative source on this matter and the complete absence of societal agreement leave these moral questions in a vacuum. One writer observes:

[A]dvocates of these theories are faced with the problem of specifying which rights or claims are sufficiently weighty to take precedence over other rights or claims. More precisely, one must decide which rights or claims justify or fail to justify abortions. Is the woman's right to decide what happens to her body sufficient to justify abortion? Is pregnancy as a result of rape sufficient? Is the likely death of the mother sufficient? Is psychological damage (sometimes used to justify "therapeutic abortion") sufficient? Is knowledge of a grossly deformed fetus, which produces severe mental suffering to the pregnant woman, sufficient?[7]

These are not merely idle questions, since various proposals to limit the right of a woman to procure an abortion encompass one or more of these considerations. Yet to couch each one of these considerations in the language of rights may be to stretch the use of rights claims beyond credibility. Does a woman have a "right" to avoid psychological damage? A "right" to avoid severe mental suffering? These states are surely desirable to avoid, but should they be elevated to the status of rights? This is only one example of the rhetorical force evident in the use of rights talk in the moral domain.

The number of different positions it is possible to adopt when rights conflict seemingly knows no bounds. The following argument purports to show that even if a woman's right to control her own body (described tendentiously as "a woman's right to free her body of parasites which will inhibit her freedom of action and possibly impair her health") does override the fetus' ("parasite's") right to life, abortion may still be prohibited.

> For if A's right is stronger than B's, and it is impossible to satisfy both, it does not follow that A's should be satisfied rather than B's. It may be possible to compensate A if his right isn't satisfied, but impossible to compensate B if his right isn't satisfied. In such a case the best thing to do may be to satisfy B's claim and to compensate A. Abortion may be a case in point. If the fetus has a right to life and the right is not satisfied, there is certainly no way the fetus can be compensated. On the other hand, if the woman's right to rid her body of harmful and annoying parasites is not satisfied, she can be compensated. Thus it would seem that the just thing to do would be to prohibit abortion, but to compensate women for the burden of carrying a parasite to term.[8]

The most common strategy pro-abortionists in the bioethics literature have adopted, however, is to deny that the fetus is a person.[9] With one singular exception, to be described shortly, those who seek cogent reasons to back up their antecedently held moral views have found it easier to move the debate to the concept of personhood than to address the sticky question of conflicts of rights. Virtually all writers who focus on the status of the fetus as a person accept the proposition that persons have rights, including a right to life.[10] Therefore, to deny that a fetus is a person (whatever else it may be) is to deny that it has a right to life. There are, then, no rights in conflict with a woman's right to control her own body, and so abortion is permissible.

Yet even that last statement oversimplifies the picture. There exists considerable disagreement about the importance of personhood for efforts to resolve the cluster of moral disputes surrounding abortion. At least the following positions can be distinguished.

1) Settling the abortion issue once and for all depends crucially on coming to some agreement about whether the fetus is a person, and if so, when in its development personhood begins.[11]

2) Since it is impossible to provide a set of necessary and sufficient conditions for personhood, and therefore impossible to secure agreement on the criteria for personhood, that issue must be seen as entirely irrelevant to arriving at a solution to the abortion controversy.[12]

3) Whether the fetus is a person is irrelevant to whether it should have legal protection; concerns about the health of the fetus create pressing policy issues regardless of whether or not the fetus is granted the status of a person.[13]

4) Settling the abortion issue has little or nothing to do with when personhood begins, since abortion may be morally justified even if it is acknowledged that the fetus is a person from the moment of conception.[14]

This last position is the most interesting for present purposes, and will occupy the remainder of this section. But before turning to a discussion of that view, a few brief observations are worth making about the above claims regarding the importance of personhood in the abortion controversy. Note that while (2), (3), and (4) all treat the issue of personhood as separable from the question of the justifiability of abortion, each draws a different conclusion. Position 4 justifies abortion even if the fetus is a person by holding that one person's rights take precedence over the rights of another person when they conflict (the rights of the mother override the rights of the fetus). Position 3 is compatible with holding that even if the fetus is not a person, it still deserves protection under the law. And position 2 claims that the abortion issue must be addressed separately from the problem of personhood, since the latter problem is insoluble.

Position 3 is the only argument discussed in this paper that addresses the question of protection of the fetus outside the narrow context of abortion. The author, an attorney, writes:

[W]e can no longer avoid some resolution of the legal status of the fetus. The potential benefits of fetal research, the ability to fertilize the human ovum in a laboratory dish, and the increasing awareness that a mother's activities during pregnancy may affect the health of her offspring create pressing policy isues that raise possible conflicts among fetuses, mothers, and researchers.[15]

Mention of these additional contexts in which the fetus may need legal protection is a useful approach since, at least in regard to in vitro fertilization and fetal health, it is not the destruction of the fetus that is at stake. On the contrary, these concerns emanate from the desire parents have for a normal, healthy infant. Although the author does not frame her argument primarily in terms of rights, her conclusion demonstrates the possibility, indeed, the desirability, of sidestepping the issue of personhood entirely:

Most legal and philosophical literature about the fetus concerns abortion, and in recent years moral philosophers have thought the critical preliminary issue in resolving the morality of abortion to be whether the fetus is a person. In *Roe v. Wade*, the Supreme Court also approached the abortion issue through the question of personhood. The Court held that the fetus is not a person, a holding that has been criticized for inadequate analysis.

I submit that whether the fetus is a "person" is irrelevant to whether it should have legal protection. The personhood debate has only obscured the decisive issues.[16]

Let us return to the position noted earlier as the one most directly relevant to the conflict of rights involved in the case of two persons and one body. There may be someone not yet familiar with the fanciful example concocted by Judith Jarvis Thomson as an analogy to the concerns of personhood and abortion. This is perhaps a better example of the ingenuity that philosophers display in cooking up bizarre cases than it is an instance of a compelling analogy, but the story goes like this.[17]

You awake one day to find yourself in bed with a famous violinist, who is hooked up to your kidneys, which he needs to sustain his own life for a period of nine months. (The Society of Music Lovers, eager to sustain the life of the violinist, has kidnapped you for this noble purpose.) After that time the violinist will have recovered, and will have no further need for use of your kidneys. The violinist is a person, and so he has a right to life. Your life is not endangered, only your freedom to move about for nine months. We are supposed to consider the violinist as an appropriate analogue to a fetus, and you and your kidneys as analogous to a pregnant woman and her life-supports for the fetus. If your right to disconnect yourself from the violinist overrides his right to life, the argument goes, shouldn't it follow that a woman's right to terminate her pregnancy overrides the fetus' right to life?

Thomson supplies additional imaginative details, but the only one possibly relevant to the analogy with pregnancy and abortion is the non-voluntary nature of the procedure. Thomson believes her example provides an appropriate analogy for rebutting the argument that a person's right to life outweighs the right of another person to decide what happens in and to her body. She concludes: "I imagine you would regard this as outrageous, which suggests that something really is wrong with that plausible-sounding argument I mentioned a moment ago."[18]

One can admire Thomson's philosophical imagination, yet reject the soundness of the analogy on a number of counts. Arguing in general against the use of artificial cases, John T. Noonan writes about this one: "The similitude to pregnancy is grotesque. It is difficult to think of another age or society in which a caricature of this sort could be seriously put forward as a paradigm illustrating the moral choice to be made by a mother."[19] Noonan's own stance regarding the concept of a person is that if you are conceived by human parents, you are human.[20] (Noonan takes the concepts of a person and that of being human to be equivalent, in contrast to others who sharply distinguish personhood from being genetically human.[21]) Noonan maintains that personhood begins at conception, thus setting a very low standard—that is, one that allows a zygote or a blastocyst to qualify as a person.

In contrast, Mary Anne Warren sets a standard for personhood that does not allow even a neonate or an infant a few months old to qualify. Warren proposes the following as "the traits which are most central to the concept of personhood, or humanity in the moral sense":

1) consciousness (of objects and events external and/or internal to the being), and in particular the capacity to feel pain;

2) reasoning (the *developed* capacity to solve new and relatively complex problems);

3) self-motivated activity (activity which is relatively independent of either genetic or direct external control);

4) the capacity to communicate, by whatever means, messages of an indefinite variety of types, that is, not just with an indefinite number of possible contents, but on indefinitely many possible topics;

5) the presence of self-concepts, and self-awareness, either individual or racial, or both.[22]

From a value stance at the opposite end of the spectrum from Noonan's,

Warren also mounts a criticism of Thomson's analogy, though not of Thomson's substantive conclusion that the rights of the pregnant woman override the right to life of the fetus. Warren says that "the Thomson analogy can provide a clear and persuasive defense of a woman's right to obtain an abortion only with respect to those cases in which the woman is in no way responsible for her pregnancy, e.g., where it is due to rape."[23] According to this view, Thomson's analogy fails because it is too weak to do the job required in the abortion argument, a job Warren herself undertakes by setting criteria for personhood that rule out the fetus.

Analogical reasoning is a powerful mode of argument, but in order for an analogy to be sound, the items compared must be similar in relevant respects. The trick is, of course, to secure agreement on which elements are relevant and which are not. Artificial cases typically appear to non-philosophers as less similar to the case under consideration than real cases might be, despite the cleverness philosophers exhibit in their feats of imagination. Accordingly, it may be useful to try out two real phenomena by way of analogy with the problem of conflicting rights posed by two persons and one body.

Two Analogies: Two Persons, One Body?

EXAMPLE 1: SIAMESE TWINS

The phenomenon of Siamese twins offers a suggestive analogy for the problem of conflicting rights where two persons are joined in one body. A range of possible cases exists, of which at least the following pose different alternatives for moral decision making.

1) The twins are connected in a manner and location that makes surgical separation possible, with both members of the pair surviving.

2) The twins are connected in such a way that only one can survive, but in order for this to be possible, they must be surgically separated and the second twin must be killed.

3) The twins are connected in such a way that both can survive if they are not surgically separated, but for surgical separation to take place, one member of the pair will die.

4) The twins are connected in such a way that both can survive only if no surgical separation is undertaken.

Let us assume, for the sake of the discussion, that any contemplated surgery is to take place soon after birth, so there is no question of either or both of the twins participating in the decision or granting or refusing consent for the procedure. Further, each of the twins must be accorded the status of personhood by parity of reasoning with the fetus. It may make that assumption easier if we add that in every one of the four hypothetical cases, the part of the anatomy the twins share is not the head; any further speculations on the anatomical construction are left to the reader.[24]

Case 1 poses no real moral dilemmas. If the twins can be separated with no great threat to the life of either, the surgery ought to be performed and no conflict of rights exists. In fact, it would be unethical not to perform a surgical separation in the event, say, that the parents of the twins wanted to reap financial gain in some fashion from the birth anomaly and refused to grant consent for the surgery. The ethical judgment that it would be wrong not to separate the twins is based on considerations of their quality of life, and on an appeal to the consequences of separating them compared to the consequences of not separating them. One could, of course, try to recast this judgment in the language of rights, claiming that Siamese twins have a "right to be surgically separated." But little is added to the moral judgment by couching it in terms of rights, and it would be a more difficult claim to defend and to justify if framed in terms of rights than if simply left as a moral statement, which can be justified by an appeal to consequences. Once the twins are successfully separated, there are then two persons and two bodies, and consequently, no more conflict of rights.

Case 2 breaks down into two additional possibilities: 2a, in which one of the pair is weaker, less viable, had additional anomalies, or some other features that make the choice of which one is to survive largely a medically determined matter; and 2b, in which each member is equally viable, so the choice of which twin should be killed is arbitrary. There remains the alternative to surgical separation in both variations—namely, doing nothing with the result that both twins die. These cases bear a clear resemblance to some examples involving a pregnant woman and fetus, since the question of a moral distinction between killing and letting die arises in both contexts; further similarities are contingent on details of the particular cases (e.g., whether the fetus is viable).

Consider 2a first. The only reasonable choices are separating the twins in a manner that involves killing the weaker (less viable, sicker, more defective) infant, and allowing both to die. The third possibility— separating the twins in such a manner that the healthier is killed in the process—is clearly irrational, and nothing further need be said about that. While there are probably few individuals, whatever their moral or religious persuasion, who would opt for the alternative of letting both twins die rather than killing one in order to save the other, many hold onto the notion that active killing is necessarily more immoral than passively allowing to die. A prohibition against active killing is the only consideration that could lead anyone to hold that the death of two infants is a morally preferable alternative to the death of one. This is precisely the type of situation the dubious "doctrine of double effect"[25] was designed to handle in abortion cases, where the life of the pregnant woman is endangered and the only way to save her is to kill the fetus. Despite the questionable reasoning in the doctrine of double effect, if it can support killing a fetus in order to save the life of the mother, so too can it justify killing one Siamese twin in order to save the other. This conclusion holds for variation 2b as well as 2a, the only difference being that in the latter case, the choice of which twin is to die is unproblematic. There is little more to be said about 2b, since if the choice of which twin should live and which should die is arbitrary, or morally indifferent, the method for choosing can be any random procedure (tossing a coin, drawing a straw).

Yet 2b remains a case of conflict of rights so long as we continue to hold that there are two persons, and that each person has a right to life. If an advocate were appointed for each Siamese twin in this case, no rational grounds could be found for an arbitrator or judge to choose between them. Moreover, it violates a person's right to life to allow that person to die when saving the individual's life is a relatively simple matter, just as much as the right to life is violated by active killing. It may be psychologically more difficult for a physician to engage in active killing than to stand by and do nothing, but the arguments holding that killing is frequently no more immoral than letting die, and is often morally preferable, are quite convincing.[26]

Does this Siamese twin analogy help in thinking about the conflict of rights that normally obtains between the pregnant woman and the fetus? Unfortunately not. It is only similar in relevant respects when both the life of the fetus and the life of the mother are at stake. In all other cases, the fetus's right to life is pitted against some other right of the pregnant woman, and so the analogy with case 2 fails to hold. Case 2 is more illuminating for an analysis of the morality of killing versus letting die, and for a rights-based versus a consequentialist analysis, than it is helpful in resolving the conflicting rights of a pregnant woman and a fetus sharing one body.

Case 3 is most like the abortion case prior to the time at which the fetus is viable. In case 3 there are two persons, each with a right to life, and one body. It seems to be very much a matter of quality of life versus sanctity of life, as that dilemma is often phrased. Even if the quality of life of two persons will most likely be relatively low, can considerations of quality of life ever override the sancitity of life? In the language of rights, the right to life itself must always take precedence over the right to a high quality of life, so the right to life of each twin overrides the right to a minimally decent quality of life for either. If life itself is valuable, then by sheer force of numbers, two lives are better than one. This holds for Siamese twins who cannot be separated without causing the death of one, as well as for a pregnant woman and pre-viable fetus.

The chief distinction between case 3 involving Siamese twins and the case of a pregnant woman and fetus lies in the length of time the two persons must remain joined in one body. In the case of the twins, that length of time is their entire lifetime; in the case of a pregnant woman, it is nine months, give or take a few days or weeks. But this distinction does not strengthen the rights of the pregnant woman against the rights of the fetus; on the contrary, the difference between being joined to another person for "only" nine months and being joined for a lifetime is staggering.

A second possible difference lies in the relative degree of lessened quality of life suffered by the pregnant woman joined to her fetus and the Siamese twins joined to one another, temporal considerations aside. Here, too, it would be very hard to demonstrate that a pregnant woman's quality of life is considerably diminished during a relatively normal pregnancy, and it is certainly nothing like the quality of life that two persons joined externally, in the manner of Siamese twins, must endure.

Fortunately, there is no need to decide here whether the quality of life of both Siamese twins who cannot be separated without causing the death of one twin is so low that it could justify surgical separation. There is no clearly objective way of deciding that, and it is a topic for a discussion of the ethics of treating defective newborns. The same observation applies to case 4, in which the twins must remain joined in one body for life if either is to survive at all. Case 4, then, poses no real conflict of rights, since either both persons in one body live, or both die. That, too, creates a troubling moral dilemma, one that occurred very recently in Illinois.[27] But just as case 1 is not truly analogous to the case of a pregnant woman and fetus because once the Siamese twins are successfully separated there are two persons and two bodies, so, too, is case 4 not a good comparison because although there remain two persons and one body, their rights are not in conflict. Either both live, or both die, so the only question is whether their joint right to life must be honored.

It is tempting to point out one further distinction between any of the Siamese twin cases and that of the pregnant woman and fetus. The twins are, after all, viable neonates, and the fetus is a fetus. But to take that step is to begin to question the assumption already granted—that a fetus is a person, and therefore has a right to life. The analogy between the conflict of rights in case 3 of the Siamese twins and a pregnant woman and fetus joined in one body is not perfect, but it may be as close as one can come to a real example, as opposed to one like Thomson concocts. The analogy suggests a solution, however, only if the right to life always overrides all considerations of quality of life—a view that many people question—and, of course, if the status of personhood is ascribed to a fetus.

EXAMPLE 2: MULTIPLE PERSONALITIES

Another situation that suggests a possible analogy can be treated only briefly, but it is instructive to consider. This is the psychiatric phenomenon sometimes called "split personality," but usually termed "multiple personality." Some years ago a movie entitled *The Three Faces of Eve*, based on a real case, portrayed the life of a woman who suffered from this disorder. There is, of course, only one body; the difficulty with the analogy is the problem of deciding how many persons there are. The analogy can be quickly dismissed by those who deny outright that "personality" and "person" could be equivalent. But that denial would be much too quick, in light of a large body of philosophical literature on the concept of a person. The particular topic under which this question falls is that of personal identity and individuation, an area of inquiry in descriptive metaphysics. Even to begin to explore that topic would lead us astray quickly. Yet some articles on personhood in the bioethics literature lend much plausibility to the view that multiple personalities may correctly be thought of as multiple persons, but with only one body. This does not, of course, require that we adopt the metaphysics of a soul inhabiting a body, since the phenomenon of multiple personalities can be described and conceptualized with no reference to souls or any other form of ontological dualism. The previously mentioned criteria for personhood that Mary Anne Warren proposes (along with similar proposals by Joseph Fletcher,[28] Michael Tooley,[29] H. Tristram Engelhardt, Jr.,[30] and other contributors to the bioethics literature) are ones that multiple personalities can often meet. Indeed, it may be easier to secure agreement that a personality, in this sense, can plausibly qualify as a person than that a zygote or blastocyst can.

The following passage, taken from a philosophical article on personal identity and individuation, describes an actual case drawn from the psychological literature around the turn of the century. The case is that of a Miss Beauchamp, who exhibited four different personalities.

> Miss Beauchamp's strikingly different personalities were individuated in the first place by reference to personal characteristics, in which they were largely opposed; also by tastes and preferences (B_1 and B_4 hated smoking, for

instance, and B_3 loved it); and by skills (B_3, unlike the others, knew no French or shorthand). Memory did not serve straightforwardly to individuate them, because their memories were asymmetrical. B_1 and B_4, for instance knew only what they were told by the investigator about the others, but B_3 knew, without being told, everything that B_4 did, and in the case of B_1 knew all her thoughts as well; she referred to them both in the third person. These remarkable and systematic discontinuities in Miss Beauchamp's behaviour, together with the violent and active conflict between her various selves, who abused and tricked each other, make the reference to different particular personalities completely natural. Thus we have individuated various personalities by reference to character, attainments and (up to a point) memories. . . .[31]

The features of Miss Beauchamp's four different personalities lend some credibility to the view that these different personalities may be construed as different persons, but in the absence of a theory of persons, it is at best a suggestion. To object that Miss Beauchamp suffered from a pathological disorder will not do, since the pathology could be described as there being four persons where there should be one (similar to birth anomalies with multiple limbs or digits, or to the multiplication of cells in a cancerous growth). As we granted the assumption, for the sake of argument, that a fetus is a person, let us grant the assumption that a personality can be a person. What follows regarding conflicts of rights?

The context in which a moral question could arise is that of therapy. If, in the effort to cure Miss Beauchamp of her disorder, her psychiatrist proposes to eliminate three of her four personalities, rendering her a being who will henceforth be one person, one body, what might any of the three personalities scheduled for extinction reply? Could B_3 claim a right to life, in the knowledge that she was one slated for elimination? Could B_4, informed of the plans by her psychiatrist, reply (in French): "Why not get rid of B_3, instead? After all, she engages in the filthy smoking habit, and will probably shorten my (her? our?) life." If there was ever a conflict of rights, where a right to life is one of the rights involved and where "two persons, one body" is an apt description, this appears to be it.

Without belaboring the analogy further, it is a simple matter to conclude that extinguishing three of the four personalities is morally permissible because Miss Beauchamp suffers from a pathological disorder. This is not the same as concluding that the various personalities cannot properly be considered persons because of the pathology. But it is to maintain that claims to the right to life by any of these personalities need not be respected. Or should they? Whatever other rights mentally ill persons may be denied, few would maintain that they lack a right to life simply because their personality is disordered in some way. Why should it be different for any of Miss Beauchamp's selves who claim a right to life, in conflict with the rights of the other three selves?

The reason it is different is this. In the case of any other mentally ill person, to eliminate the person involves destroying the body. But Miss Beauchamp's body would not be destroyed in the process of eliminating three of her four personalities. If she was formerly four persons, one body, following successful treatment she will be one person, one body. But herein lies the point of departure with the pregnant woman and the fetus. When a fetus is destroyed, a body is destroyed (there is as yet no personality, in any sense of that term). But if we deny the analogy between the case of multiple personalities and that of a fetus and pregnant woman on grounds that the fetus and the woman have bodies, but the several personalities in the psychiatric cases do not, then we have abandoned the premise with which we began: two persons, one body.

Conclusion

No rights are absolute, not even the right to life. One difficulty of using the language of rights in a moral framework is that conflicts of rights are especially hard to resolve. Even among those who accept a general framework of rights, disagreements occur over whether the right to life must always supersede all other rights (recall the position of Thomson, apart from her violinist analogy, and the argument about compensating someone in lieu of respecting that person's right). When rights conflict, whether there are two persons and one body, or two persons and two bodies, a stalemate is likely. Then the conflict must be arbitrated or adjudicated by some means that takes account of values other than the conflicting rights of the parties involved. In ethics, there is a perfectly sound approach to a wide variety of moral conflicts between persons: an appeal to the consequences of acting one way rather than another. The much maligned and oft-misunderstood theory of utilitarianism offers a reasonable alternative to the effort to pack every moral quandary into the bin of rights. Applying the utilitarian principle to the problem of two persons, one body, in the case of pregnant woman and fetus yields a very different solution than an approach based entirely on rights. A consequentialist approach is not only practically easier to manage; it also reaches what is probably the correct moral solution.

Notes

1. Chief representatives of this school in the history of philosophy are Immanuel Kant and G.W.F. Hegel, along with writers in the natural law tradition; in

twentieth century philosophy, see W. D. ROSS, THE RIGHT AND THE GOOD (Clarendon Press, Oxford) (1930); and among contemporary American philosophers, *see*, J. RAWLS, A THEORY OF JUSTICE (Harvard University Press, Cambridge, Mass.) (1971); and R. DWORKIN, TAKING RIGHTS SERIOUSLY (Harvard University Press, Cambridge, Mass.) (1977).

2. Jeremy Bentham, one of the early utilitarians, wrote:

> *Natural rights* is simple nonsense: natural and imprescriptible rights, rhetorical nonsense,—nonsense upon stilts. But this rhetorical nonsense ends in the old strain of mischievous nonsense: for immediately a list of these pretended natural rights is given, and those are so expressed as to present to view legal rights.

   Bentham, J., *Anarchical Fallacies, reprinted in* HUMAN RIGHTS (A.I. Melden, ed.) (Wadsworth Publishing Co., Belmont, Calif.) (1970) at 32.

3. J. S. MILL, UTILITARIANISM (1863).

4. For the view that goodness is a simple, unanalyzable property, which is apprehended by means of a special, moral intuition, *see*, G.E. MOORE, PRINCIPIA ETHICA (Cambridge University Press, Cambridge, England) (1903).

5. For a discussion of this claim, *see, e.g.*, Thomson, J.J., *A Defense of Abortion*, PHILOSOPHY AND PUBLIC AFFAIRS 1(1):47-66 (1971).

6. Noonan Jr., J.T., *An Almost Absolute Value in History*, THE MORALITY OF ABORTION (J.T. Noonan, ed.) (Harvard University Press, Cambridge, Mass.) (1970) at 57.

7. Beauchamp, T.L., *Abortion*, in CONTEMPORARY ISSUES IN BIOETHICS (T.L. Beauchamp, L. Walters, eds.) (Dickenson Publishing Co., Encino, Calif.) (1978) at 193 [hereinafter referred to as CONTEMPORARY ISSUES].

8. Tooley, M., *Abortion and Infanticide*, PHILOSOPHY AND PUBLIC AFFAIRS 2(1):37-65 (1972). Tooley does not subscribe to the view stated in this argument, since he denies that the fetus is a person, and hence, that it has a right to life. That value stance is implied by Tooley's use of the term "parasite" in referring to the fetus.

9. *Id.*; Warren, M.A., *On the Moral and Legal Status of Abortion*, MONIST 57(1):43-61 (January 1973); Engelhardt Jr., H.T., *The Ontology of Abortion*, ETHICS 84(3):217-234 (April 1974); J. FLETCHER, HUMANHOOD: ESSAYS IN BIOMEDICAL ETHICS (Prometheus Books, Buffalo, N.Y.) (1979).

10. An exception is Joseph Fletcher, *supra* note 9, who has little use for rights talk in ethics, and whose moral arguments are strongly consequentialist.

11. Proponents of this position are Tooley, Warren, Engelhardt, and Noonan. *See also* Brody, B., *Abortion and the Law*, JOURNAL OF PHILOSOPHY 68(12):357-69 (1971); Brody, B., *Abortion and the Sanctity of Human Life*, AMERICAN PHILOSOPHICAL QUARTERLY 10(2):133-40 (1973).

12. English, J., *Abortion and the Concept of a Person*, CANADIAN JOURNAL OF PHILOSOPHY 5(2):233-43 (October 1975); Wertheimer, R., *Understanding the Abortion Argument*, PHILOSOPHY AND PUBLIC AFFAIRS 1(1):67-95 (1971).

13. King, P.A., *The Juridical Status of the Fetus: A Proposal for Legal Protection of the Unborn*, MICHIGAN LAW REVIEW 77(7):1647-87 (August 1979).

14. Thomson, *supra* note 5.
15. King, *supra* note 13, at 1647.
16. *Id.* at 1687.
17. Thomson, *supra* note 5, at 48-49.
18. *Id.* at 49.
19. Noonan Jr., J.T., *How to Argue About Abortion* (Ad Hoc Committee in Defense of Life, Inc.) (1974), *reprinted in* CONTEMPORARY ISSUES, *supra* note 7, at 210.
20. Noonan Jr., J.T., *An Almost Absolute Value in History, supra* note 6, at 54.
21. Representative writers are Tooley, English, Engelhardt, and Fletcher.
22. Warren, *supra* note 9, at 55.
23. *Id.* at 50.
24. This writer did not perform research, for the purpose of this article, on Siamese twins and surgical separation. Therefore, technical details are omitted from the discussion, but there are known cases falling into all four categories delineated here.
25. For a good discussion of this doctrine, *see* Foot, P., *The Problem of Abortion and the Doctrine of the Double Effect*, OXFORD REVIEW 5(5):5-15 (1967).
26. *See, e.g.*, Goodrich, T., *Morality of Killing*, PHILOSOPHY 44(168):127-39 (1969); Fletcher, G.P., *Legal Aspects of the Decision Not to Prolong Life*, JOURNAL OF THE AMERICAN MEDICAL ASSOCIATION 203(1):119-22 (January 1, 1968); Bennett, J., *Whatever the Consequences*, ANALYSIS 26(3):83-97 (1966); Dinello, D., *On Killing and Letting Die*, ANALYSIS 31(3):83-86 (1971); Fitzgerald, P.J., *Acting and Refraining*, ANALYSIS 27(4):133-39 (1967); Rachels, J., *Active and Passive Euthanasia*, NEW ENGLAND JOURNAL OF MEDICINE 292(2):78-80 (January 9, 1975).
27. For a legal and ethical analysis of the case of Siamese twins born in Illinois in 1981, see Robertson, J.A., *Dilemma in Danville*, HASTINGS CENTER REPORT 11(5):5-8 (October 1981).
28. J. FLETCHER, *supra* note 9.
29. Tooley, *supra* note 8.
30. Engelhardt Jr., H.T., *supra* note 9.
31. Williams, B.A.O., *Personal Identity and Individuation*, PROCEEDINGS OF THE ARISTOTELIAN SOCIETY, Vol. 57 (1956-1957), *reprinted in* ESSAYS IN PHILOSOPHICAL PSYCHOLOGY (Doubleday & Co., Garden City, N.Y.) (1964) at 343.

Chapter 13

Comparative Legal Abortion Policies and Attitudes Toward Abortion

Bernard M. Dickens

INTRODUCTION

A study claiming to compare legal abortion policies and attitudes toward abortion must necessarily be selective, since the range of jurisdictions open to analysis is wide, and the historical depths behind national laws are often profound. Fortunately for this endeavor, Professor Charles H. Baron has undertaken the task of conducting a historical review of the legal concept of personhood; accordingly, the treatment of historical materials in this paper will be very brief, and confined to generalities. Further, the comparative presentation will focus particularly upon legal systems akin to that of the United States, whose laws are drawn from an origin in the English common law and the British Commonwealth, and secondarily upon European experience.

There is a rich anthropological literature describing and explaining the role of abortion in primitive or preliterate societies,[1] including reference to the oldest known abortifacient recipe, which is Chinese and believed to date from 2723–2696 B.C.[2] Sacred literature has frequently mentioned abortion; for instance, the religious texts of Hinduism (1500–1000 B.C.), Zoroastrianism (1000—600 B.C.), Taoism (about 500 B.C.) and Buddhism (about 500 B.C. and later) have discussed the issue.[3] For purposes of this most brief of historical surveys, it may be justifiable to step over the Babylonian Code of Hammurabi (1728 B.C.) and the practices of the ancient Greek and Roman civilizations in order to briefly address the issue of abortion in early Christian and related teachings.

It cannot be claimed that early Christianity presented new insights into biology and embryology. Rather, it drew upon the perceptions of its time, and while as a matter of doctrine abortion was condemned, it was defined by reference to earlier concepts. Critical to prevailing reasoning was speculation as to the time of commencement of human life. It was generally accepted that the fetus did not begin to live until some time after conception; indeed the Book of Genesis may have appeared to be in that tradition in relating that God made Adam out of the dust of the ground, and only some time after the body was completed was life breathed into it.[4] Along the same line, Aristotle had concluded that the life of a male fetus commenced at about 40 days after conception, and that of a female fetus at about 90 days;[5] Hippocrates determined the two periods at 30 and 42 days respectively. The Stoics believed animation to occur only at birth, but the later Roman view set the period at 40 and 80 days after conception for the male and female fetus respectively. Later still the time was settled in civil law as 40 days from conception for both sexes.[6]

In Christian theology, animation was related to theories of ensoulment. Saint Augustine distinguished between embryo inanimatus and embryo animatus,[7] the latter being endowed with a soul, whose destruction was tantamount to murder.[8] While the distinction was not accepted in all of the earlier church canons, it was accepted by Gratian in his *Decretum* (circa 1140), who concluded that abortion is not murder if it occurs before infusion of the soul into the fetus. Commentators upon Gratian accepted that animation occurred 40 days after conception for a male fetus, and 80 days for a female.[9] Causing abortion before that time may have been culpable, but it was not murder.

Jewish law reflects similar concern with distinctions based upon the age of the fetus. It has been observed that "prior to 40 days after conception, a fertilized egg is considered nothing more than 'mere fluid'. . . . However, after 40 days have elapsed, fashioning or formation of the fetus is deemed to have occurred . . . [and] a woman who aborts after the 40th day following conception is required to bring an offering just as if she had given birth to a live child."[10] Jewish law does not equate a fetus to a human being,[11] and indeed requires "a 30-day post partum viability period for adjudicating various Jewish legal matters pertaining to the newborn,"[12] reflecting not only accommodation of premature birth, but also the historically high rate of neonatal mortality.

Islamic jurisprudence is expressed in a variety of schools which identify different legal incidents and sanctions attaching to abortions occurring at different times. An Islamic scholar who enjoys international respect in population epidemiology, Dr. Abdel R. Omran, has explained the significance to the Islamic tradition of three successive 40-day periods leading from fertilization to ensoulment.[13] The first period regards the conceptus as "a drop," comparable perhaps to the notion of "mere fluid" under Jewish law. The second period recognizes "a clot of blood," and the third "a piece of flesh," after which ensoulment occurs. An Islamic legal scholar has suggested that "the various books on jurisprudence are unanimous in forbidding abortion after animation, i.e., after the completion of the fourth month of pregnancy, unless abortion is badly needed. . . . Before animation, however, the scholars' views differ and vary in the details concerning 'allowance,' 'disfavour,' and 'prohibition'."[14]

Classical doctrines, distinguishing by gestational age between male and female embryos, developed at a time when detection in utero of embryonic gender was impossible, and thus could have served only to affect punishment or compensation after abortion had occurred rather than any prospective purpose. Such doctrines were consistent, however, with an approach dependent upon perceived phenomena. This approach was shared by the historic English common law, which was influenced by the significance of "quickening," the first perceived sign of fetal movement. Bracton, writing in the early part of the thirteenth century, said that abortion after animation was homicide,[15] meaning by animation the moment of quickening.[16] Later authorities such as Coke, while quoting Bracton and noting Fleta, denied criminal liability for homicide after quickening. Coke observed: "If a woman be quick with childe [sic], and by a Potion, or otherwise Killeth it in her womb; or if a man beat her whereby the child dieth in her body, and she is delivered of a dead childe, this is a great misprision, and no murder."[17] Thereafter, Hawkins wrote that procuring the abortion of a quick child amounted to a common law misdemeanor,[18] as opposed to a more severely punishable felony. Sir William Blackstone in his celebrated *Commentaries,* published in 1765 for a lay readership, explained that "life . . . begins in [the] contemplation of law as soon as an infant is able to stir in the mother's womb,"[19] and contrasted Bracton's severe view of the offense with Coke's view, noting that "the modern law doth not look upon this offence in quite so atrocious a light."[20]

The first English legislation contrary to the common law misdemeanor of procuring abortion was enacted in 1803,[21] and was innovative in that it introduced punishment even when the stage of quickening had not yet occurred. Section 1 of the law reflected the common law in defining the offense of acting "to cause and procure the Miscarriage of any Woman then being quick with child," but in contrast to the common law declared that offenders "be Felons, and shall suffer Death." Section 2 dealt with acting to procure "the Miscarriage of any Woman not being, or not being proved to be, quick with child," and such an offense was a felony punishable with fine, imprisonment, or whipping.[22] In *R. v. Scudder*,[23] it was held a complete defense to an indictment brought under section 2 to show that the woman was not pregnant, although this decision was at variance with an earlier case, *R. v Phillips*,[24] which considered the offense to consist in the intent with which the accused administered a substance to a woman, whether or not she was actually pregnant.

The 1803 Act was superseded by a similarly worded Act in 1828,[25] but this was repealed in 1837, by the Offenses Against the Person Act.[26] The 1837 Act abandoned the distinction between women quick and not quick with child, and sought to punish anyone who acted with the intention of procuring a miscarriage, irrespective of pregnancy. This historically important distinction was thereby removed from the law of England and of the jurisdictions influenced by English legislation.[27] In 1837, Lord Macaulay presented a draft code of criminal law to the Indian Law Commissioners, which was enacted in 1860 as the Indian Penal Code,[28] and which remains to this day the law of many Commonwealth Asian jurisdictions[29] and of northern Nigeria. Perhaps influenced by Scottish law,[30] this code prohibits acting with intent to procure the abortion of a woman who is "with child."[31] The English legislation of 1861,[32] however, which set the pattern for much of the British Commonwealth in the present century, punishes a woman unlawfully involved in her own abortion while "being with child," but, subject to that, punishes "whosoever, with intent to procure the miscarriage of any woman whether she be or be not with child," acts toward that end, other than upon an approved indication.[33]

The United States Supreme Court, in its landmark decision in *Roe v. Wade*,[34] traced the history of abortion management by religion and law, commencing at the time of the Persian Empire, and progressing to the significance of "quickening" in the common law, noting that this was taken usually to occur during the sixteenth to the eighteenth week of pregnancy. The Supreme Court noted that until the middle of the last century, the law in effect in all but a few of the United States was the English common law, where procuring abortion before quickening was not a crime. When states initially introduced legislation after mid-century, they tended to punish abortion before quickening considerably more leniently than if it were procured after quickening. However, by the late nineteenth century, that distinction was no longer drawn and increasingly restrictive laws were enacted, with increasingly narrow exceptions for the preservation of the woman's life or health. The Supreme Court observed in 1973 that "at the time of the adoption of our Constitution, and throughout the major portion of the nineteenth century, abortion was viewed with less disfavour than under most American statutes currently in force."[35]

The Texas legislation challenged in *Roe v. Wade* was struck down because it "makes no distinction between abortions performed early in pregnancy and those performed later, and it limits to a single reason, 'saving' the mother's life, the legal justification for the procedure." [36] The

Court structured acceptable law in terms of the time of gestation when action was proposed, distinguishing the stage prior to approximately the end of the first trimester, the subsequent stage up to viability of the fetus, and the stage subsequent to viability. In this last stage, abortion may be regulated and even proscribed, except where necessary for the preservation of the life or health of the mother. [37] The Supreme Court thus gave more emphasis to an approach based upon time factors than to one based upon specific indications for inducing termination of pregnancy. In taking this direction, the Court was faithful to historic common law perceptions of the importance of the stage of fetal development to the abortion decision. The Court gave secondary emphasis, however, to the direction which legislatures, particularly of English-speaking countries and jurisdictions, have tended to take in seeking to balance the permission and the prohibition of abortion. A survey of legislated provisions, which aims to identify the issues legislatures have tended directly and indirectly to address, follows.

MODERN LEGISLATED ABORTION INDICATIONS

When legislatures have designed enactments under which abortion may legitimately be sought and undertaken, they have almost invariably acted against a background of prohibitory law. That law may have been based upon legislation or legal judgments, the true scope of which was untested. Accordingly, some of the more conservative modern legislated reforms claiming to liberalize the availability of legal abortion may have only made explicit the grounds upon which the procedure was legitimate under the implicit provisions of the previous law. The new legislation may have changed the clarity rather than the license of the law, and may indeed have added conditions not formerly existing. [38] Most commonly, however, legislation has introduced novel specific indications upon which abortion might lawfully be undertaken. A number of these indications may be available restrictively, particularly by reference to the stage of fetal development. Thus, while the more life-threatening or health-threatening indications might be available at any time during pregnancy, the more accommodating or elective indications might be available only during the earlier stages of pregnancy.

The following survey lists a number of the indications to be found in modern legislation, and addresses a number of their features.

STRICT NECESSITY

While modern legislation invariably expressly accommodates abortion to prevent danger to a woman's life or grave risk to her health, this indication almost invariably existed under pre-existing law. Despite the dogmatism of traditional legal prohibitions of abortion, its legitimacy has almost always been recognized to preserve a woman's life or to preserve her permanent health against serious danger. Whatever resolution religious doctrine may have offered to a conflict between the values of the life of the fetus and that of its mother endangered by continuation of pregnancy, secular laws addressing that conflict have accepted the priority of the mother's life. When such laws consisted more in recitals of doctrine than in recorded judgments producing case precedents, the issue of justified abortion did not have to be specifically addressed. Legal discussion centered upon the legitimacy of ending a child's life in the course of delivery, when its head or limb was protruding from the mother's body, rather than at an earlier time, reflecting perhaps the underdeveloped state of knowledge of medical causation and prognosis.

As laws and particularly law reform came to be more systematically approached, the conditions and exceptions of law-enforcement became clarified. In 1846, for instance, the Criminal Law Commissioners in England reflected upon the absolute-sounding prohibition of abortion expressed in the 1837 legislation[39] in light of provisions in other countries' codified penal laws,[40] and recommended the following addition to the abortion law: "Provided that no act. . . shall be punishable when such act is done in good faith with the intention of saving the life of the mother whose miscarriage is intended to be preserved."[41] This humane provision had been enacted in 1828 in New York State, whose legislation excused abortion if it "shall have been necessary to preserve the life of such mother, or shall have been advised by two physicians to be necessary for such purpose."[42] Although this latter provision tended to disappear as state laws became increasingly restrictive, preservation of maternal life remained an indication for legal abortion.[43]

It is an interesting feature of comparative jurisprudence that in many of the jurisdictions that follow the common law tradition, the defense to a criminal charge of the necessity to save human life has been established through abortion cases, following the seminal English decision in 1938 in *R. v. Bourne.*[44] The judge in that case extended life-preservation to physical and mental health-preservation, observing that:

> [I]f the doctor is of opinion, on reasonable grounds and with adequate knowledge, that the probable consequence of the continuance of the pregnancy will be to make the woman a physical or mental wreck, the jury are quite entitled to take the view that the doctor . . . is operating for the purpose of preserving the life of the mother.[45]

While this case has been cited with approval in the United States,[46] its major impact has been upon abortion cases in the British Commonwealth, where it has been widely followed and never repudiated. It was immediately followed in the West African Court of Appeal,[47] and subsequently in New Zealand, [48] the Australian states of Queensland,[49] Victoria[50] and New South Wales, [51] in Canada,[52] Fiji,[53] the Eastern African Court of Appeal[54] and Zambia.[55] Further, the only Scottish legal authority in support of necessity as an exculpatory plea is concerned with the crime of abortion,[56] and section 240 of the Penal Code of Kenya,[57] which deals with medical necessity, provides:

> A person is not criminally responsible for performing in good faith . . . a surgical operation upon any person for his benefit, or upon an unborn child for the preservation of the mother's life, if the performance of the operation is reasonable, having regard to the patient's state at the time. . . .[58]

THE THERAPEUTIC INDICATION

Most legislation reforming abortion law recognizes a therapeutic indication going beyond mere necessity to preserve life or to protect health against grave risk. The British Abortion Act of 1967, for instance, illustrates such legislation in providing in section 1(1) (a) that abortion may be performed when:

> [T]he continuance of the pregnancy would involve risk to the life of the pregnant woman, or of injury to the physical or mental health of the pregnant woman. . . greater than if the pregnancy were terminated.[59]

This recognizes that the condition of pregnancy itself bears risks, and is not designed to allow those risks alone to serve as an indication for lawful abortion, since that would create in effect a legal right to abortion on request. The risk of injury to health that justifies abortion need only be "greater" than if pregnancy were terminated, however, and not necessarily considerably greater. Further, section 1(2) provides that in making an assessment of greater risk of injury to health from continuance of the pregnancy, "account may be taken of the pregnant woman's actual or reasonably foreseeable environment."

The British legislation probably represents a more liberal application of the therapeutic indication than is commonly enacted. Many legislatures have preferred to require therapeutic justifications to be more compelling than a mere health advantage of abortion over continuation of pregnancy. They speak not of risk of "injury" to the pregnant woman, but of her "danger" or "serious danger" from continued pregnancy. Further, they may be more accommodating of therapeutic abortion earlier in pregnancy than later, when an indication closer to strict necessity may alone be permissible. The law of New Zealand presents such an indication, in providing that abortion is unlawful unless:

> in the case of a pregnancy of not more than 20 weeks' gestation . . . the continuance of the pregnancy would result in serious danger (not being danger normally attendant upon childbirth) to the life, or to the physical or mental health, of the woman or girl, and that the danger cannot be averted by any other means. . . .[60]

THE FETAL OR EUGENIC INDICATION

Although there is an obvious sense in which abortion may not be considered as serving the benefit of the damaged unborn child,[61] many jurisdictions permit abortion in anticipation of serious handicap in a child which may be born. This type of provision may be supported by data on the high incidence of spontaneous abortion of severely abnormal fetuses, since if live birth is unlikely, abortion simulates rather than opposes nature, and may be better induced to minimize risk to the pregnant woman. Nevertheless, a discomfort that fetal indications may be relatively minor, and ethical questions regarding what degree of handicap, disadvantage, or abnormality should suffice for legal termination of pregnancy, cause legislatures to define fetal or eugenic indications by reference to serious conditions. The intention is to permit neural tube defects, central nervous system disorders, gross physical abnormalities, and major damage to several sense organs, to serve as fetal indications for abortion. British legislation, for instance, which appears quite liberal on its therapeutic indication, applies the test that "there is a substantial risk that if the child were born it would suffer from such physical or mental abnormalities as to be seriously handicapped."[62] It is of interest that abnormality is expressed for the child in the plural, suggesting that a single abnormality such as a cleft lip or palate might not suffice.[63] Even this test of serious handicap leaves some questions, however, since abortions are performed upon results of amniocentesis which disclose Down syndrome (mongolism), even though affected children born alive show a wide range of capabilities, and are handicapped to different degrees.

Not all enactments contain a fetal or eugenic indication in express terms. In Canada, for instance, the only ground for legal abortion is that "continuation of the pregnancy. . . would or would be likely to endanger [the female's] life or health."[64] Abortions may be undertaken, however, when it is shown that a woman's fear of fetal abnormality, of giving birth to a severely abnormal child, or of having to rear a seriously handicapped child, would likely endanger her physical or mental health.[65] It may be doubted that abortion practice differs greatly in this regard from that in Britain.[66]

JURIDICAL INDICATIONS

The juridical indications of rape and incest are normally accommodated under strict necessity, therapeutic, and fetal indications, and tend not to be separately identified. The common law defense of necessity to terminate pregnancy was recognized in the *Bourne* case,[67] which concerned a rape victim. Apart from Commonwealth jurisdictions adopting the Indian model,[68] few contain a clear indication for abortion of rape. Further, India's Medical Termination of Pregnancy Act of 1971,[69] has a therapeutic indication rather than a specific rape indication, but included in the statute are Explanations, and Explanation I of the indication provides that:

> Where any pregnancy is alleged by the pregnant woman to have been caused by rape, the anguish caused by such pregnancy shall be presumed to con- stitute a grave injury to the mental health of the pregnant woman.

The imperative form "shall be presumed" is curiously at variance with the lack of forensic support for the allegation. This may be contrasted with the law of Cyprus, where pregnancy may be terminated "following a certificate of the appropriate police authority supported by a medical certificate whenever this is possible, that the pregnancy was caused by rape. . . ."[70] The New Zealand provision more neutrally permits its therapeutic indica- tion to be applied by taking into account "the fact [where such is the case] that there are reasonable grounds for believing that the pregnancy is the result of rape."[71]

While compassion may compel accommodation of a rape indication for abortion, it is beset by legal dilemmas and individual problems of credibility and often aggravated by victims' reluctance to complain to police and other public authorities. Legal definitions and tests may reduce rape to, for instance, indecent assault, such as where the assailant is not guilty by reason of insanity, is below the age of 14,[72] or is the victim's estranged but not judicially separated husband.[73] Further, the application of legal tests to establish rape by, for instance, identifying a suspect and concluding a trial, will often frustrate any speedy relief for a rape victim. Accordingly, action may have to be taken upon the basis not of rape *per se*, but of the woman's distressed condition due to her conviction that she has been outraged and made pregnant. This belief affects her disposition, physical tolerance, and mental composure, and may be accommodated under the physical or mental health indications which most modern legislation includes.[74]

The incest indication raises no fewer problems of principle, since it seems to rest upon a historic abhorrence and taboo, and a belief in dysgenic effects of consanguineous procreation, which are more critically received today than they once were, even with our improved knowledge of the operation of recessive genes. Apart from raising difficulties in defining the prohibited degrees of union, [75] the indication is unclear as to whether it responds to eugenic considerations, to feared exploitation of females,[76] or to anticipated sociomedical considerations affecting family functioning. Since pregnancy by incest as opposed to by rape results from voluntary conduct on the female's part, the indication raises the special question of whether the female is entitled to relief not available to others also pregnant by voluntary conduct.

SOCIAL, SOCIOMEDICAL AND SOCIOECONOMIC INDICATIONS

A narrow ground of legalizing abortion is for preservation of life and health, but "health" is not clearly defined. The concept of health may be restrictively understood to center upon life-threatening conditions, so that the exemption from criminal liability for procuring abortion will be conservatively applied. On the other hand, the health exemption may be liberally applied, by reference to the description of "health" presented in the Preamble to the Constitution of the World Health Organization, to which almost all countries subscribe. This provides: "Health is a state of complete physical, mental and social well-being and not merely the absence of disease or infirmity."[77] Accordingly, social and family factors may have an impact upon health of which the law of abortion may take note. The British Abortion Act of 1967 not only authorizes the procedure when "the continuance of the pregnancy would involve risk. . . of injury to the physical or mental health of the pregnant woman or any existing child of her family, greater than if the pregnancy were terminated,"[78] but adds that, in determining such risk of injury to health, "account may be taken of the pregnant woman's actual or reasonably foreseeable environment."[79]

Even where legislation is restrictively expressed, it may seem that recognition of a health-centered therapeutic indication for abortion may legitimately permit a physician to take account of social and socioeconomic considerations. For instance, when the Canadian Parliament was reviewing the law in 1969, it was aware of the British enactment of 1967, and its reforms expressly declined to follow the approach of the British model; the resulting legislation was intended to be conservative.[80] Nevertheless, the significance of social and socioeconomic considerations to health was acknowledged in a subsequent governmental explanation wherein the Parliamentary Secretary to the Minister of Justice explained that:

> The danger for the pregnant woman's life or health is the only criterion in this matter. If it is proven medically that financial, social or other circumstances endangered or would probably endanger the mother's life or health, a certificate [for abortion] may be given; but the decision must be based on reasons of real danger to life or health, and not on social or financial factors as such.[81]

Thus, legal propriety of abortion may be influenced by the breadth of medical sensitivity and vision, which may range from a cellular to a social or socioeconomic perspective of danger to health.[82]

FAMILY INDICATIONS

The nature of a family's functioning may be of sociomedical significance, and regard may be paid to this under therapeutic or social indications, as has been seen above, particularly in the setting of British legislation. The law of Cyprus has an exceptional provision, however, which specifically addresses the risk of breakdown of family structure. Section 169A(b) of the Criminal Code deals with pregnancy following rape, certified by an appropriate police authority, and permits termination not on grounds of the rape itself, but only "if the pregnancy was not terminated, serious breakdown would be caused to the social position of the pregnant woman or to her family environment."[83] Underlying this provision is the local dilemma of pregnancy by rape where assailant and victim are identified with different communities of the Greek-Cypriot and Turkish-Cypriot populaton. In other jurisdictions, the incidence of pregnancy crossing ethnic or racial divisions might, of course, be considered insofar as it may be accommodated by mental health, social, or sociomedical indications.

CONTRACEPTIVE INDICATIONS

While many jurisdictions seem anxious to promote recourse to contraceptive means in the hope of reducing unplanned pregnancies and the related call for abortion, there is an unwillingness to contain in legal form a fertility control package in which a diligent acceptor of contraceptive services may have access to an abortion service as back-up insurance against contraceptive failure. The closest approach to this position appears in India's legislation,[84] which recognizes an orthodox therapeutic indication but says in Explanation II that:

> Where any pregnancy occurs as a result of failure of any device or method used by any married woman or her husband for the purpose of limiting the

number of children, the anguish caused by such unwanted pregnancy may be presumed to constitute a grave injury to the mental health of the pregnant woman.

Left unstated is the comparable if not greater anguish an unmarried woman may experience. However critically one may reflect upon this legislative approach, it appears to offer an inducement to contraceptive practice. Other jurisdictions, however, have not adopted such an indica-iton since it frequently raises difficult questions about reliability of contraceptive means used, and personal conscientiousness. A further policy issue may be that a family planning agency able to offer this insurance might lose its own incentive to improve services and technologies.

REQUEST

While many jurisdictions in Europe have adopted legislation permitting abortion simply upon the request of the pregnant woman, they tend invariably to limit this right by reference to the duration of pregnancy. Countries with a simple request indication for abortion that is limited by gestational age include: Austria (three months), Bulgaria (ten weeks), Denmark (12 weeks), the German Democratic Republic (first trimester), Italy (90 days), Norway (12 weeks), Sweden (18 weeks), the U.S.S.R. (12 weeks) and Yugoslavia-Slovenia (ten weeks).[85] Only China imposes no time limit upon its request indication, and Tunisia (three months) appears to be the only non-European, non-Commonwealth jurisdiction to have legislated such a provision.[86] The only Commonwealth country whose law permits abortion upon request is Singapore, where legislation controls the procedure by reference not to indications but to qualifications of physicians, the hospital or other institution involved, and the woman's citizenship or residency.[87]

Legal recourse to abortion on request, available in the United States since *Roe v. Wade* was decided in 1973, is not confined to citizens of the jurisdiction. Accordingly, women of adequate means from jurisdictions not permitting abortion on request or on other appropriate indications may be able to travel to the United States for the purpose of terminating their pregnancies. Women from Bermuda, the Bahamas, Barbados and other West Indian jurisdictions, as well as from Mexico, Central and South America, Australia, and New Zealand frequently do so. Of Canadian resident women having abortions, one in six will use a facility in the United States.[88] Access to legal abortion on request is possible by this means because abortion laws tend not to create extra-territorial crimes,[89] although some abortion laws may bind citizens of jurisdictions following the European tradition in which criminal laws apply not to the territoriality of conduct but to the nationality of the actor.[90] In jurisdictions applying territorial criteria, however, not only may it be lawful to travel elsewhere to have an abortion lawful where performed but not permitted by the jurisdiction of the woman's nationality, citizenship, or residence, but it may also be lawful while at home to arrange such a journey without offending local law, in much the same way as one may arrange to visit the gaming facilities of Las Vegas or Atlantic City while in a jurisdiction where such gambling is unlawful.

IMPLEMENTATION PROVISIONS

It is usual for jurisdictions enacting laws that permit abortion to include provisions concerning not only gestational periods, but also the qualifications of personnel conducting the procedures, and the facilities in which they may be performed. A number of examples will be briefly considered below to show the issues involved, without making extensive reference to illustrations drawn from particular enactments.

An understanding of the interaction of such provisions may be gained by considering the Abortion Act of 1974 of the Republic of Singapore.[91] The Act provides the general legal setting for abortion, but relies upon subordinate law in the form of ministerial regulations to supply fine tuning, including the administrative refinements of physicians' qualifications, institutional approvals, and record keeping, which keep the system operable in the context of changing resources and pressures. Under Singapore's law an applicant for abortion must make a request to a registered medical practitioner, and express her consent to pregnancy termination in writing. The procedure can be performed only in a government-maintained hospital, maternity home, or clinic, or in an institution specifically approved for performance of abortions by the Minister for Health. An applicant must be a citizen or wife of a citizen of Singapore, or must have been a resident of Singapore for four months immediately preceding the performance of the abortion, except where the procedure is necessary to save her life. She must be no more than 16 weeks pregnant, although she may be aborted up to 24 weeks of pregnancy provided that the physician possesses specified and more advanced surgical or obstetric qualifications. After 24 weeks of pregnancy, an abortion may be procured only if it is necessary to save the life or to prevent grave permanent injury to the woman's physical or mental health. Where the treatment undertaken consists solely of use of prescribed drugs without any surgical operation or procedure, the physician does not require the specified higher qualifications, even if pregnancy exceeds 16 weeks, and the procedure is not restricted to a government hospital or to an approved institution. The fee for termination of pregnancy in a government facility is set at a low level.[92]

GESTATIONAL LIMITS

It has already been noted that many jurisdictions make different requirements to implement laws permitting abortion, related to the stage of advancement of pregnancy. At early stages, requirements for the procedure may be relatively less demanding, but later in pregnancy legal provisions may center upon only a strict necessity indication, where the woman's life itself is at risk. Even legislation authorizing abortion only early in pregnancy may have to accommodate late abortion on grounds of necessity. This pattern was confirmed in English law long before liberalization of prohibitive abortion law was considered. The Infant Life (Preservation) Act of 1929 [93] gave protection to a child in the course of delivery, that is, after birth commenced spontaneously or by induction (so that the abortion law ceased to apply) but before the child had completely proceeded alive from the mother's body so as to be a human being, protected by, for instance, the homicide law.[94] Section 2(1) recognized that the child's death could be caused, for instance, by craniotomy or collapsing the head, when this was done "in good faith for the purpose only of preserving the life of the mother."

Requiring that more highly qualified medical personnel and more advanced medical facilities attend terminations of more advanced pregnancies is appropriate not only because the medical procedures involved may be more hazardous for the woman, but because the fetus may be not only viable, but alive when taken from the mother.[95] While there is no general duty to perform legal abortion so as to maximize the opportunities for fetal survival,[96] the child may be born alive, and thereby acquire a legal right to appropriate medical care.[97]

QUALIFICATIONS OF PRACTITIONERS

Statutory provisions governing both quantity and quality concern physicians involved in determining the appropriateness of and performing abortions. In Indian law, for instance, a single physician need only satisfy himself upon existence of a legal indication for abortion where pregnancy does not exceed 12 weeks' duration, while if it does but is under 20 weeks' duration, there must be a second medical opinion.[98] While legislation commonly demands specialist experience or qualifications of physicians who terminate more advanced pregnancies, for obvious reasons, little recognition is given to the consideration that very early abortions may safely be performed, for instance by menstrual aspiration,[99] by nurses or paramedical personnel acting alone.[100] In part this may be because means of reliable early detection of pregnancy are not widely available, and such practices may be classified as contraception or nonabortive menstrual therapy in which such personnel may lawfully be involved. It has recently been recognized, however, that where a physician is exempted from criminal liability for terminating a pregnancy, nurses share that protection when carrying out instructions and routine related functions, even if they manage the actual stage of the woman aborting. [101]

APPROVAL PROCEDURES

Physicians are always expected to act, particularly regarding abortion, conscientiously and in good faith. Good faith may be established by recourse to a second medical opinion, unless the urgency of the circumstances makes such recourse hazardous or impossible.[102] A sizeable number of national laws reflect this by formally requiring a second, and sometimes a third, medical opinion. In Canada and Zambia, three medical opinions are required, but in rather different circumstances. Under Canada's Criminal Code, there must be certification by a therapeutic abortion committee composed of at least three physicians, none of whom may perform abortions in any hospital.[103] In Zambia's legislation, two medical opinions supporting that of the initial physician are required, including one from a practitioner who "has specialized in the branch of medicine in which the patient is specifically required to be examined."[104] It is clear that approval procedures of this nature can obstruct patient access to services. In Canada in 1977, it was found that, for a number of reasons, "the procedure provided in the Criminal Code . . . is in practice illusory for many Canadian women,"[105] although World Health Organization statistics showed that in 1971 there was one physician for every 600 Canadians. In Zambia,under 1972 legislation, three physicians including a specialist must be involved in each abortion decision; however, there is only one physician for every 8,110 inhabitants.

   Legislation genuinely seeking to make abortion services available as a health measure, rather than as a limited exception to criminal liability, tend to minimize approval procedures. In Singapore, for instance, five years experience with such a procedure resulted in its abolition. Nevertheless, a number of Eastern European countries have boards primarily of nonphysicians to consider cases, making clear that a social rather than a purely medical assessment is being made.[106] Rather exceptionally, in Bolivia judicial approval is required.[107]

MEDICAL FACILITIES

It has been seen that terminations of more advanced pregnancies may be confined to better equipped facilities, except in circumstances of emergency. Apart from taking into account health considerations, however, a number of jurisdictions confine all abortion procedures to government facilities, or to specifically approved private facilities. This tends to be done in order to achieve general quality control, and to achieve equitable access to services by controlling profiteering in the private sector of health care.

Experience in a number of jurisdictions shows that licensing procedures can generate a plethora of regulations supporting, and supported by, a weighty enforcement bureaucracy, and that they may leave considerable uncertainty about whether a particular procedure was or was not legal because of the status of the facility in which it was performed. Experience in a number of countries has caused them to simplify their licensing procedures. For instance, Singapore did so regarding drug-induced abortions, as did Britain in authorizing termination of pregnancies of under 12 weeks' duration in private day-care centers. At the other extreme is New Zealand's massively cumbersome Contraception, Sterilisation, and Abortion Act of 1977,[108] an Act so complicated that the national Abortion Supervisory Committee it created recommended amending legislation within eight weeks of the legislation coming into force.[109]

THIRD PARTY CONSENTS

Although general patterns may be apparent in legal provisions on consent to a woman's abortion required from such persons as her husband, her parents, a guardian or a comparably responsible person, those provisions tend to exist under the jurisdiction's general law rather than in its abortion legislation. Such provisions tend to have originated with the local cultural and historic system, reflecting sensitivities that are part of indigenous expectations of family functioning and of the place of the individual. They are not derived from more modern rationalizations of optimal allocation of health resources. Legal provisions in this area are conditioned by the prevailing social environment, with the result that laws in countries favoring a wide measure of individual and particularly female autonomy permit women to opt for abortion free from restraint by a husband,[110] while those in more paternalistic cultures make the woman's consent a necessary but not necessarily a sufficient condition for performance of abortion. Regarding legal minors and the disabled, interesting priorities are shown in the Indian law, section 3(4) of which provides that:

(a) No pregnancy of a woman, who has not attained the age of eighteen years, or, who, having attained the age of eighteen years, is a lunatic, shall be terminated, except with the consent in writing of her guardian.

(b) Save as otherwise provided in clause (a), no pregnancy shall be terminated except with the consent of the pregnant woman.[111]

Consent provisions may also interact with approved indications for abortion. Where this is lawful only upon a strict necessity or a therapeutic indication, there may be less room for a third party veto, but where grounds less related to the woman's health exist, third parties may be able to play a bigger role in decision making. Most jurisdictions disclose many unresolved issues, such as whether a parent can authorize the abortion of an unemancipated child who is ambivalent about terminating her pregnancy, decision making affecting adult and minor retardates, and the role of a husband and an unmarried biological father. These issues reflect the general state of development of medical consent law in the jurisdiction, however, rather than issues raised by its particular abortion legislation. Similarly, the general law will govern whether a self-appointed representative may litigate on behalf of an unborn child against a hospital[112] or the pregnant woman herself.[113]

CONSCIENTIOUS OBJECTION

Legislation which is expressed primarily in terms of historic prohibition, with a narrow exception for preservation of a woman's life or health, tends not to elaborate positive provisions for the performance of abortion, beyond providing that the medical basis of applying the exception from criminal liability is adequately established.[114] However, legislation designed around the delivery of abortion services commonly recognizes that particular health professionals may have conscientious objections to the procedure and may abhor involvement.[115] Several laws provide that health personnel with religious or other conscientious objections to induced abortion per se (as opposed to objections based on the features of an individual case) may be exempted from participation. The British Abortion Act of 1967, for instance, provides in section 4(1) that:

> [N]o person shall be under any duty, whether by contract or by any statutory or other legal requirement, to participate in any treatment authorised by this Act to which he has a conscientious objection: . . . Provided that in any legal proceedings the burden of proof of conscientious objection shall rest on the person claiming to rely on it.[116]

Section 4(2) adds the limitation that:

Nothing in subsection (1) of this section shall affect any duty to participate in treatment which is necessary to save the life or to prevent grave permanent injury to the physical or mental health of a pregnant woman.[117]

The substance of this provision is repeated in the Abortion Act, 1974 of Singapore,[118] but section 6(2), which provides that the burden of proving conscientious objection rests on the person invoking that exemption from involvement, adds that "that burden may be discharged by such person testifying on oath or affirmation that he has a conscientious objection to participating in any treatment to terminate pregnancy." The implication is that legitimate objection must be based upon a general philosophy, so that it cannot be invoked against procedures in, for instance, a public hospital by a person prepared to have involvement in abortions in a private facility.

Such conscience clauses cover surgeons and other physicians, nurses, and most likely auxiliary health personnel. It is unclear, however, whether they are confined to abortion-related procedures such as inducing abortion by surgical or other means, clearing up an operating room and disposing of products of conception, or whether they extend to administering general or local anesthetics, giving routine postoperative care, or even serving meals to abortion patients.

Whether a physician with a conscientious objection must inform a woman eligible for legal abortion of this objection, and refer her to another physician who does not share the objection, is a matter primarily addressed in codes of medical ethics rather than in abortion legislation. It would also be addressed in the general law on medical malpractice, negligence, and abandonment.

CITIZENSHIP OR RESIDENCY

Some jurisdictions with legislation providing for the provision of abortion services have been apprehensive of attracting women from other jurisdictions in their region. For example, the state of South Australia in 1969 pioneered liberal access to abortion in Australia and New Zealand, but did not want its major cities to become national or regional abortion centers, because of fear of acquiring an unsavory image and of unduly relieving other governments of their responsibility of facing the abortion issue. South Australia's law therefore provides that, with an emergency exception, abortion services are not to be provided to "any woman who has not resided in South Australia for a period of at least two months before the termination of her pregnancy."[119] This wording has at times been loosely construed to cover women who, for instance, had lived in the state for two months during childhood, or who resided there for a total of two months made up of accumulated separate days or weekends. When Singapore took a similar regional initiative in 1974, its legislation stated, again with an emergency exception:

> No treatment . . . shall be carried out . . . unless the pregnant woman is a citizen of Singapore, or is the wife of a citizen of Singapore or unless she has been resident in Singapore for a period of at least four months immediately preceding the date on which such treatment is to be carried out.[120]

This type of provision may appeal to a jurisdiction in the West Indies, for instance, which wants to legislate for abortion without attracting un-welcome visitors. The same result has been achieved, however, in a number of jurisdictions, through confining such services to government hospitals and excluding nonresidents from their services or certain of their services except in emergency cases.

REPORTING REQUIREMENTS AND CONFIDENTIALITY

Jurisdictions with developed publicly funded health services invariably require notification to government of hospital and other health pro-cedures for quality-control, fiscal accountability, statistical, demographic and, for instance, epidemiological purposes. Abortion procedures are not exceptional in that regard, but they have tended to attract reporting requirements peculiar to themselves, often expressed in specific legislation on abortion availability. Liberalized abortion provisions often appear wary of the risk of abuse, not least when procedures are authorized in private health facilities. They therefore require documentary evidence of reg-ularity of abortions performed under their auspices, often in complex and sometimes idiosyncratic detail. Further, where governmental hospitals and other such facilities are involved, there may be an incentive to have compelling documentary evidence of propriety, for fear of scandal and political accountability. Contravention of reporting requirements is usually an independent offense, and does not affect the lawful status of the procedure performed.

Balancing detailed requirements of the information to be submitted to government are equally detailed requirements of the protection of confidentiality such information is to receive. This may be governed by general provisions on protection of government data, but legislatures often recognize the special sensitivity of abortion information, and its potential for harmful misuse. Accordingly, provisions may be enacted not only on information to be given, but also on the nature and duration of its storage. Further, laws may specify that information is not to be given; in New Zealand, for instance, no report of an approved abortion shall include the name or address of any patient.[121]

POPULATION POLICIES AND ABORTION LAWS

Standing back from the particular provisions of particular legislation, and reflecting upon a nation's history of abortion law reform, one may gain a view of an underlying population policy. Clearly, the law on abortion must not be taken in isolation from laws on contraception and sterilization, nor from social programs instituted by legislation including financial allowances and tax advantages related to family size. National legislation may positively promote family limitation by, for instance, withholding financial allowances in grant or tax-relief programs upon birth of a child beyond a determined number for a family, or may favor population growth by rewarding the birth of each additional child. Family planning including abortion legislation may reflect the direction taken by national policy.

Historical instances may illustrate how such legislation may be employed to serve an overall national population goal. In post-Revolutionary Russia, for instance, legal abortion was allowed as an expression of the emancipation of women, with a slight limitation being introduced in 1920 on grounds of ensuring medical safety. In the mid-1930s, the danger of war with Germany and Japan was perceived and associated with those nations' military postures and related population perceptions. Recollection of the many millions of their population who perished in World War I remained fresh in the memory of Russia's leaders. Their acute consciousness of an imminent need for military and civilian manpower and population reserves resulted, in 1936, in explanations of the harmful effects of abortion upon women's health and its prohibition, except on clear medical and eugenic grounds. Further, literature on contraception disappeared from Russian bookshops.[122] In 1955, when the external dangers had been overcome,[123] abortion again became legal, subject only to limitations tied to gestational age and qualifications of attendant personnel.[124] Under current pressures of a low birth rate, an aging population, and a higher proportion of population growth in Soviet Central Asia, there are signs of an anti-abortion movement.[125]

Recourse to abortion law to affect population size and composition has been a characteristic of Eastern European practice. In September 1957, for instance, Romania followed the lead of the Soviet Union and issued a decree making abortion available on request. Within a few years, it had become the major means of fertility control in the country, and the birthrate showed steady decline. By October 1966, the government was alarmed to find the birthrate too low to realize the national socioeconomic plan of development, and restricted availability of abortion by new legislation.[126] The birthrate rose quickly, and eventually leveled off slightly above the rate of neighboring Eastern European countries. It has been observed that the Romanian restrictive abortion policy of 1966 represents one of the most effective reported attempts to influence fertility at a national level by changing access to means of fertility control, without accompanying changes in social structure.[127]

More recently, Czechoslovakia responded to awareness of low birth-rates and an increasingly older population by adopting pronatalist policies, including the restriction of abortion services, which appear to have succeeded in reversing fertility decline.[128] After the Second World War Czechoslovakia had a relatively high birthrate, associated with lowered age of marriage, introduction of financial family allowances and improved maternity benefits. In the 1950s, however, the birthrate declined, but the government was ambivalent about a conservative response because of its alarm at the rising rate of illegal abortion and associated maternal deaths. In 1958, that problem was alleviated by legislation permitting induced abortion under controlled conditions, but because the country lacked an infrastructure to deliver alternative family planning services, the legal abortion rate climbed from 32 percent of all pregnancies in 1958 to 40 percent in 1960.[129] Contraceptive pills and the I.U.D. were not introduced in the country until 1965. By 1968 Czechoslovakia had the lowest birthrate in Europe. Inducements were increasingly offered to encourage bigger families, so that today Czech family allowances may be the most generous in Europe, but in 1973 the step was taken to enact new abortion provisions rendering such medical services less available.[130] As an exception to the national free health care system, for instance, a fee ranging from 200 to 800 Cz. crowns is charged for an abortion, although it may be waived in special cases.[131]

Abortion applicants under the new provisions must usually act during the first 12 weeks of pregnancy upon general indications, although a 24-week period may be allowed upon a fetal or eugenic indication, since this may not be detectable until later in pregnancy. The woman has to go before a three-member district commission, usually consisting of a gynecologist, a social worker, and a member of local government. About 94 percent of applications are granted,[132] but an appeal against refusal may be taken to a regional commission. The procedure can be distressing, and a Czech gynecologist who helped to plan the system has expressed a fear that women who have experienced it may prefer recourse to illegal abortion.[133] Nevertheless, almost half of unintended pregnancies in the country are ended by officially recorded abortion.[134]

The position in Poland has been rather different from that in Czechoslovakia,[135] since the historic and revived significance of the Catholic Church has had a conditioning influence upon popular pronatalist sentiments. Poland has had a long official tradition of involvement with family planning practice, originating before the Second World War, due to the tendency of the Polish people to have a high rate of fertility, and of harmful illegal abortion. Following severe population loss between 1939 and 1945, Poland became strongly and successfully committed to rebuilding population numbers, so much so that its birthrate peaked in 1951 at 31 births per 1000 population, and Poland retains the highest birthrate (20 per 1000) and population growth rate in Eastern Europe.[136] Indeed, too rapid population growth in the mid-1950s was associated with economic difficulties, and the government began to educate its citizens about the negative effects of a high birthrate. In 1956, abortion was legalized, and fully subsidized if done in government facilities.[137] This move, together with increased availability of contraceptives brought down the birthrate to such an extent that the government again became concerned, and since the early 1970s, it has tried to stimulate more rapid population growth,[138] although it has so far resisted heavy pressure to repeal or restrict its abortion legislation.[139] Poland therefore presents a contrast with the Russian and Czechoslovakian experiences with using abortion legislation to contain national population growth.

Experience in Hungary runs closer to the Czechoslovakian experience, and was influenced by comparable dynamics. Abortion was legalized in 1956 upon liberal conditions, contributing to such a decline in the birthrate that, in 1962, Hungary's rate of population growth was the lowest in Europe, and it continued below replacement level until 1973.[140] In that year, population policy measures were adopted to encourage births, including new legislation intended to reduce access to legal abortion.[141] A committee now has to consider applications, although single women, those aged over 40 (until 1979, the age was over 35), and those who have three living children have a right to abortion.

The deliberation with which governments in these Eastern European countries have employed their abortion laws to seek effects designed to serve national policies stands in sharp contrast to the use of governmental power in the United States. The Supreme Court, in *Roe v. Wade*, established that under the U.S. Constitution, government has only a very limited entitlement ability to intervene in the privacy of personal decisions about reproductive matters. In the Eastern European jurisdictions, individual reproductive capacity is considered a public resource, which is amenable to governmental management once realized by conception. In identifying fetal viability as the point at which the state's interest in potential life becomes compelling,[142] the Supreme Court marked a boundary protecting human beings from state power to use or dedicate their bodies to the service of a public purpose.

APPROACHES TO SPONTANEOUS ABORTION

The attention the law has come to give to prevention of fetal loss through induced abortion has not been apparent regarding spontaneous abortion. Reduction of the incidence of high-risk pregnancy and spontaneous abortion may be achieved by appropriate maternal health care, but an individual's refusal or failure to take or to render such care rarely attracts legal penalties when fetal loss results, and public authorities willing to spend considerable resources upon forensic inquiries into induced abortion may feel no comparable obligation to incur expense to deter spontaneous fetal loss. Welfare, educational, and nutritional programs for pregnant women may not exist, or may easily fall under budgetary cuts. In part, this passive response may be explained historically by undeveloped means to detect early fetal wastage, and by passive acceptance of high rates of infant mortality after birth.[143] In modern times, it has been reinforced by awareness that much spontaneous loss of conceptuses involves nonviable fetuses which could not have been born alive, or fetuses which are grossly defective.[144] Spontaneous abortion represents nature's way of achieving human quality control. It has been estimated that 40 percent of human pregnancies end in spontaneous miscarriage, over half before pregnancy is recognized.[145]

Historic interpreters of the English common law, such as Bracton, assessed unlawfully inducing abortion after quickening as a homicide,[146] and modern legislators continue to consider that up to life imprisonment is an appropriate sentence,[147] as it is for homicide by murder or manslaughter. In Canada in 1975, for instance, a Supreme Court judge observed that "Parliament regards procuring abortion as a grave crime which carries with it the same maximum penalty as noncapital murder."[148] This exposes an anomaly, however, since if unlawfully inducing abortion at any stage of pregnancy is considered in law tantamount to causing death, then experiencing or inadvertently causing spontaneous abortion might be expected equally to involve experiencing or causing death, but no comparable sense of death is apparent, except perhaps where an advanced fetus is concerned. Jurisdictions in the United States do not uniformly recognize wrongful death claims on behalf of viable fetuses,[149] and those which do tend to consider viability the crucial precondition of the claim.[150] In common law jurisdictions outside the United States, live birth is the essential precondition of standing to sue,[151] although claims may usually then be allowed for prenatal injuries. It is not clear that such claims are properly described as covering fetal injuries, since the governing legal principle may apply equally regarding behavior before conception resulting in a litigant's injury after birth.[152] If the wrongful act prevents live birth, however, no claim is recognized on behalf of the stillborn child although the mother's prenatal loss may be compensated in litigation brought on her own behalf, as may that of her husband if he is the biological father.[153] Similarly, since attempts to sue on behalf of an unborn child to enjoin or otherwise prevent the mother deliberately inducing abortion have not been allowed by courts of any significance,[154] such a claim brought in order to reduce risks of spontaneous abortion cannot be expected to be successful.

Official registration of spontaneous abortion or stillbirth, which may include quite different information from that registered for live birth, tends to be limited to the more advanced stage of gestation. The application of registration requirements can lead to considerable local variations in practice,[155] but vital statistics registers tend to present some useful still-birth information.[156] Registration criteria vary between jurisdictions, however, despite recommendations for international uniformity.[157] Representative of modern provisions may be the The Vital Statistics Act of Ontario,[158] which requires stillbirth registration when the fetus was delivered dead after an estimated 20 weeks' gestation, or when it weighed 500 grams. This coincides with standard medical dictionary definitions of abortion and stillbirth, although such measures pay no definitive regard to the distinction between fetal viability and nonviability. The English Infant Life (Preservation) Act of 1929[159] includes a rebuttable presumption of viability at 28 weeks' gestation, but medical evidence may now set viability earlier in most cases. Nevertheless, for registration purposes the English law consistently provides that a stillborn child is "a child which has issued from its mother after the twenty-eighth week of pregnancy and which did not . . . breathe or show any other signs of life."[160] Earlier abortions are not registered as such, although induced abortions must be reported to the Minister of Health under the Abortion Act of 1967.

Disposal of the abortus, whether of an induced or spontaneous abortion, is also not controlled by clear legal provisions. Most legal systems punish the infliction of indignity upon a human corpse, but, perhaps with the exception of an abortus lost in the course of birth, an aborted fetus may not have this protection.[161] It has been observed that "embryos that are spontaneously miscarried prior to viability are not baptized by any Christian denomination"[162] (and accordingly do not have to be buried in consecrated ground), and this may historically have denied Western legal systems an incentive or means to develop principles in the area. In Britain in 1971, the Lane Committee was established to review the operation of the Abortion Act of 1967, and it questioned many hospital authorities on disposal of therapeutically aborted fetuses. Replies showed that incineration was most common, although waste disposal units were frequently mentioned, as was the possibility that materials might be sent to human genetics and other laboratories. Large fetuses, resulting from late hysterotomies or abortions after viability, were treated as stillbirths or neonatal deaths, and although some might be sent to the mortuary, many were incinerated or sent to laboratories. Products from vacuum aspiration were not filtered in about half of the cases, and always filtered in about a quarter.[163] Some hospital authorities mentioned staff distaste for handling fetuses and fetal material,[164] but none mentioned parental objection.

The Lane Committee supported the recommendation made in 1972 by a departmental Advisory Group chaired by Sir John Peel, which addressed the research use of fetuses and fetal material. Their report surveyed and generally approved fetus and fetal material usage in research, but the group recommended that, where human tissue donation legislation was inapplicable, parents be given an opportunity to declare their wishes about disposal of the fetus.[165] This is a more sympathetic approach than has been taken by courts in the United States, where it has been held that there is no implied term in the hospital-patient relation preventing incineration of a stillborn fetus without prior permission.[166] Similarly, a mother's claim failed when she could not show a hospital had been wanton, willful or malicious in losing the body of her prematurely born child.[167] Because at common law a human corpse is not generally considered to be property,[168] a proprietary action would probably have failed as well.[169]

Abortion and Contraception

Since historically there were no reliable means to detect pregnancy much before quickening occurred, it was natural that quickening should occupy the concern of the law on abortion, and that the point of commencement of pregnancy is no more than a notional moment from which subsequently perceived events are measured. Modern medicine offers early means to diagnose pregnancy with reliability, and has established a catalogue of related signs from which pregnancy may be reliably inferred. Few systems of legislation on abortion have had recourse to such medical data, however, to refine commencement of pregnancy. Indeed, in that illegal abortion can be committed in many jurisdictions whether the woman acted upon is pregnant or not,[170] the time pregnancy commences is inconsequential. This separation of legal norms and biological and medical information has become aggravated in light of developing knowledge of contraceptive means. Some techniques may be shown to obstruct not fertilization of an ovum, that is, conception, but its subsequent implantation in the uterus, which is the condition of its natural future growth. Historically conditioned prohibitive abortion legislation may endanger the legal propriety of modern contraceptive techniques.[171]

Both preconception applications of drugs and intrauterine devices, and "hindsight" or "morning after" applications of drugs and, for instance, menstrual therapies to obstruct or prevent implantation, may raise difficult questions with uncertain answers under abortion legislation, particularly when it focuses upon the intent with which a person acts upon a woman whether she is pregnant or not. Intent to achieve abortion and intent to achieve contraception may not be separated by much, where the suspected operation of some modern contraceptive means is concerned.[172] Defeat of the Comstock laws in the United States[173] is recent enough to leave a memory of restrictive legislation on contraception itself. In jurisdictions where contraceptive practice has only the grudging license of inhospitable law, realization that abortion law may obstruct contraception is not necessarily offensive.

A step towards separation of abortion from contraception has been taken in New Zealand. The Royal Commission of Inquiry into Contraception, Sterilisation and Abortion in New Zealand reported in 1977 that "a doubt exists as to whether certain devices and techniques are contraceptive or abortifacient."[174] After reviewing medical data on the process of reproduction, common techniques used as contraception and likely future methods, and looking at definitional problems under the abortion law, as well as the status of the unborn child, the Commission concluded: "The fetus has a status from implantation which entitles it to preservation and protection."[175] That status, however, was found not to confer an absolute right to life, lest "a greater value might be placed on fetal life with its potential still unformed than on human life with full conscious development."[176] The legislature acted upon many of the Commission's findings, and New Zealand's law against the deliberate procuring of miscarriage now provides that:

> the term "miscarriage" means
>
> (a) The destruction or death of an embryo or fetus after implantation; or
> (b) The premature expulsion or removal of an embryo or fetus after implantation, otherwise than for the purpose of inducing the birth of a fetus believed to be viable or removing a fetus that has died.[177]

In establishing that protected human life commences at implantation, New Zealand has recognized the unquestioned legality of contraceptive means which prevent implantation, such as a drug and an I.U.D., but the status of menstrual aspiration remains unclear and may have to be resolved in practice upon the basis of the clinical facts of particular cases. More legal accommodation may be given to this technique under abortion legislation modeled on the Indian Penal Code,[178] since this defines unlawful conduct only where the woman is "with child"; New Zealand's law follows the English model of condemning action whether the woman is pregnant or not. It may therefore appear that for a conviction of unlawful abortion under Penal Code systems, the prosecution must prove beyond a reasonable doubt that the woman was with child—that is, pregnant.[179] Where menstrual aspiration is undertaken within six weeks of the last menstrual period, that may not be possible, not least in view of the limited medical technologies which may be commonly available in jurisdictions where the Penal Code applies. Further, use of such a technique may not be limited to physicians. This may explain how in Bangladesh, whose law is the unaltered Penal Code of 1860, paramedics in public clinics have undertaken menstrual regulation procedures by vacuum aspiration up to nine weeks after the woman's last menstruation, in apparent legal safety.[180]

LEGAL STATUS OF THE FERTILIZED (IN VITRO) OVUM

The successful development of in vitro ("test tube") fertilization in such countries as England, Australia, and, more recently, the United States will create additional legal problems when a fertilized ovum is placed to grow not in the uterus of the genetic donor, as has been the case so far, but of another woman.[181] Modern experience of so-called surrogate motherhood may anticipate only a number of these problems, since the mothers in publicized cases have been incubating their own ova.[182]

What may be described as "ordinary" in vitro fertilization has already had two impacts upon abortion law, however—first in showing that fertilization and implantation have quite separate significance, the latter being more instrumental in establishing pregnancy,[183] and second in showing legitimate wastage of early fertilized ova. Wastage occurs in the general development of the technique, as it does when a particular fertilized ovum develops abnormally in vitro; if it develops abnormally after implantation, of course, the regular abortion legislation is applicable. Pre-implantation wastage is not unlawful abortion under the legislation of England and the Australian states, since their laws refer to intending to procure the miscarriage of "any woman." The laws actually refer to any woman, whether she is or is not with child.[184] It appears, however, that three possible positions can exist, namely: (1) the woman is clearly pregnant, (2) it is uncertain whether the woman is or is not pregnant, and (3) the woman is clearly not pregnant, and that English and Australian laws apply to positions (1) and (2) but not to (3).[185] A woman turns to in vitro fertilization, of course, because of her inability, while fertile, to become pregnant. Accordingly, since before implantation of the fertilized in vitro ovum one cannot intend to procure the miscarriage of any woman who is or who may be pregnant, wastage of the fertilized ovum is not unlawful abortion.

This exposes the question of what legal status the fertilized in vitro ovum has. It is not a human being, since this requires life after emerging from the body of the mother.[186] The ovum which emerged was clearly living, and was of human origin and human potential, but this has never been claimed in itself to be a human being, any more than is a sperm. As against this, however, courts in the United States have ordered intrusive procedures against mothers for protection of unborn children,[187] and a fertilized in vitro ovum may appear to come within this category. There may seem to be severe limits including time constraints upon the extent to which intrusive orders should apply, and to order almost nine months of gestation may appear excessive, but the cases involved imposing blood transfusions upon Jehovah's Witnesses, who may have feared eternal consequences.

Two recent biomedical developments make it more urgent that the legal approach to the status of the ectogenetic fetus be resolved. Fetal surgery ex utero is now a prospect with possible legal consequences that, upon removal from the mother, the fetus becomes a human being[188] and retains that status upon replacement in utero, that the fetus has temporary human being status but resumes fetal status upon replacement, or that it retains fetal status while ex utero even while satisfying traditional legal tests of becoming a human being. Even if this last consequence is preferred, it may compel giving not less status to the fertilized in vitro ovum, which is also destined to be placed in utero.

The second development may, however, counter the thrust of this reasoning. Fertilized ova in Melbourne, Australia, have been frozen and stored,[189] and a plan to set up banks of frozen human embryos[190] has prompted a government investigation in the United Kingdom.[191] Posthumous use of frozen sperm leading to birth of a child well over a year after the genetic father's death is already a reality, but the frozen sperm would have the status of property. It must be asked if a frozen embryo would be property per se; the question of whose property it would be if it is property will not be pursued at present. Indications favoring property status come from both principle and experience. In principle, a substance of no value is not legal property.[192] When it becomes useful, however, a demand may arise which creates or exposes scarcity, and scarcity begets value, which the law concretizes in the recognition of a proprietary interest. No theoretical limits can be set upon how far the law may go in recognizing new property interests. Historically and in present times, value creating property could be not only economic, but also decorative, sentimental, and spiritual. A healthy embryo could well be useful to, demanded by and a scarcity to a number of women, who would value its implantation into them very profoundly.

Experience comes, such as it is, from the case brought against the Columbia Presbyterian Medical Center by Mrs. Del Zio.[193] The plaintiff was involved with Dr. Landrum Shettles in seeking in vitro fertilization, when her fertilized in vitro ovum was deliberately destroyed by a third party. Mrs. Del Zio was awarded $50,000 in damages by a United States federal court jury for deliberate infliction of emotional distress. The present interest of the case, however, is that the trial judge allowed a claim for damage and loss of her *property* to go to the jury. The jury made no award on the claim, but the fact that the judge apparently considered it appropriate to go to the jury may be significant.

Whether sperm donors are selling a product or a service may be a matter for resolution under human tissue donation or anatomical gift legislation.[194] Commercial sperm banks exist in the United States, however, and legal principles govern how they acquire, hold and distribute their stock in trade. Both they and those who receive material from them are free within the law to dispose of it as they wish. Recipients will probably attempt insemination, which may fail, with resulting wastage. When they succeed, however, human life results. This may furnish a legal model for fertilized in vitro ova. If some are to grow into human beings, others may have to be lost in the cause. Had restrictive legislation, for instance on abortion, prevented the research and its clinical application which has resulted in "test tube" births, it would have denied the resulting children their lives.

CONCLUSION

The sociopolitical issue underlying the abortion law of different jurisdictions is whether the result of the law represents or accommodates the authentic spirit of the people whom the law governs. This paper has attempted to illustrate how various jurisdictions have located themselves at points on the continuum between prohibiting abortion through legislation of comprehensive criminal penalties, and uniformly permitting or decriminalizing the practice without regard to the stage of pregnancy reached. Modern legislative approaches tend to favor identification of legal indications upon which pregnancies may be medically terminated, the facilities and personnel which may be engaged for the purpose, and often the application of appropriate provisions to different gestational stages. The judicial approach taken by courts in the common law tradition, such as the U.S. Supreme Court, tends to be not to implement an abortion policy stated in such positive provisions, but to determine the scope of negative legislation or customary law in the context of broader, constitutional principles directed toward individual liberty.

The power of the individual to resist intrusions of the state into major decisions in the individual's life is perhaps more celebrated among the population of the United States than among people elsewhere. Experience from Eastern Europe in particular shows how state population policy is advanced by variation of law on reproduction, to execute both positive and negative population policies. The law is regarded primarily as an instrument to advance policy, rather than as an embodiment of important values and priorities. The U.S. Supreme Court in *Roe v. Wade* reinforced individual immunity against reproductive direction by the state, through application of the fundamental constitutional right to privacy before a fetus achieves viability, and in *Doe v. Bolton*[195] the Supreme Court recognized the legal right to abortion after fetal viability where maternal life or health are endangered.

This prioritization of values, founded upon the U.S. Bill of Rights, may, of course, be changed by resort to constitutional processes. A reordering of priorities cannot be viewed in isolation, however, since it would affect more than a single issue. Within the medicolegal field alone it has been observed that the law on contraception, promotion of life by new technologies of human conception, private and public duties to resist spontaneous abortion and, for instance, provision for the unborn through grants and services for welfare-dependent and other pregnant women, would be affected by affording a new status to the unborn. The radical change in relations between the state and the individual which such different prioritization would betoken is the change against which elevated constitutional barriers have been created in the United States. Indeed, in *Roe v. Wade* the Supreme Court observed the erosion of individual constitutional rights since the late nineteenth century under restrictive legislation on abortion.

The Supreme Court's comparison on the plane of the nation's history is different from comparison with options currently applied in other jurisdictions in managing the social, ethical and legal issues presented by the desire for safe induced abortion. A comparative perspective may serve, however, to locate the existing legal order in a relevant context, and to present scenarios for possible reform.

NOTES

1. For an earlier study of modern times, see G.DEVEREUX, A STUDY OF ABORTION IN PRIMITIVE SOCIETIES (Julian Press, New York)(1955) (prevention of

birth in 400 preindustrial societies); *see also* Hawkinson, *Abortion: An Anthropological Overview* in LIBERALIZATION OF ABORTION LAWS 122 (A.R. Omran ed.)(Univ. of North Carolina, Chapel Hill)(1976).

2. F. TAUSSIG, ABORTION: SPONTANEOUS AND INDUCED at 31-32 (Kimpton, London)(1936).

3. *See* Hawkinson, *supra* note 1, at 124.

4. *Genesis* ii, 7.

5. This and the following information is found in G. WILLIAMS, THE SANCTITY OF LIFE AND THE CRIMINAL LAW (Knopf, New York)(1958) 140-144 [hereinafter cited as Williams].

6. This was accepted by Galen; *see* WILLIAMS, *id.* at 142.

7. Apparently following the Septuagint reading of *Exodus* xxi, 22. This may, however, have been "a crucial mistranslation" from the Hebrew; *see* I. JAKOBOVITS, JEWISH MEDICAL ETHICS (Bloch, New York)(1975) at 174.

8. Saint Augustine appears, however, to have an ambivalent record on the issue; *see* W. REANY, THE CREATION OF THE HUMAN SOUL, 83-86 (Benziger, Encino, Ca) (1932), and R.J. HUSER, THE CRIME OF ABORTION IN CANON LAW 15 (Catholic University of America Press, Washington, D.C.) (1942).

9. WILLIAMS, *supra* note 5, at 143.

10. F. ROSNER, MODERN MEDICINE AND JEWISH LAW (Yeshiva University, New York) (1972) at 66-67.

11. Compatibly with English Common law, where a "human in being" meant one born alive separate from the body of the mother; see the discussion in Commonwealth v. Edelin, 359 N.E.2d 4 (Mass. 1976).

12. F. ROSNER, *supra* note 10, at 68-69. "[T]he unborn fetus, although not a person, does have some status. . . the fetus may be considered as a 'partial person.'" *Id.* at 72. *See also* Skolnick, *infra* note 143.

13. A.R. Omran, *Abortion in the Natality Transition in Muslim Countries,* in ISLAM AND FAMILY PLANNING, vol. 2, 340 (I.R. Nazer, H.S. Karmi and M.Y. Zayid, eds.)(I.P.P.F. Middle East and North African Region, Beirut) (1974).

14. Makdur, *Sterilization and Abortion from the Point of View of Islam,* in ISLAM AND FAMILY PLANNING, vol. 2, 271.

15. BRACTON, DE LEGIBUS ANGLIAE, Bk. III (De Corona) 121 (circa 1250) [hereinafter cited as Bracton].

16. This may appear from FLETA, EPITOME OF BRACTON, Bk. I, Ch. 23 (De Homicidio) (circa 1290).

17. COKE, INSTITUTES OF THE LAWS OF ENGLAND, Third Part 50 (1628-1644).

18. HAWKINS, PLEAS OF THE CROWN, Bk. I, Ch. 3 (1716).

19. W. BLACKSTONE, COMMENTARIES ON THE LAWS OF ENGLAND, vol. 1, 129 (1765).

20. *Id.* Blackstone treated the offense as a common law misdemeanor; *see also* the precedent for an indictment for the offense at common law in CHITTY, CRIMINAL LAW, vol. 3, 797-98 (1816), drawing on a case in 1802 from the Crown Office, Mich. Term 42 Geo. III.

21. Lord Ellenborough's Act, 43 Geo. III c. 58.

22. Transportation to the Plantations (that is, Virginia) had ended with American Independence in 1776.

23. [1828] 1 Mood. 216.
24. [1811] 3 Camp. 76.
25. Lord Lansdowne's Act, 9 Geo. IV, c. 31.
26. 7 Will. IV & 1 Vict. c. 85.
27. In an unrelated case in 1838, R. v. Wycherley, 8 C & P 262, where a woman sentenced to death was able to plead that she was "quick with child" in order to escape execution, Baron Gurney observed that "quick with child" meant only having conceived, and that had quickening already occurred, she would have been "with quick child." This distinction, which may have been drawn to save the convicted woman's life, had not appeared in the context of abortion law.
28. India Pen. Code, c. 45.
29. *See* Dickens and Cook, *The Development of Commonwealth Abortion Laws*, INTERNATIONAL AND COMPARATIVE LAW QUARTERLY 28: 424,426 (1979).
30. Lord Macaulay's three draftsmen were Scottish. On Scot law on abortion, see H.M. Advocate v. Anderson [1927] Scots L.T. 651, and H.M. Advocate v. Semple [1937] Scots L.T. 48, 239.
31. Section 312 of the Penal Codes of India, Jammu and Kashmir, Bangladesh, Pakistan, Malaysia, and Singapore, and section 303 of the Penal Code of Sri Lanka.
32. The Offences Against the Person Act, 1861, 24 & 25 Vict. c. 100.
33. On indications for lawful abortion, see infra note 44.
34. 410 U.S. 113 (1973).
35. *Id.* at 140.
36. *Id.* at 164.
37. *Id.*
38. On the conservative reform of Canadian law, for instance, see Dickens, *Legal Aspects of Abortion*, in ABORTION 16 (P. Sachdev ed.)(Butterworths, Toronto)(1981).
39. *See supra* note 26.
40. Including no doubt the 1837 proposal which in 1860 became the Indian Penal Code, *see supra* notes 27-29. This punished procuring miscarriage "if such miscarriage be not caused in good faith for the purpose of saving the life of the woman."
41. British Parliamentary Papers—Reports, Commissioners, 1846, 24, 42 (Art. 16).
42. N.Y. Rev. Stat., pt. IV, c. 1, Tit. II, Art. 1 § 9, at 661, and Tit. VI, § 21, at 694 (1829), cited in Roe v. Wade, *supra* note 34 at 719.
43. *Id.* at 140.
44. [1939] 1 K.B. 687. Although this case only involved an interpretation of the law by a trial judge, the impact of the case in the British Commonwealth may be compared to that caused in the United States by Roe v. Wade.
45. *Id.* at 694, *per* Macnaghten, J.
46. *See* Commonwealth v. Wheeler, 53 N.E.2d 4, 4-6 (Mass 1944); *see also* Roe v. Wade, *supra* note 34, at 138.
47. R. v. Edgal, Idike and Oiogwu, 4 W.A.C.A. 133 (1938) on appeal from the Southern States, Nigeria. The court noted that "The judge was not making

new law, he was merely expounding what in his view had always been the law, i.e. what was the common law of England"; at 136.

48. The King v. Anderson, [1951] N.Z.L.R. 439 and R. v. Woolnough, [1977] 2 N.Z.L.R. 508 (C.A.).

49. R. v. Ross and McCarthy, [1955] Queensl. St. R. 48 (C.C.A).

50. R. v. Davidson, [1969] Vict. R. 667.

51. R. v. Wald, 3 N.S.W. Dist. Ct. R. 25 (1971).

52. The *Bourne* principle was confirmed in the Supreme Court of Canada abortion case of Morgentaler v. The Queen 53 D.L.R. 3d 161 (1975).

53. R. v. Emberson, Criminal Case No. 16, 1976, resulting in conviction since no *Bourne* type of defense was found to exist.

54. Mehar Singh Bansel v. R., [1959] E.A.C.A. 813, a manslaughter appeal from Kenya arising from abortion.

55. The People v. Gulshan, Lusaka High Court (Criminal Jurisdiction), March 19, 1971; three physicians were acquitted.

56. G.H. GORDON, THE CRIMINAL LAW OF SCOTLAND (Green, Edinburgh)(1967) at 381.

57. Stats. Ken., c. 63.

58. The same appears verbatim in, for instance, section 285 of the Criminal Code Act 1974 (cap. XXII) of Papua New Guinea, reflecting the rather eclectic application of codes of criminal law by the historical administrators of British dependent territories.

59. U.K. Stats. 1967, c. 87. Enacted by the United Kingdom legislature, this Act applies only to Britain, and not to Northern Ireland.

60. Crimes Act, 1961, No. 43, § 187 A(1). Section 187 A(2) permits account to be taken of the female's age being near the beginning or end of the usual child-bearing years, and of reasonable grounds to believe pregnancy is the result of rape.

61. Courts in the United States almost uniformly reject the so-called "wrongful life" claim of a child that its mother was wrongfully denied her option of abortion; *see* Turpin v. Sortini, 174 Cal. Rptr. 477 (1982).

62. *Supra* note 59, at §1(1)(b).

63. Such condition might be disclosed by modern techniques of prenatal screening such as fetoscopy; although such genetic condition might well be associated with other abnormalities.

64. Criminal Code, R.S.C., 1970, c. C-34, s. 251(4)(c).

65. In this setting, results of prenatal monitoring may be an important basis for not terminating the pregnancy, rather than for abortion, as is often the case in the United States.

66. Physicians discuss their experiences without noting differences in their abortion legislation; *see Report of an International Workshop*, Special Issue, PRENATAL DIAGNOSIS (December 1980).

67. Bourne, *supra* note 44.

68. *See* R.J. COOK AND B.M. DICKENS, ABORTION LAWS IN COMMONWEALTH COUNTRIES (World Health Org., Geneva) (1979) at 71.

69. Stats. Ind. 1971, No. 34.
70. Criminal Code, c. 154, §169A(b). This Code amendment was introduced in 1974 (Law No. 59) following conflict between the Turkish army and the Greek Cypriot population.
71. Crimes Act, 1961, No. 43, §187A(2)(b).
72. At common law, a male aged below fourteen years is irrebuttably presumed incapable of sexual intercourse; *see* R. v. Groombridge, 7 C & P 582, 173 E.R. 256 (1836).
73. Few jurisdictions have followed the practice of a number of states in the U.S. of enacting spousal rape laws.
74. In the Bourne case, *supra* note 44, however, the defendant made clear that he would not have aborted the rape victim had she been feebleminded or of "prostitute mind," and the judge excluded such a woman from those whose pregnancy following rape might lawfully be terminated because the pregnancy would not have affected her mind; *see* B. DICKENS, ABORTION AND THE LAW 43 (MacGibbon & Kee, London) (1966).
75. Illustrated by the case of In re May's Estate, 305 N.Y. 486, 114 N.E.2d 4 (1953), where a Jewish uncle-niece marriage was lawfully contracted in Rhode Island when it would have been void in New York, where the parties were domiciled and returned to live.
76. New Zealand's incest indication, for instance, considers incest along with other sexual offenses against vulnerable females such as the severely subnormal; *supra* note 60, §187A(1)(b), (c) and (d).
77. The W.H.O. Constitution further states that "The enjoyment of the highest attainable standard of health is one of the fundamental rights of every human being."
78. U.K. Stats. 1967, c. 87 §1(1)(a).
79. U.K. Stats. 1967, c. 87.This wording is repeated verbatim in section 3(3) of India's legislation; *see* Stats Ind. 1971, *supra* note 69.
80. *See* Dickens, *Legal Aspects of Abortion, supra* note 38.
81. Gilles Marceau, 119 Can. Parl. Deb., H.C. 5103 (April 22, 1975).
82. In some cultures, for instance, the value of a bride may be related to sexual innocence and childlessness, and to years of schooling which pregnancy and child rearing would abbreviate, so that a physician may address a patient's pregnancy in the light of its social effects upon her. *See* J.B. AKINGBA, THE PROBLEM OF UNWANTED PREGNANCIES IN NIGERIA TODAY 102-3(1971).
83. Criminal Code, c. 154 §169A(b).
84. Stats. Ind. 1971, No. 34. Regulations in a number of jurisdictions, such as Czechoslovakia, may allow abortion upon failure of intrauterine contraception; *see infra* note 130.
85. Information from the United Nations Fund for Population Activities' SURVEY OF LAWS ON FERTILITY CONTROL, PART II (1979) [hereinafter cited as Survey].
86. *Id.*
87. The Abortion Act, 1974 (No. 24 of 1974).

88. REPORT OF THE COMMITTEE ON THE OPERATION OF THE ABORTION LAW (Canada) 80 (1977) [hereinafter cited as REPORT].
89. *See generally* the discussion in Findlay, *Criminal Liability for Complicity in Abortions Committed outside Ireland,* 1980 IRISH JURIST, 88.
90. *See generally* the Harvard RESEARCH ON INTERNATIONAL LAW (1935), Jurisdiction with Respect to Crime.
91. The Abortion Act, 1974, (No. 24 of 1974).
92. In 1979, it was set at five Singapore dollars.
93. 19 & 20 Geo. V, c. 34.
94. *See supra* note 11.
95. A pre-viable fetus may also be born "alive."
96. *Compare* Colautti v. Franklin, 439 U.S. 379 (1979) (Pennsylvania statute held unconstitutional by the Supreme Court).
97. For consideration of what medical care is appropriate, see A.R. HOLDER, LEGAL ISSUES IN PEDIATRICS AND ADOLESCENT MEDICINE (Wiley & Sons, New York) (1977) at 107 [hereinafter cited as HOLDER].
98. Stats. Ind., 1971, No. 34, § 3(2).
99. *See Bangladesh: Menstrual Regulation Performed by Paramedics Found Safe,* INTERNATIONAL FAMILY PLANNING PERSPECTIVES 6:151 (1980).
100. See the discussion in LePoole-Griffiths, *The Law of Abortion in Ghana,* UNIVERSITY OF GHANA LAW JOURNAL 10:103 (1979).
101. Royal College of Nursing of the United Kingdom v. Department of Health and Social Security, [1981] 1 All E.R. 545 (House of Lords).
102. Hong Kong's Offences Against the Person Ordinance (c. 212), §47A(4) is exceptional in requiring two physicians to approve abortion in circumstances of a life-threatening emergency; this is not completely explained by the small size and high population density of the territory, where two physicians may be easily assembled.
103. Criminal Code, *supra* note 64, § 251(4), (6). It follows that at least four physicians may have to be involved, including one to examine the woman and make a recommendation, three to serve on the committee, and one to perform the procedure. The latter physician may have made the initial recommendation, but that is very unusual.
104. Terminination of Pregnancy Act, 1972 (No. 26 of 1972) § 3(1) (Zambia).
105. *See* REPORT *supra* note 88, at 141.
106. *See* Survey, *supra* note 85.
107. *Id.* at 47.
108. N.Z. Stats., 1977, No. 112.
109. *See* the Contraception, Sterilisation, and Abortion Amendment Act 1978, N.Z. Stats. 1978 No. 5.
110. *See* Paton v. Trustees of B.P.A.S., [1978] 2 All E.R. 987 in England, precluding a right of spousal veto under British legislation, upheld in Paton v. U.K. by the European Commission of Human Rights; *see* HUMAN RIGHTS LAW JOURNAL 1:324 (1980).
111. Stats. Ind. 1971, No. 34.

112. *See, e.g.*, Dehler v. Ottawa Civic Hospital, 101 D.L.R. 3d 686 (Ont. 1979)(refusing a stranger representative status on behalf of unborn children scheduled for abortion).

113. See the recent South African case of Christian League of Southern Africa v. Rall [1981] (2) S.A. 821 (0), refusing status of curator ad litem for an unborn child of an unmarried mother seeking abortion.

114. The implication of this may be that physicians are bound by legal duties to assist patients to obtain abortions which are legally available and which they want; see the discussion in Zimmer v. Ringrose, 124 D.L.R. 3d 215 (Alta. C.A., 1981), at 227.

115. There is evidence, for instance, that in the southern provinces of Italy, more than seven out of ten obstetricians and gynecologists have officially declined to provide services under the liberal 1978 law; see Filicori and Flamigni, *Legal Abortion in Italy, 1978-1979*, FAMILY PLANNING PERSPECTIVES 13: 228 (1981).

116. U.K. Stats. 1967, c. 87.

117. This necessary limitation may explain why conservative legislation, such as exists in Canada, *supra* note 38, has no conscientious objection provision.

118. The Abortion Act, 1974 (No. 24 of 1974).

119. Criminal Law Consolidation Act, 1935-1966, §82a(2).

120. The Abortion Act, 1974, § 3(3).

121. N.Z. Stats. 1977, No. 112,§§36(2) and 45(2).

122. See the discussion in H. MANNHEIM, CRIMINAL JUSTICE AND SOCIAL RECONSTRUCTION (Paul, Trench, Trubnem & Co., London) (1946).

123. The military defeat of Japan appears itself to have had an effect upon that country's population control policies, including liberalization of abortion practice.

124. *See* Decree of the Supreme Soviet of the U.S.S.R., November 23, 1955: "On the Repeal of the Prohibition of Abortions." *See also* Instructions of the Ministry of Public Health of the U.S.S.R., November 29, 1955: "On the Procedure for Performing Artificial Interruptions of Pregnancy."

125. *See* M. Ryan, *Letter: The Anti-Abortion Campaign*, BRITISH MEDICAL JOURNAL 283:1378 (1981).

126. Decree No. 770, September 29, 1966 of the Council of State, *see* INTERNATIONAL DIGEST OF HEALTH LEGISLATION 18:822 (1967).

127. Berelson, *Romania's 1966 Anti-Abortion Decree: The Demographic Experience of the First Decade*, POPULATION STUDIES 33:209 (1979).

128. T. FREJKA, FERTILITY TRENDS AND POLICIES: CZECHOSLOVAKIA IN THE 1970s (Center For Population Studies, Working Papers, No. 54, 1980).

129. White, A.C., *A Long Campaign*, PEOPLE (IPPF) 7:20 (1980) at 21 [hereinafter cited as White].

130. Regulations of the Czech Ministry of Health, May 16, 1973 (Sbírka zákonů No. 71/1973), Regulations of the Slovak Ministry of Health, May 16, 1973 (Sbírka zákonů No. 72/1973).

131. SURVEY, *supra* note 85, at 53.

132. WHITE, *supra* note 129, at 22.

133. Dr. Miroslav Vojka, *quoted in* H. SCOTT, DOES SOCIALISM LIBERATE WOMEN? (Beacon Press, Boston) (1976).

134. *See* INTERNATIONAL FAMILY PLANNING PERSPECTIVES 7:62 (1981).

135. *See* White, *supra* note 129.

136. White, A.C., PEOPLE (IPPF) 9:32 (1982).

137. Law of April 27, 1956 on the Conditions of the Termination of Pregnancy (Dziennik Ustaw 1956, issue 12, No. 6).

138. Mazur, *Contraception and Abortion in Poland,* INTERNATIONAL FAMILY PLANNING PERSPECTIVES 7:79-80 (1981).

139. *See* White, *supra* note 136.

140. Wulf, *The Hungarian Fertility Survey, 1977,* INTERNATIONAL FAMILY PLANNING PERSPECTIVES 12:44 (1980).

141. Ordinance No. 4 of December 1, 1973 of the Minister of Health (Magyar Kozlony, No. 80, p. 836); *see* INTERNATIONAL DIGEST OF HEALTH LEGISLATION 25:332 (1974).

142. Roe v. Wade, *supra* note 34, at 164.

143. It has been observed that "When infant mortality rates were high in Europe, parents tended to become only minimally attached to their infants, and the death of an infant was not an occasion for deep or prolonged grief"; Skolnick, *The Limits of Childhood: Conceptions of Child Development and Social Context,* LAW AND CONTEMPORARY PROBLEMS 39:38, 48(1975).

144. It has been estimated that 54 percent of spontaneously aborted fetuses are abnormal; *see* Kajii, *et al., Banding Analysis of Abnormal Karyotypes in Spontaneous Abortion,* AMERICAN JOURNAL OF HUMAN GENETICS 25:539 (1973).

145. R.W. Erbe, *Genetic Disorders,* in THE HORIZONS OF HEALTH, H. Wechsler ed. (Harvard Univ. Press, Cambridge) (1977).

146. Bracton, *supra* note 15.

147. Up to life imprisonment is imposable under the law of the United Kingdom, *supra* note 32, s. 58, and of Canada, *supra* note 64,§251(1).

148. *Per* Dickson, J. in Morgentaler v. The Queen, *supra* note 52, at 206. This statement may misrepresent the law, since life imprisonment for noncapital murder was the minimum sentence.

149. The first case allowing a wrongful death action for an unborn (though clearly viable) child was Verkennes v. Corniea, 38 N.W.2d 838 (Minn. 1949).

150. *See* HOLDER, *supra* note 97, at 69.

151. Dehler v. Ottawa Civic Hosp., *supra* note 112.

152. This was seen in Renslow v. Mennonite Hospital, 351 N.E.2d 870 (Ill. 1976).

153. Awards to husbands may be small, since a husband has no right to a child-bearing wife; *see* Murray v. Vandevander, 522 P.2d 302 (Okla. 1974) (involved wife's nonconsensual sterilization).

154. *Supra* notes 112, 113. A family court in Nova Scotia, for instance, interpreted a child welfare law to permit appointment of a guardian ad litem for an unborn child in Re Simms and H. 106 D.L.R. 3d 435 (1979), but this is contrary to *Dehler, supra* note 112, which was upheld by the Ontario Court of Appeal, 117, D.L.R. 3d 512 (1980).

155. *See* I. Chalmers, *Evaluation of Perinatal Practice: The Limitations of Audit by Death*, in CHANGING PATTERNS OF CHILD-REARING (R. Chester, P. Diggory and M. Sutherland eds.) (Academic Press, London)(1981) at 39.

156. *See generally*, Kleinman, *The Continued Vitality of Vital Statistics*, AMERICAN JOURNAL OF PUBLIC HEALTH 72:125 (1982).

157. *See* recommendation in the ninth revision of the INTERNATIONAL CLASSIFICATION OF DISEASES (World Health Organization, Geneva) (1978).

158. R.S.O. 1980, c. 524, §1(v).

159. *See supra* note 93.

160. Births and Deaths Registration Act 1953, 1 & 2 Eliz. 2, c. 20, §41.

161. *See* the High Court of Australia case of Doodeward v. Spence 6 C.L.R. 406 (1908) (involved property interests in a two-headed stillborn child exhibited in a circus).

162. J. FLETCHER, THE ETHICS OF GENETIC CONTROL (Anchor Press, Garden City, N.Y.) at 140.

163. REPORT OF THE COMMITTEE ON THE WORKING OF THE ABORTION ACT (Chaired by The Hon. Mrs. Justice Lane), Vol. 1, 260 (Cmnd. 5579, 1974).

164. This may have been reduced because of the "conscience clause"; *see* text, *supra* at note 116.

165. THE USE OF FETUSES AND FETAL MATERIAL FOR RESEARCH: REPORT OF THE ADVISORY GROUP, 12 (HMSO)(1972).

166. Hembree v. Hospital Board of Morgan County, 300 So.2d 823 (Ala. 1974).

167. Brooks v. South Broward Hospital District, 325 So.2d 479 (Fla. 1975).

168. The "no property" rule has a rather insubstantial basis; *see generally* Skegg, *Human Corpses, Medical Specimens and the Law of Property*, ANGLO AMERICAN LAW REVIEW 4:412 (1975). For a case where a property interest was considered, *see* Long v. Chicago, R.I. and P. Railway Co., 86 P. 286 (Okla. 1905) at 291, and Doodeward v. Spence, *supra* note 161.

169. *See* Dickens, *The Control of Living Body Material*, UNIVERSITY OF TORONTO LAW JOURNAL 27:142 (1977).

170. *See supra* notes 30 and 33, and accompanying text.

171. *See generally* V. Tunkel, *Modern Anti-Pregnancy Techniques and the Criminal Law*, 1974 CRIMINAL LAW REVIEW 461.

172. In Britain, the Minister of Health has recently approved "morning after" pills, taken within 72 hours after intercourse, on the grounds that they are not abortifacient since pregnancy commences at implantation; *see* PEOPLE (IPPF) 9:33 (1982).

173. *See* Griswold v. Connecticut, 381 U.S. 479 (1965) and Eisenstadt v. Baird, 405 U.S. 438 (1972).

174. CONTRACEPTION STERILISATION AND ABORTION IN NEW ZEALAND: REPORT OF THE ROYAL COMMISSION OF INQUIRY 92 (1977).

175. *Id.* at 192.

176. *Id.*

177. Crimes Act. 1961, No. 43, §182A.

178. India Pen. Code, §312.

179. Queen-Empress v. Ademma, [1886] Indian L.R. 9 Madras 370.
180. *See supra* note 99. The view that criminal conviction may be imposed for attempted abortion (Penal Code, §511) is resisted by the House of Lords' ruling in an English case which may be influential that there is no unlawful attempt in pursuing an end impossible to achieve; *see* Haughton v. Smith, [1975] A.C. 476.
181. *See* B.M. DICKENS, MEDICO-LEGAL ASPECTS OF FAMILY LAW (Butterworths, Toronto) (1979) at 69. A woman scheduled for hysterectomy has already received another woman's fertilized ovum; *see* Abel, *The Legal Implications of Ectogenetic Research,* TULSA LAW JOURNAL 10:243,247(1974).
182. *See* Mady, *Surrogate Mothers: The Legal Issues,* AMERICAN JOURNAL OF LAW & MEDICINE, 7:323 (1981).
183. *See supra* note 172, where "test tube" experience was cited in justification.
184. See text, *supra*, between notes 32 and 33.
185. Laws based on the Indian Penal Code apply only to position (1); *see supra* note 28.
186. *See supra* note 11.
187. *See* Raleigh Fitkin-Paul Morgan Memorial Hospital v. Anderson, 201 A.2d 537 (N.J. 1964).
188. *See supra* note 11.
189. *See* [1981] REFORM 129 (The Law Reform Commission of Australia), and AUSTRALIAN LAW JOURNAL 55:314 (1981).
190. It has been reported that, in an in vitro fertilization birth in Calcutta, India, the fertilized ovum had been frozen and stored for 53 days before implantation; see R. SCOTT, THE BODY AS PROPERTY (Viking Press, New York) (1981) at 215.
191. Reported in *The Globe and Mail (Toronto),* Feb. 11, 1982. On proposed guidelines on in vitro fertilization to be drawn up by the Central Ethical Committee of the British Medical Association, see *The Times (London),* Dec. 23, 1981.
192. *See supra* note 169, at 180.
193. The case appears unreported, but its background is discussed in D. RORVIK, IN HIS IMAGE, ch. 8 (J.B. Lippincott, Philadelphia, and Pocket Books, New York)(1978). The trial result was reported in *The Globe and Mail (Toronto),* August 19, 1978.
194. On general principles of blood donation, see Perlmutter v. Beth David Hospital, 123 N.E.2d 792 (N.Y. 1954).
195. 410 U.S. 179 (1973).

Chapter 14

The Impact of Religious Beliefs on Attitudes toward Abortion

Sidney Callahan

Do religious beliefs have an impact on attitudes toward abortion? It could be argued that they do not, since persons without any religious beliefs are found on all sides of the current debate over abortion, and perhaps more to the point, religious believers of every different persuasion can be found advocating all the possible positions on the troubling question. Thus, goes one argument, religious belief per se does not determine or imply a person's attitudes toward abortion; one still must move once more to basic philosophical debates concerning principles, politics and personhood.

Yet a case can be made for the thesis that religious beliefs do have an impact on attitudes toward abortion. Religious beliefs, I argue, affect what questions are asked, which hypotheses are focused upon, and, in addition, predispose adherence to certain positions rather than to others. Moreover, religious beliefs will undoubtedly make a difference in how persons' attitudes toward abortion are formed. Besides influencing what positions are adopted and how they are arrived at, religious beliefs will often influence a person's actual behavior. While no individual case can be predicted perfectly, certain patterns recur with enough frequency to be fairly convincing that religious belief does have an impact on abortion attitudes.

But before embarking on my arguments, some limitations have to be set. Religious beliefs have had a thousand and one various incarnations across every culture and throughout human history. No one can take on all religions at once. To narrow the discussion, let us focus solely on the present-day American scene. Even with this limitation one must employ strictures. If Oriental and American Indian and other influences are left to one side, there is still an enormous pluralism manifested in the Judeo-Christian religious tradition of America. Do all these different manifestations of traditional western religion have enough in common even to be discussed together, much less lumped together under the rubric of religious beliefs? Perhaps so, if the very broad brush of psychology is used. To do this one must ignore the anguish that such a sketchy picture will give to theologians, historians, philosophers and others interested in the separation of ideas and in the making of distinctions about particulars.

ATTITUDES AND RELIGIOUS BELIEF

One psychological approach employing a very broad definition of religious beliefs or religious sentiment can be found in a work of distinguished psychologist Gordon Allport, who writes in defense of religious development:

> The developed religious sentiment, therefore, cannot be known in terms of its many empirical origins. It is not a mere matter of dependency or of reliving the family or cultural configuration; nor is it simply a prophylaxis against fear; nor is it an exclusively rational system of belief. Any single formula by itself is too partial. The developed religious sentiment is the synthesis of these and many other factors, all of which form a comprehensive attitude whose function it is to relate the individual meaningfully to the whole of Being.[1]

Allport further says, along with many other commentators, that while religious belief can be reasoned and rational, it must also go beyond the intellect and engage faith and love. Religious beliefs must in a sense be held as "morally true" as well as "metaphysically true."[2] This is much the same distinction as that made by Cardinal Newman between "real" and merely "notional" assent.[3] While all persons may have ultimate intellectual presuppositions by which they live, religious belief for many is "a synthesis of all that lies within experience and all that lies beyond."[4] The *whole* personality is involved in relating to the *whole* of reality.

Attitudes, by contrast, are usually seen as directed toward specific objects. While everyone agrees on the centrality and importance of attitudes, there have been many arguments over how to conceptualize and define them.[5] Most psychologists agree that while attitudes are specifically aimed at discrete entities, they are quite complex in composition. These dimensions are the familiar cognition, affect, and conation of traditional philosophy. While attitudes include some thinking, feeling, and willing, some analysts have lately seen the liking-disliking or affective component as the most important.

Measuring attitudes is a complicated endeavor. Many different methods have been devised and employed, each possessing certain advantages and disadvantages. Longstanding controversies over the correct definition and measurement of attitudes are matched by two other ongoing debates over whether a person's set of attitudes toward different things are related in some patterned way, and whether or how attitudes are related to behavior.[6] To make these controversies over attitudes more concrete, think of the problem of how we can find out what people's attitudes toward abortion really are. Are persons' attitudes on abortion related to their attitudes on other issues? Then again, even more pragmatically, will a person's attitudes toward abortion predict actual behavior?

If one could answer all the above hard questions, one might then be ready for the deeper and more complicated controversies over how attitudes can be changed. Each major psychological theory of attitude change reflects assumptions about human nature as well as a specific view about attitudes. Some theories stress personality needs that attitudes serve, especially the unconscious ones. Some theories stress behavioristic conditioning with reward and punishment; some stress cognitive factors and the individual search for rational consistency. Research conducted within each theoretical framework seems to give some validity to each approach.[7] For that matter, anyone who carefully analyzes a good commercial advertising campaign, particularly when it is selling a political candidate, will conclude that Madison Avenue also places its bets on the use of all theories at once. It also seems that people trying to change other people's attitudes on abortion are employing simultaneously every different approach to attitude change. We see a wide range of efforts, including: the providing of information and statistics; rational arguments that appeal to rational consistency; veiled and less veiled appeals to fear and prejudice; and finally, of course, we get to the display of coat hangers, roses, and fetuses in bottles.

This brief treatment of the nature of attitudes and religious belief brings us to the question of a connection between the two. How can we find out if there is a relationship between religious belief and attitudes toward abortion? One research strategy is to do survey research of a representative sample of the population. Other approaches involve studying self-selected activists in the pro-life or pro-choice movement, either with survey methods or interviews or some combination of the two. While such studies have been few and present many problems, some patterns do seem to emerge. According to Donald Granberg, a sociologist who is a leader in such investigations, "there is ample reason to suppose that one's position on abortion is affected by one's religious affiliation, beliefs and involvement."[8] In his landmark study of almost 900 pro-choice and pro-life abortion activists, Granberg found that 87 percent of the pro-life group members reported that religion plays a "very" or "extremely important" role in their lives, compared to only 20 percent of the pro-choice group. Ninety-five percent of the pro-life group members attend religious services more than once a month, compared to only 19 percent of the pro-choice members. Atheists and agnostics are also significantly more represented in the pro-choice activist group. Certain patterns of denominational differences also appear; Jews, Episcopalians, Methodists, Presbyterians, and Unitarians are more likely to be among the pro-choice activists, while Catholics, Lutherans, Baptists, and Mormons are more likely to be members of the pro-life group. As Granberg comments on his results: "It is difficult to imagine data that might more convincingly demonstrate that religion is a very important factor in determining attitudes about legal abortion."[9]

Of course, correlation does not prove causation, since some third factor may be the cause of the observed relationships. But, the pattern of findings does prove suggestive and seems to point to some real relationship. In a sense, surveys study phenomena from the outside; they do not illuminate what might be the inner connection or structural relationship between religious belief and abortion attitudes. Content analysis and in-depth interview studies may soon provide further understanding.[10] For the present, as a participant observer in the debate, I think it is possible to intuit how certain religious configurations can have an impact on abortion attitudes. In order to understand truly these deep structures one must leave behind the prejudiced caricatures of religion which so many non-religious persons hold. Many intellectuals in the liberal community, formed for the most part in an earlier era of confident positivism, have been guilty of simplified stereotypes. For them, especially if they are pro-choice, religious belief would correlate with pro-life positions since religious people, particularly Catholics, are known to be anti-sex, anti-women, anti-liberty and so enslaved in superstitious obedience to religious authority that they cannot begin to think for themselves.

It is of course true, as Gordon Allport astutely points out, that in many cases religious development and growth are arrested. Indeed, "some of the arresting forces leave the individual with an infantile form of religious belief, self-serving and superstitious."[11] Religion can serve neurotic needs and basically be a defensive maneuver. But it is also fair to take seriously Allport's analysis of unbelief.

> Unbelief, while it may be the product of mature reflection, may also be a reaction against parental or tribal authority, or may be due to a one-sided intellectual development that rules out other areas of normal curiosity. We find many personalities who deal zealously and effectively with all phases of becoming except the final task of relating themselves meaningfully to creation. For some reason their curiosity stops at this point.[12]

A serious attempt to understand how belief might make a difference must refrain from using stereotypes derived from immature unbelievers about immature believers. In any argument the focus should be on the best and most mature examples of a position, and this is true in trying to understand how certain religious ultimate presuppositions affect abortion attitudes.

THE BENEVOLENT CREATOR

Perhaps the primary and most relevant ultimate presupposition of religious belief is the affirmation of a benevolent Creator who has created the universe. No believer in the Judeo-Christian tradition could go along with the idea of an evil creator deceiving or torturing humankind; they cannot assent to the despairing cry in Shakespeare's *Lear,* "We are to the Gods as flies to wanton boys, they kill us for their sport." When the question arises as to why there is something rather than nothing, the religious believer affirms that a good God has created a good universe out of gracious benevolence and love. This belief undergirds a basic affirmation of life; believers not only "accept the universe" with Margaret Fuller, they also gratefully celebrate all that is seen and unseen as a good gift from the Creator. The particulars may be dim and perhaps unknowable, and arguments rage over questions of processes or the measure of immanence versus transcendence, but basic benevolence at the core of reality is assumed.

The belief in benevolence and the response of gratitude influence the acceptance of life as a good. Life is a precious gift and is better, far better, than the absence of life. There is an ultimate presupposition in favor of fruitfulness, abundance, and procreation as God-like which influences where a person begins any discussion of life issues such as abortion. Moreover, human life is considered the most special and blessed form of life we can know. For the believer, humankind is made in the image of God and given stewardship over the good creation. If this be "speciesism" from an animal liberationist point of view, so be it. Humankind, with its special powers and responsibilities, is to imitate God in creating—by work in the world and by procreation. Thus, in any debate over bringing life into the world a religious believer will be more likely to cast the question as one of "Why not?" rather than "Why?"

Another important influence in religious belief is the affirmation of purpose and meaning in God's creative enterprise. All of this process is going somewhere; there is a meaning to the flow of events. Instead of meaningless absurdity or the despair of hopelessness, the believer affirms that there is a story being enacted which is going to have a happy ending, come hell or high water, fire or ice. The religious believer is committed to a teleological approach since this is God's story. Here, of course, is where the Judeo-Christian tradition separates into two streams. Christians affirm that the main event in the drama has already happened while Jews are still waiting for a more convincing plot intervention. Among Christians, too, there has been much bloodshed over other disagreements about the story line. Just how detailed is the script? Are the actors basically good? Are they depraved or simply wounded in nature? Does the Author welcome revisions and improvisations by the actors? Could it be that this story is a group effort, the Author and players creating the plot together with only the last act and final exit lines already written?

Theologians argue and will continue to argue over the correct interpretations of God's nature and will, but for the ordinary Christian believer, a two-fold message comes through. There is meaning in what humans do since there is a purpose in the world; individuals are free and responsible participants and at the same time borne along in God's providence. The whole wide world is in God's hand, but people must also do their part by faith and ceaseless good works. Whatever may be the origin of chance events or accidents or unplanned occurrences, the Christian believer affirms that it is possible to transform whatever occurs into part of the plan, into God's purpose, into some meaningfulness in the long run. Therefore, there can be little justification for judging all involuntary things as negative occurrences. Christians are charged to be able to respond properly when events occur and not simply to exert control on behalf of personal agendas. No matter how hard one works to control and bring order into existence, surprises and untoward events will occur and should be accepted as part of the challenge of a religious life. The man suddenly fallen among thieves, the stranger who arrives at the gate, the person in need who requests aid—all are unexpected opportunities to respond.

When the accidental occurrence or unplanned event is a pregnancy, even more significance can be granted and more of a positive response can be made. Those believers who affirm the Incarnation and believe that God became human through a pregnancy and birth can give a special affirmation to these life processes of the body. The body is seen as a temple of the Lord which shall be resurrected at the last day. Salvation of everyone came through an obscure hidden beginning in a mother's womb. The implication of this belief in the humanizing of Deity and the divinization of humanity, in a Lord truly divine and truly human, is profound. In addition to benevolence, purposiveness and meaningfulness, the natural processes of the human species have been blessed and incorporated into the ongoing plan of salvation. Thus you must feed, clothe, nurse, restore, and deeply respect the integrity of the body which is "for the Lord." Sexuality is given as a good gift for the purpose of procreation and unity. The reproductive processes which created the Saving Life once and creates new individual lives destined for eternal existence therefore becomes most valued. Unfortunately, at times the significance invested in these processes verges on a return to the pagan mystique of worshipping Nature and fertility. But even when reverence and respect do not flourish into romantic excess, there is definitely a Christian predisposition present to deeply affirm biological reproduction processes. This reverence may help explain why so many believers are more likely to take a genetic position in the debates over when human life begins. Even the mysterious unknown hidden moments in which a uniquely new individual life begins are clothed with dignity and significance.

A belief in purposiveness and meaningfulness of events in the universe also affects the sense of time and how one values the developing embryo at any one stage or point in time. If the flow of time comes from a beginning and is moving toward some end, then the future potential of a developing life invests the embryonic beginnings with value. The achieved level and stage of human development may be slight, but the potential future development also counts for a believer taught to hope for and meditate upon final ends and transformations. Christianity is all about transforming unlikely specimens of humanity into meaningful actors in a benevolent drama of Grace. The present moment in time, which implies the present stage of development, only makes sense if it is invested with its past origins and potential future. Every manifestation of life is from God and is going to God. Many believers cannot help but live within a two-dimensional consciousness of time—our human perspectives and God's perspective.

The two-dimensional perspective regarding time is matched by the two-dimensional view of values. What God values, and who God chooses, may be very different from that which human wisdom would advise. A belief in the radical transcendence of God implies a possible difference in point of view. Certain worldly achievements and success may be foolishness in the eyes of God, and what is seen as foolish and lowly may be God's choice. Christians are regularly taught that "the last will be first in the Kingdom," that the world may be turned upside down, with the poor and handicapped in positions of honor.

Along with this admonition to see and value differently from the world comes the impetus to defend, champion, and succor those who will be ignored when the counsel of worldly wisdom is followed. The poor, the lepers, the maimed and deformed, the dying, the prisoner, the hungry, the sick, women and children—all the helpless and suffering are special in God's sight and so the special concern of believers. Therefore, it seems that a concern for the unborn is but an extension of this concern for the helpless, the hidden powerless ones of the earth. One basis for this different valuing is the conviction that the unseen is as real as the seen. Reality is not simply what humans decide to construct or construe as real. The fact that one cannot see the embryo does not alter the conviction that empathy and concern should be extended. In psychological terms, one could say that religious believers are constantly exhorted not to let "perception capture the field," and told to cultivate "object permanence"—i.e., things still exist when we are not looking at them.

Furthermore, a religious emphasis on human equality under God results in discounting physical differences between embryonic developing life and mature forms of adult life. The mutilated leper or the aged, withered and sick person also differ physically, but may be no less human in God's eyes. Different races, from time to time, have been denied humanity, and women also have been regarded as less than fully human. The argument that the fetus is treated as women once were motivates the many feminists who are pro-life and active in such movements as Feminists for Life, or Pro-Lifers for Survival—an anti-nuclear group who carry the argument further. Interestingly enough, there are different configurations in pro-life attitudes toward abortion.[13] My own pro-life convictions are those of a socialist, pacifist, Quaker-influenced tradition, manifested in the left-wing liberal Catholic tradition in the work of the Berrigans and the *Catholic Worker*. From the feminist pro-life pacifist viewpoint, all the arguments asserting the value of women's development in the face of male power and hostility to feminine equality can be made on behalf of the fetus. Affirmative action is needed to protect women, the unborn, and all human beings from nuclear proliferation and violence. Consciousness must be raised on behalf of the powerless. In a pro-life feminist position, it is asserted that women of all people should not identify with a traditional male aggressor and attack fetal life as insufficiently developed. After all, women were once thought to be so different and undeveloped that their rights and participation in the larger world were denied. Pregnancy is not a disease to which women are subject, nor does it render women so different from men that they are disqualified from participating in the male world. The male body is not the norm. Thus faced with a choice between men and women, this kind of feminist chooses women; and faced with a conflict between women and the fetus, the choice is made for the fetus for the same reasons. In tragic conflicts and choices, one must give the benefit of the doubt to the more powerless and renounce violent solutions. Accordingly, most feminist pro-lifers are not only for the Equal Rights Amendment, but also against capital punishment, against nuclear arms, against the draft, for redistribution of income, and other pro-life left-wing causes. Perhaps the most important feminist pro-life demands are for family allowances, health care, day care, and the end of society's virtual abandonment of women and children. The religious believers among them see themselves living out a consistent Christian point of view which must challenge the status quo and the expedient utilitarian values so embedded in a world indifferent to suffering.

SUFFERING

The question of suffering is, of course, the crux of the matter. In all pro-life positions the problem remains that one also inflicts suffering by supporting the claims of the fetus. For the most part, women choose abortion in order to avoid suffering—their own, their family's, and sometimes (as in the case of birth defects) the suffering of the potential child. How can religious believers who believe that they are called to love their fellow beings and sacrifice for their well-being as God loves and gives, how can they be willing to inflict so much suffering in the defense of fetal life? Those who believe that the fetus may suffer pain in the process of abortion, especially in late abortions using saline solutions, can answer that in a sheer calculus of suffering, fetal pain will outweigh the social and psychological suffering which drives women to choose abortion.[14] Others will espouse the argument that psychological and social suffering, even the suffering of economic deprivation, is relative in that it is a human construct. As a socially constructed reality such suffering is capable of being adjusted and changed by social interventions. In this argument, sociopsychological pain cannot be given as much weight as the definitive ending of a human life which will end both physiological life and a potential psychological and social life. Besides, say some, women still suffer psychologically and physically when they do have readily available and institutionalized access to abortion. They decide in anguish and ambivalence; their health can be harmed from abortions (especially repeated abortions), and they suffer the loss of their potential child, which they may mourn.

But it is still the case that many, many women regularly choose abortion as the way of lesser suffering, so the problem of suffering cannot be bypassed. Dealing with the question of why there is suffering is a central problem for all religious believers in a benevolent Creator, and has been since Job. Christian approaches to suffering can be complex. Some suffering seems to be justly related to the free and evil choices made by a person who receives commensurate punishment in this life. Other suffering seems totally disproportionate to the individual's misdeed or lapse which precipitates it. Much more suffering is endured by completely innocent persons and this is absolutely unjust and unfair. On the other hand, the evil prosper or at least escape unscathed. The world as we know it is grotesque in the overwhelming suffering regularly visited upon innocent people. One Christian response to all this unbearable injustice has been to say that on the last day a just reckoning will be made. The good will be rewarded and comforted—every tear will be wiped away—and the evil will be denounced and punished.

In the interim, where daily life takes place, Christians have the example and comfort of the unjust suffering and death of God as incarnate human being. This suffering of the Innocent One has won the ultimate victory and transformation of all creation; all are to be liberated from sin and death forever. This liberation and example enjoin all Christians to liberate, heal, reconcile, and relieve the suffering of everyone whenever possible. However, when suffering cannot be relieved, or when it is freely taken on for the sake of others, the suffering will not be meaningless. Pain and suffering can be used in the ongoing transforming work still to be done to bring forth the Kingdom. Human suffering is given meaning by being joined to Christ's suffering and used to serve the good of all. Christians are thus to relieve the suffering of others, to avoid suffering, but when necessary, to bear suffering patiently in the belief and hope that such endurance will be used in God's plan. The Good News is that suffering, like death, has been ultimately defeated, but on the way to the Parousia suffering can have meaning and be used.

Yet how can one tell the difference between necessary and unnecessary suffering? When suffering cannot be avoided, it is obviously necessary. However, suffering may also be necessary in order to avoid doing evil, or to avoid letting wrongs be done to others, especially those who cannot protect themselves and are the least members of the human community.

COMMUNAL INFLUENCE

Another influence of religious belief upon attitudes arises from most religions' thoroughly communal perspective. All individuals are God's children; thus, they are united as brothers and sisters, and intimately interconnected. The imagery used in religious language and worship confirms this unified view of the human species. Individuals are seen as knit together in one body, co-heirs of Adam and Eve and, in a body, redeemed by the new Adam. All are related in their humanity, and all are also related to the rest of creation in ecological interdependence. Thus, to refute the famous image used in abortion debates, it is impossible for one to suddenly wake up and find oneself connected to a violinist because everyone *already is* connected to each other in physical, psychological, and spiritual ways. These interconnections are seen to impose noncontractual obligations and duties; such pre-existing mutual relationships also predispose persons to be more willing to compel others for the common good. With this communal view, there is less responsiveness to appeals for privacy and more remembrance that privacy has its negative aspect, as in deprivation or privy council. Certainly no human life can be the private property of others; thus, parents cannot claim the unborn or a neonate as their private property. In a real way, the communal religious sense of membership in God's family works against the claim of the biological family to control and dispose of its individual members. Such considerations have worked against the power of the patriarchal male in the family in order to champion women's emancipation and children's rights; and now the loyalty to the larger community predisposes many to support the claims of the fetus against family indications.

In summary, I see the impact of one's religious beliefs upon one's abortion attitudes to be powerful but indirect. Religious belief provides a worldview with certain horizons, groundings, and contexts which will predispose a person to take certain positions before the particular argument is begun. Presuppositions are made about the ultimate reality of benevolence, purpose, meaning, equality, Divine Incarnation, suffering, and communal unity. Such assumptions will often result in a predisposition to take a pro-life stance in the abortion debate. The religious believers who take a pro-choice position would, following my hypotheses, take rather different positions on some of these ultimate presuppositions. The pattern of denominational differences on abortion would follow other differences. Less literal believers in the Incarnation, or God's providence, for example, might emphasize the social construction of meaning or controlling for the quality of life as more important than affirmatively responding to an involuntary pregnancy. If one sees religion primarily as a process of constructing symbolic meanings for individual growth and self-realization, then it would make sense to grant the individual the right and duty to construct for herself the meaning of a particular pregnancy and then to act accordingly. The individual as active moral agent is given more weight than the interdependencies of community or transcendent realities.

Finally, it should be noted that while persons with religious beliefs may differ about what they believe, they are much alike in how they come to their positions on abortion. Religious belief has an impact on the processes involved. First of all, while religious belief means that you may always have to say you're sorry, you never have to ask that old philosophical question, "Why be moral?" Believers are sure that God is on the side of moral action and demands it of those who believe. The problem is finding the moral course of action and discerning God's will. Here religious believers, like everyone else, must use good sense and the rational powers allotted to them. But believers will also pray for guidance, both individually and collectively, and hope for answers. In dilemmas and moral conflicts believers are enjoined to pray and "wait on the Spirit"; believers in every communion are also ready to inform their consciences by consulting their own community's tradition and teachings. Certain religious traditions claim more clout or authority for their traditions or teachings than others, but no member of a religious group would be likely to ignore their own religious resources for guidance in making difficult decisions.

There is also a great motivating force inherent in religious belief to keep believers struggling and wrestling with the abortion question. Most believers are convinced that in some fashion they will be held accountable for their actions. Whatever the particular convictions about Heaven or Hell, some ultimate confrontation is envisioned in which the action or inaction of one's life will be judged. If one will be judged as to whether one is a doer of the word and not a hearer only, continuing action is called for here and now. The stakes in the abortion conflict are serious; either one is in a sense contributing to the slaughter of the innocents, or one is imposing needless suffering and more burdens upon struggling women. The energy impelling the movements on both sides of the abortion conflict is quite understandable. Persons are trying to bring their political actions into accord with their central beliefs and attitudes.

In such an emotionally charged climate, one traditional Christian teaching needs to be stressed and reemphasized. Religious believers are explicitly told to love their opponents and to strive patiently to be peacemakers. If this teaching were to be observed by all, it would surely have an important impact on abortion attitudes. Mutual respect, charity and reconciliation are much needed in the troubled and troubling debate over abortion.

NOTES

1. G. W. ALLPORT, BECOMING: BASIC CONSIDERATIONS FOR A PSYCHOLOGY OF PERSONALITY (Yale University Press, New Haven) (1955) at 94 [hereinafter cited as Allport].
2. R. M. GREEN, RELIGIOUS REASON: THE RATIONAL AND MORAL BASIS OF RELIGIOUS BELIEF (Oxford University Press, New York City) (1978).
3. J. H. NEWMAN, GRAMMAR OF ASSENT (Doubleday & Co., Garden City, N.Y.) (1955) at 86–94.
4. Allport, *supra* note 1, at 97.

5. McGuire, *The Nature of Attitudes and Attitude Change*, in HANDBOOK OF SOCIAL PSYCHOLOGY, Vol. III (G. Lindzey and E. Aronson, Eds.) (Addison-Wesley, Reading, Mass.) (2nd ed. 1969) at 136–314.

6. M. FISHBEIN, I. AJZEN, BELIEF, ATTITUDE, INTENTION, AND BEHAVIOR (Addison-Wesley, Reading, Mass.) (1975).

7. L. S. WRIGHTSMAN, K. DEAUX, SOCIAL PSYCHOLOGY IN THE 80s (Brooks Cole Pub. Co., Monterey, Calif.) (3rd ed. 1981) at 326–377.

8. Grandberg, D., *The Abortion Activists*, FAMILY PLANNING PERSPECTIVES 13(4):157–163 (July/August 1981).

9. *Id.* at 160.

10. For example, Kristin Luker of the Department of Sociology at the University of California, San Diego, is conducting research on worldviews of those active in the pro-life and pro-choice movements.

11. Allport, *supra* note 1, at 96.

12. *Id.* at 97.

13. Meehan, M., *The Other Pro-Lifers*, COMMONWEAL 107(1):13-16 (January 18, 1980).

14. Noonan Jr., J.T., *The Experience of Pain by the Unborn*, HUMAN LIFE REVIEW 8(4):7–19 (1981).

Audience Discussion

Henry W. Strobel, Moderator

CAROLINE WHITBECK, PH.D. (Institute for the Medical Humanities, Galveston, Texas): I think we must recognize that women often undergo abortions at great risk to themselves because they have no other options. In fact, 84,000 women around the world die every year as a result of unsafe abortions.[1] Indeed, they may take such risks for the benefit of others, often including their existing children. The moral dilemmas faced by such women are similar to the grim choices faced by many women who must choose between the welfare of the fetus she carries and that of existing children. In this state, the only referral hospital is in Galveston. A pregnant woman who is poor and living in the Texas Panhandle, who has to get medical care for an existing child, must decide whether she is going to take an automobile trip of 700 miles or more and risk inducing labor and have a premature delivery in order to take care of her existing child. She must balance off the risk to that fetus and the risk to the child. It would be absurd to say that the solution to her dilemma is simply to put the fetus's welfare above all else. Indeed I suggest that the rest of society has some moral obligation to relieve her of the burden of such dilemmas.

A very interesting survey was published in *Life* magazine last fall revealing women's attitudes toward abortion.[2] It found that most women believe that the woman should make the decision regarding abortion, so that it should be legally permissible in a great variety of circumstances for a woman to have an abortion. When women were asked whether it would be morally right for them themselves to have an abortion under the same circumstances; however, the majority of them said it would not. What I think women are saying is that women are competent to make moral decisions, and should be the ones to make the decisions about abortion, but that women will often decide that, all things considered, it would be morally wrong to have an abortion. If we are concerned about feticide, then we should be trying to remove the conditions that force women to resort to abortion rather than trying to remove the possibility of safe legal abortions, forcing more women to resort to illegal abortions.

If we wish to bring in religious values, we must first confront the sexism in those values. Within the Judeo-Christian heritage, women have often been viewed as property—first the property of their fathers and then the property of their husbands. In Deuteronomy 22, we are told that a woman is to be stoned if her male relatives cannot prove that she is a virgin when she marries, but that, as the examples of Abraham and Isaac show, husbands are excused for giving their wives for the sexual use of other men, and fathers, like Lot and the father in Judges 19, are approved for offering their virgin daughters to be raped to forestall the rape of their male guests. Furthermore, we find Paul, in I Corinthians, saying that woman is not made in the image of God the way man is, that woman is only necessary as a means to the existence of men. Paul says that woman stands to man as man does to Christ. To be worthy of consideration as a moral position, a religiously based pro-life position must not relegate women to the status of property, but must recognize women's capacity to make moral decisions governing their own lives.

SIDNEY CALLAHAN (Conference Faculty): I guess what you are saying is that I am not taking the suffering seriously enough. You mean that the suffering of women has to be weighed more seriously. Yet, we live in a system in which there is much suffering. We cannot change that; if you take a pro-life position, you are going to have to add this suffering. I suffer over that. I take that seriously. This is what I meant when I said that a religious person always has to be willing to repent. Suppose you have taken the wrong position and you have laid a burden on people who now suffer under it. In the final judgment you have been working for the wrong thing. But I think I understand your question as "How can you change the system?" This is where I think differences come in. I, by the way, am a democratic socialist. I do think that you can change the system and that we must make a more communitarian system with redistribution of all resources. It is interesting that some other socialist women have had second thoughts about abortion too. Just because the woman has been thought of as property, we then cannot go to the next stage and make the fetus property. What we have found is that people are not property and have to be given equal rights.

How do you change a system if something is horrible and you have a way of keeping the status quo going, which in this case is abortion, as the solution to these horrible things. By giving in, aren't you just reinforcing the system? Nobody is ever going to change the problems if there is a solution that has already been available. I mean, will people really work harder on birth control and contraception and make it more available along with education if they have abortion available? The whole question about the law is something that I find very difficult to struggle with. The law is supposed to be a teacher as well as an order-keeper in a certain way, and the teaching function of the law may be an important one that we have overlooked. I certainly am not an expert on the function of the law, but my intuitions are to try and determine if there is some way that the law can be a teaching force without necessarily being punitive, particularly toward women. I haven't worked that out and so I have no answer.

UNIDENTIFIED PARTICIPANT: May I ask Professor Dickens if any other country has a law similar to that in the United States permitting abortion with few limits, and whether fetal rights are recognized here in the abortion decision at any time before birth commences?

BERNARD DICKENS (Conference Faculty): China has a law comparable to that in the United States, under which there are few limits upon abortion, except those designed to protect maternal life and health, for instance, against unskilled or contraindicated treatment. In the United States, fetal rights have been recognized by the Supreme Court from the point of fetal viability. From then, the interests of the fetus weigh in the balance, although they are not necessarily decisive, depending upon the terms of the state laws and, for instance, the countervailing interests advanced by the pregnant woman. Her interest in protection of her physical and mental health against medically agreed-upon risk of danger may prevail over fetal interests, if the perceived danger appears sufficiently compelling. After fetal viability, unlike before that stage, a reason beyond the woman's wish and request must exist for pregnancy to be terminated.

ROBERT M. FINEMAN, M.D., PH.D. (University of Utah Medical Center, Salt Lake City): Suppose it were possible to perform an early "abortion" on a woman who did not desire to carry her pregnancy to term and not kill the fetus but deliver it alive. The fetus could then be placed in some sort of guarded environment where it would grow to weigh six or seven lbs. This would alleviate or obviate a lot of problems I think we are having because the child would be kept alive. Do you know any religious proscriptions which would prevent such action?

SIDNEY CALLAHAN: I do not know that it ever came up, but I wonder because sometimes the argument is given by people who say, "I could never bring the baby to term and then give it away—I could not stand to do that. Therefore, I will have an abortion now rather than to do this." Now, the question is would the mother have the same kind of feeling about giving consent for this if it were not this sort of intimate growing within her own body. That would be an interesting question psychologically.

RUTH MACKLIN (Conference Faculty): The feasibility of this depends on advances in present technology, which we should not rule out, given how fast things are moving in a variety of fields. But I thought the question focused on the religious features of it, and it is interesting that in your answer, you speak only of the psychological aspects. The two fields, religion and psychology, blended so nicely in your talk; but now the question is really focusing on the religious thing, and I wonder why the question was thrown to me.

HENRY W. STOBEL, PH.D. (Professor of Biochemistry, University of Texas Medical School, Houston, Texas): Since no one seems to have any religious reason why that could not be done, are there any psychologists, philosophers, or lawyers here who would object or who can think of reasons to object?

SIDNEY CALLAHAN: I think an interesting analogy is in Huxley's *Brave New World* where any talk about wombs and birth was a dirty word. Also, if you think about the evolution of parenthood and reproduction, that is the way it used to be: organisms put eggs in the sea and they all floated around or eggs were laid and left someplace. But the whole development of parenthood, in vivo parenthood, has been for the parent to be able to protect and nurture the offspring. Now, I guess a crucial question would be, could you really insure protection and nurturing in this artificial womb.

UNIDENTIFIED PARTICIPANT: One of the basic problems we have here between the "pro-abortionists" and the "anti-abortionists" is a large amount of money, time, and energy taking care of an issue which will never be resolved probably at any level—even at the law level. But we have an issue that goes on in this country every day which was brought out by the woman from Galveston. I work at two hospitals in Houston—the county as well as a private hospital—and if a patient referred to the private hospital has insufficient funds, even if there is an imminent probability of delivery, she has to go to the county hospital. However, county hospital will not accept her because she has a husband who is working and making too much money to be considered there. Moreover, frequently there is no place in the neonatal intensive care facility. There are a lot of babies at 26, 27, and 28 weeks around the Houston area who do not survive because they cannot get the proper care. My question is, how do we attack this particular problem which I consider perhaps more important than the abortion issue.

SIDNEY CALLAHAN: I am for socialized medicine, which is probably really popular in Houston. No, redistribution of resources seems to me to be an easy ethical problem but a horrible political problem, which is what we are facing right now in this country. I think that there is obvious injustice.

There should be more equality of outcome. The idea that we have equality of access is ridiculous and I am totally in favor of some sort of change in redistribution, but I think it has to be done more through the political processes.

RUTH MACKLIN: I am glad that the opportunity to disagree with my colleague on this panel and personal friend, Sidney Callahan, is not only on the religious issue. Although I share the principle that redistribution would be a fine thing, and on the political spectrum I am right where Sidney is, nevertheless, it would be practically impossible to bring about changes in the allocation of our country's resources through the political process. Even allocating an increased amount over what we now have in any area is not going to be an easy problem to solve, given the difficulties that we face on every front with distribution of resources. Allow me to say one quick word that encompasses both of these remarks by way of a response in ethics. If it shows a lack of answers, it doesn't mean we should give up on an approach based on ethics; but this is one of few cases of the sort I mentioned earlier in which a rights approach is really in conflict with a consequentialist approach. Surely a consequentialist approach would argue against removing a fetus or trying to keep alive a conceptus or blastocyst or zygote, partly because of financial reasons and partly because there may not be enough parents to go around for these abortuses. So a consequentialist analysis on ethical grounds would argue against the proposal that an alternative to abortion might be trying to sustain the life of a conceptus to term. The rights-based approach, however, would yield a different answer because, if indeed, the right to life overrides other types of rights, then the rights-based approach would yield a different moral solution than a consequentialist one. No single answer is then given by ethics or ethical theory just as, I think, Sidney pointed out there is no single answer given by religion. One has to move carefully in order to make some distinctions regarding what ethical theory is to be used, just as one must specify which religious perspectives one is talking about.

BERNARD DICKENS: I would expect that there is some consensus regarding the instances where infants born prematurely at, for instance, 26, 27, or 28 weeks gestation, fail to survive because they cannot be admitted to hospitals, and others where threatened spontaneous abortion cannot be prevented because patients have insufficient funds to cover treatment in private hospitals, but too much income for eligibility for admission to publicly funded hospitals. Where a child is born alive and viable, but is at risk through prematurity, and a woman wants to resist threatened spontaneous abortion, both pro-life and pro-choice forces should be agreed regarding the need for appropriate medical care. Perhaps they could usefully join forces to apply political pressure on state government to limit the avoidable loss of wanted children.

JEANNE E. FRIEDEN, R.N. (Arizona Right to Choose, Phoenix, Arizona): I want to ask a couple of questions of Professor Dickens and one of Dr. Callahan. I am from Phoenix, Arizona, and I feel like perhaps I have been out in the desert in more ways than one. I have been a little shocked by what some people have said today. One is, Dr. Dickens, you said in answer to a question that throughout the United States abortions are legal on demand for the full-term of the pregnancy—I believe that is the way you answered the question from that other gentleman. Is that right, was that your answer?

BERNARD DICKENS: Not for the full duration of the pregnancy. Some state laws have permitted intervention after fetal viability. From that point, state interests are legitimate, and laws may require that the interests of the fetus have to weigh in the balance, even though they may not necessarily be decisive. The United States Supreme Court has acknowledged state authority in trying to preserve the interests of the viable fetus.

JEANNE FRIEDEN: Well, I think the United States Supreme Court was clear that only during the first three months is the state prohibited from interfering. Secondly, you said something about a law prohibiting abortions in Cypress and Turkey—about family indications? In Arizona, we have a state representative, Ratliff, who at one time said he thought all abortions ought to be illegal except in the case where a white woman was raped by a black man and it sounds very similar. I can't believe, I mean we all thought that was a completely ridiculous statement on his part and I know it got national attention. Are you saying that there is such a similar racist kind of law in existence somewhere in the world today?

BERNARD DICKENS: In Cyprus, the law permits account to be taken in case of rape of the harm to family reputation of a woman belonging to the Greek-Cypriot or to the Turkish-Cypriot community bearing a child fathered by a member of the other community. The law does not simply protect women of one community against involuntary impregnation by members of the other. It protects each community against such acts caused by the other.

JEANNE FRIEDEN: Oh, I see, it's an equal protection argument. I also have a question for Dr. Callahan. As a member of an anti-nuclear group in Arizona as well as Arizona Right to Choose, I have not met any feminists who were anti-choice or "pro-zygotes" as I call them, since I feel that I am pro-life and so I do not want to call the opposition "pro-life" because I feel it is a misnomer. I would like you to explain if you are of the position that birth control devices such as the IUD should be illegal for women.

SIDNEY CALLAHAN: I am not sure how the IUD works, but I certainly am for birth control and contraception when it is the woman's body that she is controlling. Otherwise I think you have problems, but I don't know enough to be sure how it works.

JEANNE FRIEDEN: I think that is a real critical point in the discussion in terms of a feminist being against abortion because the extreme anti-abortion position would say that life begins at the moment of conception which would prevent use of IUDs and prevent the use of minipills. An IUD prevents implantation and the minipills in about 40 percent of women act to prevent implantation, not ovulation. So with the two major forms of effective birth control eliminated, if you are saying that those are not going to be allowed and abortion is not going to be allowed . . . One of the problems—I mean aside from the problem of lack of control over my body—another sort of likely scenario is the overpopulation that in this day and age might seriously lead to a nuclear war. I mean, I am not saying that in a provocative way: I think that is a serious problem. I would like to address how you feel about those contraceptive issues.

UNIDENTIFIED PARTICIPANT: Well, just a minicomment at this stage. The young lady was correctly shocked and I am sorry that the gentleman from Canada is incorrect. The United States Supreme Court in *Roe v. Wade*[3] and *Doe v. Bolton*,[4] its companion case, allows for abortion right up to the moment of birth. During the first three months, the decision is left to the woman and her attending physician. During the second three months, the only permissible regulations are those that seek to protect maternal health. Regulations designed to protect the pre-viable fetus are not permitted. In the last trimester, beyond viability, abortion can be, it is not mandated, proscribed by the state if the mother's life or health is in danger. The key word here is "health". In *Doe v. Bolton*, health is defined by the Supreme Court to cover almost anything, including the age of the woman, her economic condition, and effectively it makes abortion available right up to birth. Now whether abortions are done or not right up to the birth is beside the point; the point is that that is what the law is in this country.

BERNARD DICKENS: I must agree, and say that my earlier observations concerning the state of the law in the United States are not inconsistent with your statement.

NOTES

1. Complications of Abortion in Developing Countries, POPULATION REPORTS, Series F, No. 7 (Johns Hopkins Univ., Baltimore) (1980) at 1.

2. LIFE 4(11):45–54 (November 1981).
3. 410 U.S. 113 (1973).
4. 410 U.S. 179 (1973).

Part Five

The Future

Chapter 15

Toward an Even Newer Genetics

Leon E. Rosenberg

The papers collected in this volume come from biologists, clinicians, lawyers, and philosophers, and address a number of issues concerned with the beginnings of human life and personhood. It should not be surprising to see clinical geneticists figure prominently in these discussions, since some of the moral and ethical dilemmas under consideration have been generated by the ability of geneticists to carry out prenatal diagnosis, to offer selective therapeutic abortion, and to initiate fetal surgery. Perhaps, in fact, I am one of only a few people who is amazed at the speed with which my professional field has generated legal and philosophic debate, and who is sometimes disoriented by its move from the dim light of the cloistered laboratory to the harsh glare of the public arena. Admittedly, I needed to be convinced that gazing into the future of genetics would be a proper way to begin to conclude the conference.

I guess I must accept the fact that genetics has become a household word. It is virtually impossible to pick up a newspaper or magazine or to turn on the radio or television set without encountering something about genetics. An almost bewildering panorama of progress is portrayed. One day we are told that recombinant DNA technology will soon provide us with unlimited amounts of medically useful hormones such as insulin.[1] The next day we learn of successes in mapping genes to specific chromosomes.[2] On a third day we find out that people at risk for premature heart. attacks due to an inherited increase in blood cholesterol can be treated with cholesterol-lowering drugs,[3] and on a fourth, that it is possible to treat surgically certain birth defects in the human fetus.[4] But scientific and medical progress is not all we hear about. There is also a plethora of disquieting news. The current Surgeon General of the United States is reported to have called prenatal diagnosis of genetic disease "a search and destroy mission." A professor at UCLA is severely criticized and disciplined for trying to treat patients with inherited disorders of hemoglobin production with recombinant DNA-containing cells. A prominent geneticist at Harvard creates a stir by taking a leave of absence to assume a managerial role in a major biotechnology company. The parents of a child with Down syndrome sue their obstetrician for wrongful birth. Given the magnitude of this media coverage, it is not surprising that genetics is a general topic of conversation at home, at the office, or in church. Given the nature of the news, it is, likewise, not surprising that geneticists are viewed by some as scientific or medical heroes, by others as unethical fame seekers, and by still others as greedy opportunists.

BRIEF HISTORY OF GENETICS

Let me emphasize that this public visibility of genetics (unprecedented, I think, in the history of the biological sciences) is a very recent phenomenon. The seminal work of the Austrian monk, Grègor Mendel, who in the 1860s described the fundamental laws of gene segregation and unit inheritance which now carry his name, went unnoticed for nearly 40 years. In turn, the contributions of Archibald Garrod, the British physician whose study of patients with inherited metabolic diseases at the turn of this century laid the foundation for modern medical genetics, were buried for another 40 years until Beadle and Tatum resurrected them in the form of the one gene–one enzyme hypothesis of gene action. In the 1950s progress began to accelerate. The discovery of DNA's double helix launched the field of molecular biology on its exciting trajectory toward an understanding of gene replication, of the genetic code, and of the control of protein synthesis. The definition of the biochemical defect in such human diseases as sickle cell anemia, phenylketonuria, and galactosemia brought medical genetics closer to clinical medicine on one side and to molecular genetics on the other. The determination of the correct chromosome constitution of human cells ushered in a new branch of medical genetics concerned with disorders caused by chromosomal abnormalities.

Even these discoveries failed to attract much public attention. They did, however, attract a number of Ph.D. and M.D. scientists to the field. I was one such M.D., who, in 1961, assumed the care of a young boy with a previously unrecognized familial disorder of amino acid metabolism. Although I had not shown any particular interest in genetics prior to that time, I became fascinated by this boy's specific problem and by the general premise that the study of inherited metabolic disorders might allow one to explore the biochemical genetics of man and, at the same time, use that information toward the diagnosis, treatment and prevention of disease. Thus, I joined the ranks of the then small number of medical geneticists and the even smaller number of geneticists specializing in the inherited metabolic diseases. What a lucky decision that was! For the past 20 years I have had the good fortune to carry out and direct laboratory research, to teach students, and to care for patients. From these several vantages I have witnessed the explosive growth of the field of genetics. It has been exhilarating to watch the molecular and cellular biologists make one spectacular discovery after another, each moving us even closer to a complete understanding of gene structure and function. It has been equally gratifying to participate in the emergence of clinical genetics as a bona fide medical specialty concerned with identifying the literally hundreds of inherited and congenital disorders that affect mankind, and with mitigating the consequences of these conditions through appropriate prevention, treatment, and counseling. And it has been startling to see genetics capture the public's eye.

RECENT INTEREST IN GENETICS

Why has public interest in genetics increased so much recently? There are many reasons. First, the very nature of the field attracts attention. Human beings are fascinated by themselves. Anything that tells them why they are different from or like one another is bound to be deemed important, and that is what genetics is all about. The field considers the mystery of our species—our evolutionary origins, our ethnic differences, our innate uniqueness. Second, people are concerned about health and worried about disease. They know that some of the most common afflictions, such as birth defects, cancer, and heart disease, result, at least in part, from genetic factors. They reason, in turn, that anything learned about genetics may improve the quality of life by reducing the impact of disease. A third reason is more tangible still. People who share with Calvin Coolidge and Ronald Reagan the view that the proper business of America is business see the scores of biotechnology companies spawned by recent genetic advances as appropriate ventures to invest in and profit from. That sector of the public responding to these facets of genetics tends to see the efforts of scientists and clinicians in the field in a positive light.

But the field attracts public attention for negative reasons as well. Some remember that Hitler used genetic slogans to carry out his heinous programs of genocide, and they fear that eugenic programs (or pogroms) could emerge from modern genetic research. Some, believing that geneticists are simply getting too close to understanding the essence of life, wish nostalgically that geneticists would just go away and leave certain marvelous events like conception, embryonic development, and birth to poets and priests. Some, addicted to the drama of larger-than-life science fiction, live in real or imagined terror that current genetic experiments could go awry and loose on our civilization strange and horrible creatures. That portion of our society responding to these real or imaginary threats tends to view genetics and geneticists with suspicion and even hostility. Taken together, they help explain why any new scientific finding or clinical application in genetics is likely to be greeted with public ambivalence.

PRENATAL DIAGNOSIS AND TREATMENT

Nowhere in clinical genetics has this ambivalence been as visible as in the area most germane to the theme of this conference—prenatal diagnosis. It is sad, but true, that medicine has very little to offer babies with a large number of genetic or congenital disorders. For example, in the era before prenatal diagnosis was possible, a couple who had a child with multiple congenital anomalies due to an extra chromosome No.18, were told that their baby would not develop normally and would almost certainly die by age one year. They were told that such chromosomal accidents are the most common reason for spontaneous first trimester abortions and that only a few such conceptions are carried to term. And they were told that they had between a one and two percent chance of having the same outcome with any subsequent pregnancy. Similarly, if a couple had a child with Tay-Sachs disease, they learned that no effective treatment existed, that their baby would die by age five years after a prolonged course characterized by neurologic deterioration, and that each subsequent pregnancy carried a 25 percent risk for recurrence of this recessively inherited disorder. Needless to say, this kind of news was crushing. Not only were their children to die, but the tragedy might recur with subsequent pregnancies. This kind of clinical situation, repeated for literally scores of conditions and for thousands of couples annually, led some couples to divorce, many to refrain from additional childbearing attempts, and all to view pregnancy with foreboding and even terror. This distressing situation has begun to change. As mentioned in earlier papers, it is now possible to withdraw a small amount of fluid from the sac surrounding the baby, to culture cells from or examine chemicals in this amniotic fluid, and to determine the chromosomal complement and something about the metabolic characteristics of the fetus.[5] This means that some couples at risk no longer are required to take their chances blindly. If they desire the information, they can know what to expect, and can make decisions based on fact rather than probability. By 1980, this kind of prenatal diagnosis was being used by more than 40,000 American women annually. The procedure has proven itself safe and reliable. Other related diagnostic modalities have appeared as well. If sampling the amniotic fluid cannot provide the answer to the question of recurrence, then sometimes an ultrasound study,[6] fetal blood sampling,[7] or direct visualization[8] can. In about 97 percent of all cases, such testing shows that the fetus is unaffected, the pregnancy continues to term, and the parents are relieved of a terrible anxiety. It is unfortunate that, in the event the fetus is found affected, the parents must choose between having another damaged child or terminating the pregnancy by abortion. That choice, I assure you, is an excruciatingly difficult one. Yet, given an affected fetus, most couples choose abortion and suffer the depression, guilt, and grief that invariably results from that choice. In their minds, abortion causes less suffering than bringing into the world another child doomed from the start to fail and die.

Others in our society find such prenatal diagnosis morally abhorrent on the grounds that it may lead to abortion which, in their view, is no different than the taking of any other life. They fear that if fetuses with trisomy-18 can be aborted today, then fetuses with less severe or trivial problems will be aborted tomorrow. They believe deeply that any life is better than no life. They profess that a society which condones selective feticide now will permit infanticide later. My personal view on this matter is well-known and will not be repeated here.[9] I raise the issue to emphasize how differently the same medical modality can be viewed and, more importantly, to remind you that prenatal diagnosis is but one kind of preventive approach offered by practicing clinical geneticists. Too often, I am afraid, clinical genetics is viewed as synonymous with amniocentesis, and genetic intervention equated with therapeutic abortion. Genetic disease can be prevented by other means as well. For instance, some couples known to be at risk will choose to adopt children, to use artificial insemination, or to refrain from procreation. Their choices should be supported as strongly, in my view, as those of individuals prepared to take their procreative risks or those wishing to use prenatal diagnostic techniques.

It is likewise too often forgotten that a growing list of genetic disorders can be treated effectively. Nearly all children in this country, for instance, are screened at birth for phenylketonuria (PKU), a metabolic disease in which the amino acid phenylalanine accumulates in the blood. In the past this metabolic derangement led regularly to severe mental retardation and to the institutionalization of most affected children. Now, a diet low in phenylalanine is prescribed in the early weeks of life and such children attain normal or near normal intellectual potential.[10] Such dietary treatment exists for at least a score of other metabolic disorders with different clinical and chemical findings. Nutritional restriction is but one mode of medical therapy. An increasing number of metabolic conditions have been shown to respond to supplements of a specific vitamin.[11] In at least two such disorders, treatment has been started in utero by administering a vitamin to the mother and allowing the placenta to deliver it to the baby.[12] More examples of such prenatal medical therapy will surely appear. Administration of hormones and drugs, too, are efficacious in certain conditions, and the more we learn about the biochemical bases of inherited metabolic disorders, the longer the list of treatable conditions becomes. For still other conditions, it is the avoidance of certain drugs or inhalants which must be prescribed. For example, patients with deficiency of the serum protein alpha-1-antitrypsin who are predisposed to pulmonary damage do better if they don't smoke cigarettes.[13] Other patients with other conditions must avoid barbiturates or sulfa drugs.

The surgeon also has an important role to play. This role may take the form of correcting heart defects, excising inherited tumors, reconstructing limb abnormalities, or repairing such defects as cleft lip and palate. As you have already read, surgery can also be carried out on the fetus. This modality has only recently been introduced, and it is too early to know how widely it will be employed. It is already clear that the human uterus can be entered by needles and even opened by incision without necessarily interrupting pregnancy. From the medical standpoint, the most complicated aspects of fetal surgery will be in determining when to operate and what kinds of lesions are truly correctable. From an ethical point of view, other issues will arise: should anyone but the parents permit or refuse such intervention? Will intervention become mandatory if shown to be effective? These questions should not deflect us from the reality that detection of genetic disease in utero need not necessarily be followed by abortion—true therapies are emerging and will increase in number and effectiveness.

GENETIC TECHNOLOGY IN THE FUTURE

Having provided you with this admittedly abbreviated and personal view of the current state of clinical genetics, let me turn to my task of predicting the future. For this discussion, "future" will refer to the next 20 years—that is, to about the year 2000. This limit will prevent the kind of frivolous speculation that open-ended forecasting encourages. Moreover, it may, if I am lucky, permit me to smile at the wisdom or to frown at the ignorance of my projections. Some of my colleagues and some members of the press speak in terms of a "biological revolution" when referring to the near future. I shall refrain from such hyperbole but I share their view that a great deal will happen during the remainder of this century. As is always the case in biomedicine, new biological information (whether basic or

applied) follows the development of new technologies; and the new techniques pertinent to genetics are unusually powerful. Let me describe a few
of them.

First and foremost is the development of recombinant DNA technology. This scientific innovation, discovered less than 10 years ago, was
largely responsible for the expression "new genetics." Although I include
prenatal diagnosis, fetal surgery, and in vitro fertilization as additional
components of such a "new genetics," recombinant DNA techniques deserve special comment.

To oversimplify, recombinant DNA technology permits one to isolate
a gene from one species and recombine it with the genes of another
species.[14] This technical feat depends on two general kinds of bacterial
enzymes: restriction enzymes (which may be thought of as chemical scis-
sors that cut genes at discrete locations) and joining enzymes (which, by
analogy, are like chemical tape for hooking up DNA segments end-to-
end). With these tools, it has become commonplace to splice a gene from a
complex organism like a human into the DNA of a bacterial plasmid,
which is a small circular piece of DNA that replicates independently of the
bacterial chromosome. The bacterium, with its recombinant plasmid, is
then allowed to do what it does best—namely, multiply rapidly—thereby
allowing the human gene to be amplified (or cloned) along with all the
other bacterial products. This technique has proven to be a uniquely
powerful tool in purifying and characterizing genes, in modifying them at
will, and in examining their expression under widely different circumstances. It promises to permit the synthesis of enzymes, hormones, and
other proteins on a scale previously unattainable, and seems to be on its
way to making great contributions in areas as diverse as agriculture and
environmental waste disposal.

I believe that recombinant DNA techniques, when employed with
other advances in cellular and molecular genetics, will make the next 20
years the most exciting ones in the history of the biomedical sciences. This
excitement will span the field from the most fundamental to the most
applied; it will influence developments in all the biological and clinical
sciences. Small wonder that recombinant DNA is as big an issue in the *Wall
Street Journal* as in the *New England Journal of Medicine*; small wonder that it
is as much a topic of conversation in the industrial board room as in the
university classroom.

A second major technologic advance has to do with transferring
genes and chromosomes from one cell to another without involving a
bacterial host.[15] It is now clear that genes from one cell can be injected into
the nucleus of another, and that under suitable circumstances, such donor
genes will be integrated into the genome of the recipient cell and be

expressed there as well. We still have much to learn about the rules which govern such gene transfer, but the rapid pace of progress makes it seem likely that the process can be understood, controlled, and used safely.

Two other techniques of note involve manipulation of cells or tissue rather than molecules. Successful in vitro fertilization of human oöcytes by sperm has been accomplished, followed by several rounds of cell division and, ultimately, by uterine re-implantation and normal gestation.[16] This has permitted couples whose infertility has resulted from blockage of the tube between the ovary and uterus to have children. Its potential, however, exceeds that. Finally, cell and organ transplantation should be mentioned, not because they are so new, but because new uses for them are at hand and are relevant to the future of clinical genetics. Transplantations of kidney, liver, and bone marrow cells, particularly, have been undertaken often enough to recommend their consideration in novel situations.

USING THE NEW TECHNOLOGY

What will these new tools provide? Let me consider their utility in a few diagnostic, preventive, and therapeutic settings. Huntington's disease is currently a familial tragedy and a geneticist's nightmare. Although we know that the disease is inherited as a dominant trait and, therefore, that each child of an affected person has a 50 percent chance of being affected, we have no way of telling the children of an affected person which of them will develop the disorder. Since clinical manifestations do not usually appear until the 30s or 40s, most affected people have had their own children before they know they have the disease. This disease pattern always leads to enormous personal and familial unrest, and not infrequently to divorce and suicide. I believe that recombinant DNA techniques will soon provide a diagnostic test for Huntington's disease. This will permit young people at risk to make decisions about marriage and family based on certainty rather than probability. Those with the gene may still, of course, decide to have their own children as they do now. Many, I think, will either adopt children or use artificial insemination or in vitro fertilization so as to avoid the 50 percent risk of passing the disorder on to each of their offspring. Artificial insemination has been available in such settings for a long time. Soon, it will be possible for a woman carrying a particular gene to consider carrying and bearing a child which is the product of her husband's sperm and someone else's ovum—perhaps that of an unaffected sister or other close relative. In this situation, in vitro fertilization provides people with choices that are currently unavailable.

A similar scenario can be described for a woman who has been shown to be a carrier for the X-linked disorder Duchenne's muscular dystrophy.

Currently that diagnosis is hard to establish until she has had an affected son. In the future, recombinant DNA-generated probes should facilitate detection of carriers. Then, fertilization with her husband's X-bearing sperm only (a technique still unattained but being actively sought) would free her from the risk of having males with the disease. In both of these settings, primary prevention—that is, prevention of conception of an affected fetus—is being employed. Let me hasten to point out that secondary prevention, by which I mean prevention of birth of an affected fetus, will not disappear in the face of new technical advances. Most chromosomal disorders for which prenatal diagnosis is now performed are not likely to yield to recombinant DNA technologies or alternative gestational strategies. Until we learn why chromosomes don't always segregate properly during meiosis, the autosomal trisomies (like Down syndrome) will still present their dilemmas for families. Whether we like it or not, therapeutic abortion will remain an important preventive option during the years to which I am looking ahead.

But it is in the area of treatment that I project the greatest changes during the coming two decades. The medical and surgical modalities now employed will be extended to more conditions and will be used with greater precision. Replacement of missing proteins such as insulin or gamma globulin will be greatly facilitated by recombinant DNA-linked synthesis. Replacement of some intracellular enzymes will also be perfected as we learn more about the specialized "zip codes" which govern the movement of proteins from where they are made to where they reside.[17] These quantitative changes will be joined by even more dramatic qualitative ones in terms of the range of therapeutic options and of the time that such options will be offered. Young children with inherited defects of circulating blood cells such as sickle cell anemia or thalassemia may be treated by transplantation of healthy bone marrow cells after their own mutant marrow cell population has been irradiated. Even more dramatically, normal genes may be inserted into their own bone marrow cells in vitro and then readministered. A wide variety of such gene replacement strategies are currently under investigation in the laboratory. Some employ transfer of single, isolated genes; others, of whole chromosomes. Some seek to transfer naked DNA; others, to insert DNA linked to specific viral vectors.

Postnatal gene replacement may, even when successful, be applicable only to certain classes of disorders—like those of circulating red blood cells. What about disorders due to defects in less accessible organs such as the liver or brain? It may be possible to use viruses with genes spliced into them to "home" to particular tissues of their affinity. On the other hand, it may be that such gene transplantation will have to be carried out during

fetal life or even immediately post-conception if healthy cells are to popu-
late a sufficient portion of the tissues to prevent disease manifestations. In
fact, injecting genes into the fertilized ovum may turn out to be one of the
easiest systems to manipulate and one in which to achieve development of
normal progeny cells in all tissues. Workers in the field agree that we know
far too little about the rules which govern where such transferred genes
go, how they become integrated into the recipient cell's chromosomes,
what balances their expression, and whether their presence can disturb
normal cellular controls, to consider human experimentation at this time.
There is still much that must be learned from tissue culture and animal
models, and there is a need for unusually disciplined self-restraint and
patience on the part of scientists in the field. Nonetheless, I believe we are
much closer to perfecting such potentially curative therapeutic strategies
than anyone would have thought possible a decade ago. We won't cure
genetic diseases by gene replacement tomorrow or next year. I think there
is a good chance that we will see such advances during my lifetime, and
that, I should add, is a far more optimistic guess than any I have been
willing to make before.

In conclusion, I wish to emphasize that the aim of these diagnostic
and therapeutic strategies is no different than those used to control and
even eradicate certain infectious diseases, which are very like genetic
diseases in that they too are passed from one person to another and even
from one generation to another. Evolution tells us that neither nature nor
nurture is static. History reminds us that mankind has never been willing
to be a passive symbiont in his world, but rather has strived to learn about it
and change it for our betterment. Nowhere has that learning process been
more rapid or exciting than in the field of genetics. Nowhere, too, is there a
field with greater promise for increasing mankind's knowledge of ourselves, for reducing the suffering caused by disease, and for improving the
quality of human life.

NOTES

1. Miller, W.L., *Medical Progress—Recombinant DNA and the Pediatrician*, JOURNAL
   OF PEDIATRICS 99(1):1 (1981); Baxter, J.D., *Recombinant DNA and Medical Progress*, HOSPITAL PRACTICE 15(2):57 (1980).
2. McKusick, V.A., *The Anatomy of the Human Genome*, AMERICAN JOURNAL OF
   MEDICINE 69(2):267 (1980).
3. Havel, Goldstein, Brown, *Lipoproteins and Lipid Transport,* in METABOLIC CON-
   TROL AND DISEASE (P.K. Bondy and L.E. Rosenberg, eds.) (Saunders, Philadelphia) (1980) at 393.
4. Golbus, M.S., *et al.*, *In Utero Treatment of Urinary Tract Obstruction*, AMERICAN
   JOURNAL OF OBSTETRICS AND GYNECOLOGY 142(4):383 (1982); Harrison,

M.R., Golbus, M.S., Filly, R.A., *Management of the Fetus with a Correctable Congenital Defect*, JOURNAL OF THE AMERICAN MEDICAL ASSOCIATION 246(7):774 (1981).

5. Golbus, M.S., *et al.*, *Prenatal Genetic Diagnosis in 3000 Amniocenteses*, NEW ENGLAND JOURNAL OF MEDICINE 300(4):157 (1979).
6. DeVore, Hobbins, *Diagnosis of Structural Abnormalities in the Fetus* in CLINICS IN PERINATOLOGY (J.B. Warshaw, ed.) (Saunders, Philadelphia) (1979).
7. Mahoney, Hobbins, *Fetoscopy and Fetal Blood Sampling* in GENETIC DISORDERS AND THE FETUS (A. Milunsky, ed.) (Plenum Press, New York) (1979) at 501.
8. *See, e.g.*, FETOSCOPY (I. Rocker and K. Laurence, eds.) (Elsevier/North-Holland, Amsterdam) (1981).
9. *Human Life Bill: Hearings on S.158 before Subcomm. on Separation of Powers, Comm. on Judiciary*, 97th Cong., 1st Sess. 48-62 (1981) (Statement of L. Rosenberg).
10. Scriver, C.R., Clow, C.L., *Phenylketonuria and other Phenylalanine Hydroxylation Mutants in Man*, ANNUAL REVIEW OF GENETICS 14:179(1980).
11. Rosenberg, *Vitamin-Responsive Inherited Metabolic Disorder*, in ADVANCES IN HUMAN GENETICS (H. Harris and K. Hirschhorn, eds.)(Plenum Press, New York 1976) at 1.
12. Roth, K.S., *et al.*, *Prenatal Administration of Biotin in Biotin Responsive Multiple Carboxylase Deficiency*, PEDIATRIC RESEARCH 16(2):126 (1982); Ampola, M.G., *et al.*, *Prenatal Therapy of a Patient With Vitamin-B$_{12}$-Responsive Methylamonic Acidemia*, NEW ENGLAND JOURNAL OF MEDICINE 293(7):313 (1975).
13. Morse, J.O., *Alpha$_1$-Antitrypsin Deficiency*, NEW ENGLAND JOURNAL OF MEDICINE, *Part I* 299(19):1045; *Part II* 299(20):1099 (1978).
14. *See* Baxter, *Recombinant DNA*, and Miller, *Medical Progress, supra* note 1.
15. McBride, O.W., Peterwon, J.L., *Chromosome-Mediated Gene Transfer in Mammalian Cells*, ANNUAL REVIEW OF GENETICS 14:321 (1980).
16. Biggers, J.D., *In Vitro Fertilzation and Embryo Transfer in Human Beings*, NEW ENGLAND JOURNAL OF MEDICINE 304(8):336 (1981).
17. Sabatini, D.D., *et al.*, *Mechanisms for the Incorporation of Proteins in Membranes and Organelles*, JOURNAL OF CELL BIOLOGY 92(1):1 (1982).

Chapter 16

The Role of Science in Moral and Societal Decision Making: The Human Life Bill as a Case Study

Daniel Callahan

When I was a child, and my parents moved about a great deal, I was given a traditional piece of advice about starting at a new school: "Find the toughest kid and make him your friend; that way no one will pick on you and everyone will be your pal." In our society, the toughest kid in the school is science. If you can get science on your side, security and perhaps prestige will be yours. At the very least, others will find it hazardous to pick on you.

What no one adequately explained to me, however, was just how one manages to befriend the toughest kid. As far as I could observe, he was in fact the one most likely to beat me up. Or sometimes there was uncertainty about just who the toughest was after all. Whichever candidate one chose to court, one was likely to be assaulted by the other claimants and their gangs.

Matters are not much clearer in the case of science. We all want science on our side, with its hard data and undeniable truths. If I want to claim that the earth is round, or state that the speed of light is 186,000 miles per second, the support and prestige of science are at my command. Should I, however, try to recruit science to buttress a belief—say, that recombinant DNA research poses dangers, or that the notion of "altruism" can be reduced to a programmed biological strategy for advantageous kinship promotion, or that busing is a fine way to promote a better education for the disadvantaged—then I will have some problems. They will take a variety of familiar forms. I will discover that the scientific evidence I can amass to support my claims will be sharply attacked by those with other, allegedly contradictory, data. Should I persist in claiming that the evidence is on my side of the case, my motives will then be impugned. My ideological biases, I will be told, no doubt account for my egregiously selective reading of the facts. Should I go so far as to support legislation based on my empirical convictions, my scientific gang will tell me that I can hardly do otherwise without flying in the face of the data. The other scientific gang will have a different message: that I am trying to impose my private values, supported by the flimsiest of evidence, on otherwise innocent citizens who should be left free to make up their own minds.

This now familiar ritual in debating moral and social issues reveals some important assumptions about the purported role of scientific evidence in the making of policy decisions. One assumption is that solid scientific evidence can and should be decisive in settling social arguments. Another assumption is that, lacking good scientific evidence, the matter reduces personal preference or ideological conviction; the issue becomes, in principle, undecidable. Of course there is a middle ground: that while the scientific evidence may not be decisive, it can be strong enough to lend credence to the beliefs of one group rather than another. Most policy issues are probably argued out on this middle ground, with all of the attendant problems of claims and counterclaims and the adducing of new evidence and counterevidence. In any case, the great prize is to have a set of moral and social beliefs that have the solid backing of the best, most unassailable science.

The abortion debate in general, and the Human Life Bill in particular, serve as good illustrations of the allure and seduction of scientific support for one's convictions. Though no one had any solid figures, a major impetus in the reform of American abortion laws in the late 1960s and early 1970s was the alleged high prevalence of illegal abortions. The estimates ranged from 250,000 a year to well over a million, and that somewhat vague range was good enough to help the cause. No less prominent, then as now, was the conviction that the unwanted child faced bleak prospects, and various studies from Czechoslovakia and other European countries were produced to provide the requisite scientific backing. That those studies were methodologically flawed in serious ways, and actually offered some counterevidence, were easily overlooked imperfections. The other side, which we have now come to call the "pro-life" position, has been no less opportunistic in finding or alleging facts to support its position. Is it not true, as a matter of simple psychological observation, that the desire for abortion is motivated by gross selfishness? that the Nazi toleration of abortion for nonaryans was the opening wedge for euthanasia and the death camps? that many doctors and others stand to make a good pack of money from legal abortion?

Both sides, moreover, have engaged in playing out hypothetical empirical scenarios. The pro-choice side, stung by charges of hypocrisy in saying they are pro-choice rather than pro-abortion, has argued that if we can provide better sex education backed by better contraceptive services, then eventually abortion rates will decline. That this has rarely if ever happened in any real society is persistently overlooked, so strong is the faith. The left wing of the pro-life group has contended that, if women were provided with greater dignity and support in their childbearing and child rearing, then abortion would also decline. Yet, there is no credible evidence from any known society to substantiate either side's claim.

It is not my purpose in this paper, however, to examine the way the different sides in the abortion debate employ empirical evidence to support their convictions. I would only observe that both sides eagerly, even desperately, seek the support of scientific data; that both sides have been willing to rely upon, and to tout, even the weakest evidence; and that both sides, in imagining ideal solutions, project a future reality for which there is little empirical support. This does not lead me to conclude, as some might, that the issues are beyond reason and logic, or that the use of scientific data is mere rationalization on both sides. It only suggests that decisive data one way or the other are hard to come by, that all the pertinent evidence is filtered through the lens of values and moral convictions, and that both sides, well aware of the status of science, feel the necessity to enlist its high credence.

The Human Life Bill S. 158,[1] as well as the hostile responses to it, offers a fine case study in the uses of science for moral, social and legal purposes. Let me briefly summarize the nature and purpose of the proposed bill. It was introduced by Senator Jesse Helms (R-N.C.) in the 97th Congress in 1981 as a proposed amendment to Title 42 of the United States Code. Its formal title is: "A bill to provide that human life shall be deemed to exist from conception." The key passage in the bill comes at the very beginning: "The Congress finds that present day scientific evidence indicates a significant likelihood that actual human life exists from conception."[2] Senator John East (R-N.C.) a sponsor of the bill, stated clearly at the hearings on the bill just what its intended and presumed impact would be:

> As I understand this bill, we would attempt to define this question of life and whether it begins at the time of conception. If the determination would be that, yes, life does commence at the time of conception, then the effect of this bill would mean that the unborn child—the fetus—is protected as a person within the meaning of the due process clause of the Fourteenth Amendment, as are all other persons under the U.S. Constitution. . . . What would I think the practical effect of it would be? I presume it would be this: the *Roe v. Wade* decision of 1973 would be vitiated—negated—because in the majority

opinion of that case it was indicated that if person included the unborn, that their decision would no longer be operative, and hence, if person is so defined, by the view of the Court in its own majority opinion, *Roe v. Wade* would be vitiated. The issue would revert to the states. The states would then have the power to deal with the issue of abortion, as they had the power to do prior to *Roe v. Wade*.[3]

The testimonies for and against the bill at the hearings were instructive, particularly on the scientific question. For one group of scientists, the time of the beginning of human life is a well-established fact. According to Dr. Jerome Lejeune:

> To accept the fact that after fertilization has taken place a new human being has come into being is no longer a matter of taste or of opinion. The human nature of the human being from conception to old age is not a metaphysical contention, it is plain experimental evidence.[4]

Dr. Hymie Gordon testified:

> Now we can say, unequivocally, that the question of when life begins—is no longer a question for theological and philosophical dispute. It is an established fact. Theologians and philosophers may go on to debate the meaning of life or the purpose of life, but it is an established fact that all life, including human life, begins at the moment of conception.[5]

In her testimony, Dr. Micheline Mathews-Roth quoted from a large number of standard textbooks in embryology, biology and obstetrics, all of which contain passages in which the authors state that human life begins at conception.[6] She then concluded that "[I]t is scientifically correct to say that an individual human life begins at conception, when egg and sperm join to form the zygote, and that this developing human always is a member of our species in all stages of life."[7]

It was noteworthy that those scientists who spoke at the hearings in favor of the view that human life begins at conception did not directly address the nature or the wisdom of the proposed amendment. That was not the case with those who denied that science can resolve the problem of the beginning of life. Dr. Leon Rosenberg stated: "I know of no scientific evidence which bears on the question of when actual human life exists . . . the notion embodied in the phrase 'actual human life' is not a scientific one, but rather a philosophic and religious one."[8] Dr. Rosenberg then went on to argue that the implications of passing such a bill could lead to the prohibition of some contraceptives, and could also stop amniocentesis.[9] In his testimony, Dr. Lewis Thomas stated:

> The question as to when human life begins, and whether the very first single cell that comes into existence after fertilization of an ovum represents in itself

a human life, is not in any real sense a scientific question and cannot be answered by scientists. Whatever the answer, it can neither be verified nor proven false using today's scientific knowledge. It is, therefore, in my opinion in the domain of metaphysics. It can be argued by philosophers and theologians and perhaps settled, but it does lie beyond the reach of science.[10]

Dr. James Neel stated that "I can find no biological basis for saying at exactly what stage in development human personhood begins. The definition of that moment is a matter of religious conviction, philosophical inclination, or legal necessity."[11]

There is no reason to think that one or the other of the opposing scientists possesses stronger scientific credentials. How, then, can there be such fundamental disagreement? One might—all too readily—say that each side wants either to define the issue of when life begins, or to leave it resolutely undefined, in order to serve its own moral views on abortion. But that is not to say anything very illuminating. It could well be that their convictions on the scientific state of affairs are the basis for their moral views on abortion in the first place. It is an unhappy characteristic of the abortion debate that each side impugns the alleged motives, secret or otherwise, of those they oppose, and so I will not engage in that kind of analysis here. It seems to me to be inherently fruitless—a clear case of the *ad hominem* argument in action. Instead, let me turn to the question of whether the beginning of human life can be understood as a scientific question. In my own testimony, I argued that the issue is not scientific, and sided with the group of scientists who took a similar position.[12] I have now had some second thoughts on the matter, and would like to pursue it further.

NATURE OF THE SCIENTIFIC QUESTION

I believe there are three general questions that might be asked in this context. (1) What is a legitimate scientific question? (2) Does the fact that not all scientific questions can be answered with precision imply that the questions are not scientific? (3) Even if it is determined that a question is not scientific, strictly taken, does it therefore follow that scientific evidence is irrelevant in coming to a prudent moral or policy judgment?

Question 1: What is a legitimate scientific question? In *The Logic of Scientific Discovery*, Karl R. Popper writes that "A scientist, whether theorist or experimenter, puts forward statements, or systems of statements, and tests them step by step. In the field of the empirical sciences, more particularly, he constructs hypotheses, or systems of theories, and tests them against experience by observation and experiment."[13] This is a standard view of the scientific method. In the case of the beginning of human life, it was argued by one side in the hearings that there is no scientific hypothesis or theory that can be tested to answer the question; there is no way, to use Popper's phrase, of testing a concept of the beginning of human life "against experience by observation and experiment."

Such assertions are open to question. Is the problem that there is no way of giving the expression "the beginning of human life" an operational definition—that is, no way of formulating a testable empirical proposition about the characteristics of "human life" that could be confirmed or falsified? But surely it is possible to do that. We could simply formulate a proposition that human life begins at conception, or at some other empirically ascertainable point during gestation, and then seek to confirm or falsify the proposition by testing it against observational data. If it is objected that there is no consensus about how "human life" or "beginning" should be operationally defined, does that then prove that the question is not scientific? Not at all, for science constantly works with systematically ambiguous and disputed concepts, and they are not considered nonscientific simply because there is disagreement on what they might mean, or how meanings ought to be stipulated. The concepts of "temperature," "time," "space," and "species" provide good examples. A standard way of handling the problem of allegedly scientific concepts is to stipulate an operational definition, and then to test the validity of the definition by the devising of testable propositions—ones that can either be confirmed or falsified. The issue of "the beginning of human life" is perfectly amenable to that treatment.

That there are constant arguments among scientists about how best to define concepts does not thereby relegate those concepts to the realm of metaphysics or religion. Zoologists have fought for decades over the defining of criteria necessary for the inclusion of specific flora and fauna into one species or another. Medical researchers argue at times about whether a certain cluster of symptoms should be classified as a disease, e.g., "Legionnaire's Disease." Continental drift theorists squabble about what is to count as a "continent," just as they contend with each other about when it can be said, for example, that the North American continent actually "began." In short, the mere fact that scientists struggle with questions of definition, and frequently disagree with each other, is not taken as evidence that the issues are nonscientific. The questions of when "life" began on earth, or when "human life" began, have never been dismissed as nonscientific questions despite the endless debates about which criteria to accept in defining both concepts. Yet they pose questions as inherently difficult and debatable as that of the beginning of individual life.

"When does human life begin?" can therefore be understood as a perfectly appropriate scientific question. The fact that there are arguments about whether the key operational characteristics ought to be genetic, or morphological, or psychological, does not by itself prove the question to be anything other than scientific. To say that, however, is not to say that the question is only scientific. More appropriately, it can be said that scientific evidence is highly relevant; the issue is in part scientific but not exclusively so. The purposes to be served by the definition and the value-laden implications of different definitions are also pertinent considerations.

Question 2: Does the failure to achieve great precision imply that the question is not scientific? Science cannot tell us when, precisely, the universe began, when caterpillars become butterflies, or when acorns become oak trees. Yet I do not believe anyone would want to claim that these are metaphysical rather than scientific questions. There would, I suspect, be some considerable agreement that what we might want to count as the "beginning" of anything, whether the human species or caterpillars, would be a function of the way we define the term. But again, that is not a sufficient reason to say that the issue is nonscientific. That there will always be boundary questions—that is, questions about borderline cases—does not conceptually undermine the validity of the enterprise.

Question 3: Even if a question is not judged to be, strictly speaking, scientific, does it follow that scientific evidence is irrelevant in a prudent moral or policy judgment? Not at all. There are many cases in which we mix our moral or policy goals with scientific evidence to achieve reasonable judgments. The notion of "risk," for example, is a scientific concept based on the statistical probability of adverse outcomes. The notion of "acceptable risk," by contrast, is highly subjective, since people differ considerably in their willingness to gamble on adverse outcomes. Nonetheless, we consider it prudent public policy to put railings on the top of high places, warning labels on poisonous substances, and brakes on automobiles—despite the fact that some portion of the population might consider those acts an infringement of their liberty, or deny that there is much risk in the first place. In those cases, the known facts are consonant with our values. The debate over the definition of death has followed an analogous course. While there has been widespread agreement that "death" is in part a philosophical concept, it is no less widely agreed that scientific evidence is highly relevant in determining what organic conditions (or lack thereof) would satisfy a reasonable definition of human death.

The key to circumstances of that kind—where the "is" and the "ought," facts and values, are merged—is that in many situations there exist tacit, widely held value assumptions; e.g., that most people prefer to live rather than to die, that they would rather protect their health than harm it, and so on. The role of scientific evidence in those situations is the simple one of showing that certain states of affairs in the world pose a threat to those values.

In many situations, however, the relationship between values and facts is more problematic. In the case of nuclear energy, for instance, we may simultaneously want two valued goods: cheap energy on the one hand, and the protection of our health on the other. But there may be little, if any, social consensus about what the proper balance between those values ought to be. The problem is further complicated by disagreement concerning the relevant scientific data—for instance, on the health hazards of low level radiation, or about the probability of a major accident or melt-down at a nuclear energy plant. Given the uncertainty concerning the values at stake, and uncertainty also about the relevant data, it is hardly surprising that there is social disagreement. In such circumstances, the most we can do is hope that those arguing the issues will make clear their value premises or preferences and how they weigh them, and that they will make honest use of the data they believe pertinent to the problem, admitting where the evidence is doubtful and where it might even be contradictory to their policy preferences.

PROBLEMS WITH THE HUMAN LIFE BILL

The Human Life Bill and its effort to make use of scientific evidence is a more complicated case. I have argued, contrary to my earlier testimony and against that of many of the scientists who testified at the hearings, that the question of when human life begins is as legitimate a scientific question as many other controverted issues in science. I would similarly argue, for the logic is no different, that the question of when personhood begins could be construed as equally scientific.

But what are the implications of that statement for the abortion debate? Not very great. Even if we are prepared to agree that the question can be understood as scientific, we have not moved very far toward solving the moral, legal, or policy problems. At the hearings, some scientists seemed to fear that if they agreed the issue of when life begins is scientific, then inevitable moral implications would follow. That is not the case. At the very least, it would not solve the problem of determining when full ethical standing ought to be accorded the developing embryo or fetus. I will not pursue this issue here; instead, I will note some other problems with the bill.

First, the bill proposes to legislate one particular definition of the beginning of human life, that of the initiation of genetic individuality.

There are other contending definitions, and it is fair to say that science has not reached a consensus on which of the competing definitions is best or scientifically most fruitful. Given that scientific state of affairs, it surely short-circuits the course of scientific debate to pass legislation based on one of many possible definitions. Put another way, it is perfectly consistent to say that the question of when life begins is scientific, but that it is still an open question, and therefore it ought not to be decided by legislative fiat.

Second, it does not seem wise to put an issue of this kind, with all of its social and legal implications, up to a legislative vote. An obvious implication is that another legislature in another era could say that the scientific evidence has changed, that life really begins only at puberty and ends at about age 65.

Third, there is an additional important complication. The necessity for law and public policy in any organized society requires the passage of legislation that necessitates the drawing of lines. Who, for the sake of disability benefits, ought to be counted as "blind" or "mentally retarded" or, for the sake of voting rights, as a "juvenile" or an "adult"? Each of those concepts, which can be given a scientific, empirical meaning, is ambiguous and a subject of contention. Nevertheless, policy purposes require that we make some kind of decision. How is this usually done? A number of considerations go into the drawing of such lines. There must be some reasonable compatibility with scientific knowledge; that is, there must be an appeal to some observable phenomena. A decision must then be made about how narrow or generous we want to be, i.e., what values are we trying to protect or foster? The consequences of drawing the line at one point or another must also be weighed.

For example, we might believe that the blind have a right to our care and financial support. We must then draw upon some empirical evidence to decide who is to count as "blind." Ought it to be those who have no vision, not even a response to light? or those totally blind in one eye only? or those who can read only if they are no farther than one inch away from a text? or those who cannot see in bright sunlight? If we have unlimited funds at our disposal, we might feel free to adopt the broadest possible definition of blindness. If funds are tight, we might adopt stricter standards. In each case, of course, one could take advantage of the various disputes over how blindness ought scientifically to be defined in the first place. Moreover, in trying to evaluate the implications of different legal or policy definitions of blindness, the social consequences of adopting a particular definition will have to be considered—for instance, the possibility of an excessive demand upon medical care or of unnecessary stigmatization. In sum, the drawing of lines in the case of blindness will call upon scientific evidence, but will make use of that evidence in the context of various policy ideals, economic limitations, and assorted other social considerations.

In the case of defining human life, or personhood, we have a similar range of issues to consider. What values do we want to serve by our definition? The pro-life group, whose aim it is to stop abortion, wants as restrictive a definition as possible, one that will protect even the newly fertilized egg. The pro-choice group obviously prefers that the definitional issue be left open so that women can make up their own minds and, thus, obtain abortions if they desire. A number of those who testified against the bill pointed out that consequences of the proposed legislation might involve not only restrictions against abortion, but also the possibility of banning some forms of contraception. This would be one important, and deleterious, consequence of the bill.

Yet is should also be recognized that to leave the question up in the air is to open the way for mere expediency, as if any criteria for the beginning of human life can be used. An unfortunate characteristic of political debate in this country is that the terms "religious," "philosophical," or "moral" often serve as code words for "subjective" or "inherently undecidable." The still warm body of positivism, with its sundering of facts and values, lingers on in the assumption that if science can provide no decisive evidence on an issue, then the matter must be left to individual choice. Yet it is obvious from many other public debates involving both scientific and moral issues that reasonable policy decisions can (and often must) be made when there is uncertainty on both fronts.

CONCLUSION

It is not inherently outrageous, as many seem to think, that the pro-life group in America seeks to ground its moral views of abortion in one possible—and plausible—reading of the scientific data. The deeper question, for political purposes, is whether legislatures should decide to go with one reading of the evidence rather than another. I believe that would be a mistake. Unlike the regulation of nuclear energy plants or the control of pesticides in which some decision, however uncertain the evidence, is necessary to protect the public health, the case of abortion presents a far less clear picture. In the latter case, the debate over the scientific evidence is far more fundamental, just as is the debate over the social desirability of legislation to restrict abortion. Few would deny that some regulation of nuclear power plants is necessary. Most of the argument there turns on how strict the regulations should be; it is a matter of drawing a line on a continuum of safety rather than the drawing of lines altogether. It is just the opposite in abortion, although some analogies may be drawn in the sense that most would agree it is pertinent and permissible to draw a line for legislative purposes in the case of third trimester abortions.

Though I have argued that the question of when human life begins can be understood as a perfectly valid scientific question, I have also argued that this belief carries little significance for the abortion debate at present. That debate turns, in great part, on what would be wise legislation in the area. Given the fact that the scientific question of when life begins is still an open question, and given the various possible consequences of this proposal, I consider the Human Life Bill a bad piece of legislation.

I would not, however, conclude that because the question of the value to be attached to early life is philosophical in nature, one position is as good as another. If the issue is one that ought to be settled at the individual rather than the state level, as the pro-choice group (of which I count myself a member) contends, then it is necessary to discuss what qualifies as a sound moral argument at that level. By and large, the pro-choice group seems highly reluctant to explore this issue. They seem to believe that since the issue is a matter of individual conscience, no more can or should be said in public about appropriate criteria for individual moral decisions. This view serves only to lend credence to the suspicion of the pro-life forces that "pro-choice" really means "pro-abortion." The political credibility of the pro-choice side is strong; it can rest its arguments on solid social and political grounds. But it has yet to establish fully its moral credibility—something that will be possible only when it is prepared to contend with the question of what counts as a responsible and moral use of the freedom made possible by *Roe v. Wade*.[14]

NOTES

1. S. 158, 97th Cong., 1st Sess., 127 Cong. Rec. 287 (1981).
2. *Id.* §1.
3. *The Human Life Bill: Hearings on S. 158 Before the Subcommittee on Separation of Powers of the Senate Committee on the Judiciary*, 97 Cong., 1st Sess. 2 (1981) (statement of Sen. East, chairman) (Gov't Printing Office Serial No. J-97-16, Washington, D.C.) [hereinafter cited as *Hearings*]. *See also* Roe v. Wade, 410 U.S. 113 (1973).
4. *Hearings, supra* note 3, at 10.
5. *Id.* at 13.
6. *Id.* at 14-16.
7. *Id.* at 17.
8. *Id.* at 49.
9. *Id.* at 51.
10. *Id.* at 73.

11. *Id.* at 78. It is not clear why Dr. Neel used the language of "personhood" in his testimony since that was not directly the issue at the hearings.
12. *Id.* at 127-131.
13. K. R. POPPER, THE LOGIC OF SCIENTIFIC DISCOVERY (Hutchinson, London) (1968) at 27.
14. Roe v. Wade, 410 U.S. 113 (1973).

Audience Discussion

Margery W. Shaw, Moderator

MARGERY SHAW: Dr. Rosenberg, do you have a response to Dr. Callahan's presentation?

LEON E. ROSENBERG (Conference Faculty): I think I would most like to remember what Dr. Callahan said last, namely, that because we say that something should be left to an individual's choice does not mean that we should fail to inquire about how such choices are made. I think this is a very appropriate place for the dialogue to continue. The whole matter of when life begins, it seems to me, carries us back beyond the beginning of our conference and gets us nowhere. Preoccupation with that very complex question has served only to make it impossible to debate the legal and political issues on any common ground.

K.C. SULLIVAN, M.D. (Southwest Women's Center, Houston, Texas): I was a medical officer in World War II for four years and had ample chance to see many of the atrocities carried out by the Germans. I might note that prestigious German doctors, many of them from universities, were dispatching many of the handicapped people before the Holocaust started. This was a eugenic abortion policy. My question is this: if we all are concerned for quality of life rather than sanctity of life, how can we be assured that the same set of circumstances will not happen in this country?

DANIEL CALLAHAN (Conference Faculty): I don't think we can ever have any assurance that it won't happen in this country. Yet, I suspect that for any moral debate one can conduct on any subject, one can find some terrible earlier precedent. Nonetheless, I do not believe, for example, that we ought to halt research in genetic engineering simply because we have experienced the misuse of genetic knowledge by the Nazis and by the early eugenics movement. There is no way of having a foolproof moral system— one that may not lead to some potential corruption. I think our task, though, is to see that that does not happen and do our best to make certain that corruption does not reappear. But, I can give no guarantee that it won't.

ROBERT M. FINEMAN, M.D., PH.D. (University of Utah Medical Center, Salt Lake City, Utah): I tend to agree with Dr. Rosenberg's statement to the Senate Subcommittee concerning life and when it begins. I disagree with Dr. Callahan's statement this morning that the answer to the question of when life begins is within the realm of science. I think that an individual's religious beliefs, whether he or she is a scientist or not, greatly influences that person's thoughts as to when life begins. At this time, I do not think the United States Congress will ever have sufficient information to determine when life begins.

DANIEL CALLAHAN: There is a great difference between what counts as a scientific statement, and what counts as true religion. They are totally separable questions and should not be confused.

UNIDENTIFIED PARTICIPANT: It was very interesting to me that Dr. Rosenberg, in his last comment, decried the deception that is often associated with this debate. Dr. Rosenberg implied that only the most severely defective children, such as trisomy-18 and Tay-Sachs, are now being destroyed by abortion after genetic screening. Is it not true that more Down syndrome children are aborted as a result of amniocentesis than both trisomy-18 and Tay-Sachs combined? The deception that is achieved by referring to only the most heinous handicaps cannot long endure in a free society. Until geneticists are willing and able to prevent the eugenic elimination of mongoloids, XYYs, cleft palates and even XX females, they will continue to come under the wrath of those who seek justice for all people, not just those who fit into the elitist concoction of genetic perfection.

LEON ROSENBERG: In no way did I mean to indicate that trisomy-18 and Tay-Sachs disease were the only genetic reasons for which therapeutic abortions are done. The statement that more abortions are carried out for Down syndrome than trisomy-18 or Tay-sachs disease is unquestionably correct. I think that is where the questioner and I would part company in terms of a legitimate dialogue.

ANNE E. BANNON, M.D. (Doctors For Life, St. Louis, Missouri): Dr. Rosenberg made the statement that some fear that a society that permits feticide now will permit infanticide later. I may be misjudging your statement, but it seemed to me that you implied that this is an insubstantial fear. For someone from Yale, you must be aware that your colleagues allowed 40 to 50 defective children to die without treatment. I think that is a little less than honest. Perhaps you will comment on that. The other question: is there a possibility that if you removed the haploid nucleus from an egg and inserted a diploid nucleus from the husband's somatic cell you would be able to produce a viable child?

LEON ROSENBERG: Let me try to answer only the last question. Studies in amphibian species would suggest that the experiment described would reconstitute a diploid organism. That was not what I was talking about. I was talking about maintaining the kind of reproduction that we practice as humans, that is, in which a haploid ovum is combined with a haploid sperm.

ANNE BANNON: If that were a possibility, then you would have a child of both parents in one sense, even though the genetic material would be only from one.

LEON ROSENBERG: I think that that is a formal possibility, but I carefully refrain from talking about cloning people, because I find that picture repugnant on all kinds of moral and ethical grounds.

ANNE BANNON: Dr. Callahan, you said that the free choice should be left to women. Do you really feel that a choice is free if the basic issue as to whether or not you have at least a biological human being at conception is clouded by rhetoric?

DANIEL CALLAHAN: Well, I suppose you could say that any issue that is clouded by rhetoric is not a free issue. But, that seems to be the case with most debates and most things in our society. When one gets into the political arena, rhetoric rules the day. I would suggest, however, that it is possible to cut through some of the rhetoric and try to deal with the more substantive issues. Then, I think one might make a free choice. Free choices are very difficult under the best of circumstances on most issues.

UNIDENTIFIED PARTICIPANT: Dr. Callahan, you seem to imply that the public policy questions with regard to the definition of blindness should be determined with regard to the resources and the consequences of the definition and I wondered if there was anything else you wanted to include or if those were the only two determinants that you think are overriding when we come to public policy questions. Also, I have another question. You stated that you feel that the question of when human life begins is an open question, and I wonder if there isn't any line that you would be willing to draw rather than just saying it's an open question.

DANIEL CALLAHAN: On the first question, there are various arguments about what constitutes blindness—from total lack of vision to some degree of impairment. There is a continuum. People in that field argue about how one ought to define the term. For public policy purposes, if one is increasing funds, or cutting funds, one could probably find some set of experts who would have a set of criteria that would play into the hands of one side or another. That goes on in lots of other fields. In the area of mental retardation, for example, who would we want to count as retarded? There is a continuum from the severely retarded to the mildly retarded and there are debates among experts about where you draw the line. That seems a characteristic of many scientific policy debates, and in fact, we do make decisions whereby one side often wins or loses, based on the appropriation and use of scientific data that is helpful to their cause. On the question of where I would draw the line on the beginning of human life, I suppose I am most attracted to the notion of drawing the line at the beginning of electrical activity in the brain. At that point, there is more fully developed potential for rationality and self-consciousness. I argued some years ago that the line ought to be drawn somewhere, probably in the vicinity of 8 to 12 weeks.

LEON ROSENBERG: I was asked where I would draw the line. I think that the temporal moment with which I feel most comfortable is when a baby can exist independently outside the uterus of the mother.

BENT G. BOVING, M.D. (C.S. Mott Center for Human Growth and Development, Wayne State University, Detroit): I appreciate Dr. Callahan's earlier point, the fact that a question has not yet been answered scientifically is not a criterion for judging whether it can be answered scientifically. His examples included when human life begins and when personhood begins. I suggest that these two questions are distinct and that the first is unanswerable, whereas the second can be answered exactly.

"When does human life begin?" is unanswerable not for lack of knowledge but because, in the present tense, it is an illogical question. Life began in the distant past and is propagated through the process of reproduction during which it is transmitted but does not begin. Therefore, asking "when" it begins is nonsense. The other aspect of the question, "When does the humanness of human life begin?" is fallacious for the same reason. (The pertinent and secure scientific facts are that human life is not propagated unless the spermatozoon and ovum that merge during fertilization are both alive and human before they meet, and before they become mature sex cells, and before sex cells develop from unspecialized cells, and before these derive from the respective parental zygotes—and so on back through preceding generations.)

"When does personhood begin?" can be answered scientifically if one accepts the standard definition: a person is a human individual. Unfortunately, most attempts to answer the question have considered only the human part of that definition. The error is not obvious, but it is fundamental. Since humanness of human life is a continuum just as the life is, it has no beginning to mark when personhood begins. More obvious is the mistake of purporting to mark the beginning of humanness by one or another single human characteristic (chromosome number, heartbeat or reflex kick). This approach has been stretched to include a variety of psychological and social characteristics even if they are of doubtful concern to a fetus (smiles, love, and an income tax deduction). Nevertheless, the one-criterion approach has the glaring fault of giving a different answer for each criterion and, therefore, no general answer. It also has the subtle but serious defect of implying nonhumanness when only one criterion is missing (abnormal chromosome number, abnormal heartbeat, paralysis or a government with no income tax). Let's face it, we have become trapped by fuzzy thinking, emotion, euphemism and cliché; we accept the concept that every person has "a" human life, his very own— discrete from the life of all other living things. If we stretch our minds a bit, using that ecological or "communitarian" viewpoint that was dawning among us yesterday, we may be able to recognize that we have something backwards. Life is something we are a part of, and instead of individuals having life, life has individuals. Life is a continuum, but individuals are discrete, and that means that we can define the beginning of personhood if we can answer the question, "When does the individual begin?"

An individual (Latin *in* = not, *dividuus* = divisible) is defined as an indivisible single entity. A human zygote or fertilized egg is not indivisible; on the contrary, it must divide if development is to continue. Therefore, a human zygote cannot be considered to be a human individual or person. Consider twins. If every human zygote were considered to be a person, then each monozygotic twin would have to be considered a half person. That seems unacceptable. Monozygotic twinning can begin as late as 16 days after fertilization. Might personhood be said to start then? No. There is a still later major division, and it is required of all conceptuses. Here I must mention that, in this meeting, the term "conceptus" has been incorrectly used as a synonym for fetus. A conceptus is everything derived from a zygote from fertilization until birth; it specifically includes two major components, the embryoblast and the trophoblast. The trophoblast forms the placenta and extra-embryonic membranes; the embryoblast forms the embryo, which develops into the fetus or unborn offspring. The two major components of the conceptus are associated during intrauterine life but are separated just after birth. That final division of the conceptus, usually by cutting the cord, frees the newborn baby from the placenta, which dies. Since the baby undergoes no subsequent divisions, it is thenceforth an indivisible single entity, an individual and person. Scientific facts, concise definitions and careful reasoning show that the beginning of personhood is marked by severance of the umbilical cord.

MARGERY SHAW: Thank you for your comments. Your last example is one concept that had not been brought up at this meeting previously.

M. SIMONE ROACH, R.N., PH.D. (Associate Professor of Nursing, St. Francis Xavier University, Antigonish, Nova Scotia): Yesterday someone made the point that we do not seem to be getting anywhere by trying to define person. Instead, what is at stake is a conflict involving fundamental concepts and values. My question is whether or not we ought to address these specific conflicts face-on. It has been held, for example, that one of the very foundation stones of our system of law and ethics in western society is the sanctity-of-life principle. It is sometimes asserted, however, that this principle is no longer a valid one in a society where secularistic humanism prevails and, specifically, that this principle is incompatible with quality-of-life considerations. I hold that the sanctity-of-life principle is not incompatible with quality-of-life considerations. I suggest that, where incompatibility is claimed, it is so because of a particular vitalistic interpretation of the sanctity-of-life principle which I do not perceive to be consistent with the root meaning of that principle. For a future symposium, there may be some merit in engaging scientists, philosophers, theologians, and professionals in dialogue, examining the significance of the sanctity-of-life principle to the issues we are dealing with, and the implications for our society of the erosion and/or denial of that principle.

MARGERY SHAW: We considered inviting some theologians to speak at this symposium but decided against it for two reasons. First, several other symposia have already been held addressing the topic from a religious viewpoint (Notre Dame University, St. Louis University, and University of Missouri at Columbia). Secondly, we would need to add another day or half-day to include representatives from among Catholic, Protestant, Jewish (orthodox, conservative, and reformed) and non-Judeo-Christian religions.

JAY L. GARFIELD (Hampshire College, Amherst, Massachusetts): Professor Callahan, you very carefully distinguished the concepts of risk and acceptable risk, pointing out that one of those was scientific and one of those was not. You did not carefully distinguish the concepts of *human* life and human *life*. This distinction is a critical one, for you wish to argue that scientific evidence regarding the onset of human life will yield decisive moral conclusions concerning the permissibility of abortion. But to bridge the fact-value gap, you equivocate on "human." There is the sense of the adjective, human, in which the natural contrast would be, say, nonhuman.

There is also the sense of the word human in which one of the natural contrasts, anyway, would be, say, inhuman or subhuman. It is clear that we have got a scientific issue in the first case. It may not be clear which scientific issue, an embryological issue, a genetic issue, an ecological issue, etc. But it seems equally clear, doesn't it, that given the second understanding of the word, human, that we have got on our hands a moral issue, or at least a metaphysical issue. And that question, while scientific evidence might be relevant in its solution, hardly seems to be the same scientific question. It also seems clear that while scientific evidence is relevant to the solution of the second question, it can hardly be dispositive in the way that it can be with respect to the first question. Could you respond to that?

DANIEL CALLAHAN: I absolutely agree on that. First, when we use a term like inhuman, that is really quite a different realm of discourse. It is a kind of metaphorical way of talking about something that we consider evil, something that violates some underlying essence of what it is to respect human beings.

DIANA ROSENBERG (J.D. Candidate): I would like to address this question to Dr. Rosenberg, in the interest of adding a little spice to our family harmony. You state in your talk that the present and likely future of genetic procedures will and do have a vast impact on humanity and health care. With the likelihood that such impact will occur and conceding possible dangers, who do you suggest place the controls on genetics?

LEON ROSENBERG: This is a very unique situation for me. I have been asked many questions by many people. I have been asked many questions by my daughter before, but never when I was on the podium and when she was in the audience at a scientific meeting. Diana, I think that genetics is not a private field for the geneticist. It is quite clear that what geneticists are going to be allowed to do in our society is going to be determined by society itself. I believe that the importance of indicating where the field is going is to allow that kind of dialogue to begin. I do not share with Dr. Callahan the view that we are the toughest kids on the block. In fact, I have never heard that appraisal before. His appraisal does, however, indicate the genesis of a number of other things that he conveyed in his remarks. In my view, science is no more the final determinant in society's use of scientific information than any of the other vantage points that have been presented during the last two days. Nor should it be.

LEWIS H. KOPLIK, M.D. (La Mesa Medical Center, Albuquerque, New Mexico): Dr. Callahan, when one considers other animal species, there are other modes of reproduction that do not involve fertilization—asexual modes. Might we learn something about human life by examining them? My question is what function does fertilization serve in the development of the individual human being?

DANIEL CALLAHAN: The primary function of genetic recombination in sexual reproduction is to establish a new genetic individuality.

LEWIS KOPLIK: But in the establishment of new life, is that essential?

DANIEL CALLAHAN: In the case of clones, there are some interesting questions, given the interaction of genetics and environment. Whether and if an individual occurs is not merely a genetic matter, but also a function of the way genes interact with the environment. That is where you get uniqueness. A clone could thus have a potential for individuality different from a similar clone. Two human clones would not necessarily be utterly identical to each other.

LEON ROSENBERG: In a formal sense, cloning an individual would in no way insure that that clone would develop in a fashion identical to the individual from whom the cell was originally obtained. That says that environment is a profoundly important determinant upon which the blueprint of genetics is played. But I don't know how that helps you answer the question you asked.

JOHN C. FLETCHER, PH.D. (National Institute of Health, Bethesda, Maryland): I would like to address a question to the entire panel based on Dr. Rosenberg's imagining a future possibility of beginning treatment for the newly fertilized embryo at risk for a genetic disorder such as thalassemia. Only suppose that enough scientific and animal work were done to make this a plausible step, I can imagine an institutional review board facing the question of what kind of respect, if any, we owe to a newly fertilized embryo following the failure of DNA insertion. That is, the scientist or the physician realizes that he or she has done the gene insertion improperly and there is no point in implanting the embryo in the mother. The generic question is what kind of respect, if any, is owed? How are we to feel towards a newly fertilized embryo who is a candidate for the beginning of gene therapy, but it doesn't work?

LEON ROSENBERG: I have no answer, John. I think that question, like so many others we have been asking, is in reality a multitude of questions. The person who tried to do the in vitro fertilization or gene replacement would feel bad because it was an experiment that hadn't worked. The fact that it was being done with human cells in the hope of providing human cure would certainly heighten the sense of failure that would come from such an experiment. But, when we carry the matter further and ask what should be done with such a failed experiment in terms of death rights, or burial, or whatever, we get into other kinds of complicated issues.

Chapter 17

Panel Discussion—
Legislating Morality:
Should Life Be Defined?

Panelists: Daniel Callahan, Clifford Grobstein,
Leon E. Rosenberg, Daniel Wikler

Margery W. Shaw, Moderator

MARGERY SHAW: The legislatures in this country have a rather sad record
of passing statutes that can be construed as legislating moral behavior and
later finding their statutes to be held unconstitutional by the Supreme
Court. Examples include legislation regarding pornography and the use
of contraceptives. On the other hand, laws banning polygamy and pros-
titution have been upheld. Our subject for the panel is whether the U.S.
Congress or any other legislative body should define human life as a
means to ban abortion. Should morality be legislated?

DANIEL CALLAHAN: On your general question—whether morality ought
to be legislated—my simple answer is, yes, of course. We do it all the time
and the real issue is deciding which morality we ought to legislate. I take it
that our laws against murder, stealing, rape, etc. embody moral points of
view and they are not merely regulatory principles. In fact, most of the law
rests on some moral foundation, so in that sense I see no problem with
regulating morality. The prudential problems are, first of all, how important is it to the common welfare that certain moral values or moral
convictions be imposed on a community? Second, there is a practical
problem of whether one can successfully legislate the morality. That is a
major problem with the abortion debate—I don't think either side can win
since the population is so strongly divided. On the specific question of
whether there ought to be a legislative definition of the beginning of life, I
have already given my answer to that in my earlier presentation—no. The
question has not been satisfactorily resolved at the scientific and philo-

sophical level. To legislate any one definition at present would be more or less arbitrarily to pick one from among a range of competing possibilities and that would not seem to me justified or wise.

CLIFFORD GROBSTEIN: I agree with much of what Dan Callahan has said but I would like to expand a bit on a couple of points. We are asked to consider "Legislating Morality: Should Life Be Defined?" I take this to mean: should legislatures define life in the interests of morality? Biologists have given a great deal of thought to defining life and appear to have become less and less enthusiastic about all-encompassing definitions. The reason is that reducing the enormous diversity of life forms, with all their complexity, interactions and beauty, to a neat and tidy commonality impoverishes the whole concept of the living world. In the specific form in which the matter has been broached in the United States Congress—defining the beginning of human life—there are comparable difficulties. Scientifically, we cannot really talk about human life beginning except in an evolutionary sense. Since human life came into existence, by whatever definition, it has persisted, it has been continuous from generation to generation. Neither the definition of life, nor of human life, is really the issue that legislatures are equipped to grapple with. They can only take cognizance of what our best knowledge reveals about the matter.

What I would like to emphasize are the important differences among a number of terms that tend to be loosely interchanged in common parlance—life, human life, individual and person. Biologically, these are interrelated but hardly equal. The nature and origin of life is entirely a scientific question in terms of objective knowledge—primarily biological. The nature and origin of human life is also a scientific question, with important biological, anthropological, sociological, legal, and religious aspects. The nature and origin of a human individual or being has the comparable range of aspects but with a significant shift of emphasis from the scientific toward the normative end of the range. That this shift raises difficulties for scientific perspectives does not mean that they can be ignored. Finally, in considering the definition of person the emphasis is very heavily at the normative end. Although there is a relevant scientific substrate, its application depends on the context and purpose of the definition to be formulated. It does not seem sound for a legislature to seek to resolve a conflict of purpose and morality by imposing an arbitrary and dubious biological definition.

MARGERY SHAW: I agree with you, Dr. Grobstein, and I think some of the lawyers who spoke to us yesterday would also agree. They pointed out that a global definition of person is not very helpful, but that if one wanted to make different definitions of persons for different legal purposes, such as for taxes, censuses, estates, corporations, etc., then the definitions could be very helpful. It is important to determine the legislative intent. Otherwise, one legal definition of "person" may be incorrectly applied in a different context.

DANIEL WIKLER: We have spoken of the different notions of a person, one being individual Homo sapiens or individual human. And then distinct from that, something which is either a moral or a psychological or some other kind of entity which may not be the same as individual human being. I think it is important to note, if only for courtesy, that the right-to-life position is that the individual human being is the relevant concept—that once you have an individual human being, this entity is deserving of good treatment and protection. So I think that a right-to-life advocate might be willing to admit that you can use the word person to refer to a conscious, rational being, or to something with awareness, but that it really doesn't matter whether you do so or not, because the moral issue is already settled once you have answered the biological question. Once you have established that there is an individual human being, you know who it is that you are supposed to protect and who it is that you are not supposed to kill. So in that sense, if that is a biological question, it seems to me there is an internal logic in this position that says: "Let's ask the scientist when you become an individual human being." Dr. Grobstein says that is a scientific question. And, once we get the data from the scientist we have supported our position scientifically. Now what is, perhaps, a question of external logic is whether or not this particular belief (namely, that individual human beings are the ones who deserve this kind of protection and respect and so on) is correct, whether it is binding on others, etc. And that, of course, is not established scientifically; it can't be. That's a moral question. So, there is a kind of scientific question in there, but there's an external question which is not scientific. And, I think what that says is that some of the rhetoric that surrounded the human life statute in the press and elsewhere was half-right and half-wrong. Scientific data may be relevant to one of the questions but clearly the question of whether Congress should enact a statute is not one that can be answered by scientists qua scientists. To that extent the human life statute and the human life amendment are tactics in a larger, moral crusade and it may be a distraction, actually, to argue endlessly as to what a person is and whether or not science supports the notion of person in the way that advocates of these measures have insisted. We are looking at a skirmish in a much larger battle, and we ought not lose sight of the larger forces arrayed and what they're ultimately trying to do.

I want to dissent for a moment from what Dan Callahan has said about legal moralism, about legislating morality. It's maybe an elaboration rather than a dissent. Legislating morality is itself, I think, a prescriptive term. It's hurled by one side at another when you want to make the other side look like they are doing something they shouldn't do. What lies behind this, I think, is a certain philosophy of government, which is sort of part of the typical American view, that the government should not tell people what kind of character to develop, what kinds of personal standards they should set. It should stay out of the business of legislating morality where we are conceiving of morality as behavior that does not involve victims. So the government should stay out of sexual behavior, it should stay out of questions about when to have a child, let's say, and a host of other questions. This is part of the standard, liberal philosophy of government. At the same time almost everybody recognizes that the government has an important role in protecting abused minorities. And there are many who count themselves on the pro-choice side who got involved in skirmishes over civil rights because the government was not protecting minorities, and they may have suffered personal injury in doing so. So, there may actually be a common philosophy of government to the two sides. Both sides would maintain, or could maintain with all consistency, that the government must not engage in legal moralism. They shouldn't legislate morality in the sense of telling people what a good life consists of, or what personal moral standards they should have. At the same time, both sides can agree that the government must—not only should or can—but must intervene to protect abused minorities from such threats as murder or killing. So, if both sides share these views I don't think it's fair for the pro-choice side to accuse the pro-life side of being intolerant. The principles upon which the pro-life side argues and the motivation they have for trying to change public policy in their direction are principles which I think implicitly have total assent from all sides.

The real question is whether or not the fetus is a being which ought to be protected in the way that the government ought to protect other disadvantaged and imperiled minorities. And, of course, it's here that there is a total divergence of opinion. If you, as pro-choice people, were as convinced as pro-life people are that fetuses deserve protection, I wouldn't be surprised to see you using pressure tactics on Congress. Compared to the things that were done to end slavery or the things that were done in the civil rights crusades, what we see in Congress, with a minority trying to get the rest of the country to obey their views, is mild. And that's why I think that ultimately the question of whether the fetus is something that ought to be protected really is the question. I think there is or can be agreement on the other questions. It's this fundamental thing that causes people not only to differ over what a woman should do about abortion, but also to define the social problem as either being on the one hand legal moralism, or on the other protection of minorities, and this dictates whether or not majority opinion should rule and a whole host of other questions that make this issue seem so intractable.

DANIEL CALLAHAN: One of my own motivations in trying to make a distinction between "human being" and "person" was perhaps my desire for an outcome that would allow women to have abortions. Hence I said to myself: "My gosh, if this kind of distinction is not possible, we can't have abortions. Therefore, let's see if I can make another move that will give me the kind of outcome I want." Was that rationalization a clever way of evading the moral issue? Well, I think that's possible, and that is the kind of thing one has to worry about morally with oneself. Was I evading the issues by trying to distinguish my way out of them? I don't know, but it seems to me in many cases we are allowed to distinguish our way out of some problems, and the question is at what point does that become an illegitimate process? I would hope that others might also be candid about the way they morally use distinctions. I have given you my candid statement of what I think may have been going on morally with me.

Let me follow up a bit on Dan Wikler's comment. I think the argument about legislating morality has in great part been an argument about what ought to remain in the private sphere and not be subject to governmental regulation. I'm struck by the fact that this debate has occurred over and over in the history of our country. What is considered "private" in one case can be seen as "public" in another—e.g., pornography. One now finds feminists, for instance, saying that these so-called private matters between consenting adults have important public consequences and pornography should be put back into the public realm. There is the question of how many children one ought to bear. The family planning movement said that ought to be a personal and private decision. In the next stage, however, along came great concern about population growth and the population explosion. Everybody said, "My God, all of these private decisions add up to important social consequences that ought *not* to be left as a matter of private decision making." I have very serious doubts about whether one can validly draw a distinction between the private and the public sphere. I simply believe that our private behaviors almost always have public consequences and that the distinction may be artificial.

MARGERY SHAW: I know this has been discussed in detail in the context of suicide. One might argue that there is a "private" right to commit suicide unless one hurts a third party. But since all of us are connected in the human community and we all have an effect on others, then suicide is a social problem as well as an individual decision.

I'm afraid that time is slipping away too rapidly and we want to leave some time for audience discussion of this important subject. Then we will close the symposium with some concluding remarks by Dr. Bentley Glass. Thank you, panel members, for your thoughtful comments.

Audience Discussion

Margery W. Shaw, Moderator

MARGERY SHAW (Conference Faculty): Dr. Grobstein began a line of thought on definitions. He talked about life and human life and human individual and he made a plea for continuing to struggle with the definition of person. Father Albert Moraczewski has discussed this subject with me in the past and we have invited him to discuss it with the audience at this time.

ALBERT MORACZEWSKI, O.P., PH.D. (Pope John XXIII Medical-Moral Research and Education Center, St. Louis, Missouri): When engaged in an interdisciplinary dialogue about personhood, we would be wise to make clear an important distinction in regard to the use of the term person. During the last two days I was listening to the way that different speakers and participants used that term. It soon became obvious that the word was not being used univocally, but analogically, so that the word conveyed different meanings for different speakers and to different listeners. Consequently, while we were assuming that we were talking about the same subject, in reality we were not; we were using the term to refer to different, even if related, realities.

I think it should be made explicit that the term person may legitimately refer to a variety of entities. For example, one can speak about a person in the legal sense—a "legal person." Our Constitution and laws generally refer to the legal concept of personhood. One result is to recognize and give the individual human certain rights: the right to vote, the right to hold public office, the right to make contracts, etc. Those would be examples of the "legal person," and this is often the sense in which the term is used in current public discussion.

Another use of the term person mentioned in our discussions here is "moral person," such as a corporation or other legally recognized entity. Ordinarily, it is a collection of individual human beings which meet certain criteria. Society agrees that the group has certain privileges and responsibilities. The reality of such a moral person is constituted by a societal fiat.

The "psychological person," or the phenomenological aspects of personhood, represents a third way in which the term person is used. In the discussions of this meeting, that usage is probably the most frequent. I think that Joseph Fletcher's "Indicators of Humanhood" represents an essay to define operationally the meaning of personhood in this sense, the psychological person: e.g., minimal IQ of 20, self-awareness, capacity to relate to others, etc. This is to look at the human person in his or her observable, measurable dimensions.

Finally, I would propose another use of the term person—the "ontological person," which is really the substrate for, and presupposed by, these other aspects of personhood. This is the human being at its very roots. Without it there would be no legal, moral or psychological aspects of personhood, but the converse is not necessarily true. Many persons find it very difficult to accept the existence of this ontological person, or to separate it, conceptually at least, from the phenomenological aspects of personhood. One reason, of course, is that personhood at the early stages of development does not lend itself to the kind of observations and measurements ordinarily used for born individuals. Yet, the existence of this ontological person is not entirely unobservable. The basic requirement is an organism—even the newly constituted one-cell human zygote—with the appropriate set of human chromosomes. Proof of the humanness of such a being is that unless prevented by genetic disorders, disease or accident, the inconspicuous, biologically microscopic person will ineluctably develop into an adult human person with the characteristic and unique properties of Homo sapiens. Now, the pro-life people, of which I am one, are talking basically about this ontological person which is rooted in the very biological being.

Dr. Grobstein mentioned in his lecture that the person has both a biological component and something beyond. I think that is true. There is that aspect of person which is biological. It is found in those biological entities that belong to a particular species, namely, Homo sapiens. But there is another component which, for want of a better term, is spiritual, nonmaterial. That component is the human spirit and is ultimately responsible for those activities which are distinctively human and which set us apart from other primates, e.g., the ability to communicate by means of a syntactical language, to develop mathematical theories, to think historically and futuristically, to form abstract concepts such as entropy, justice, etc.

Those abilities may not be always exercisable, such as during sleep or coma, or they may not yet be expressed because the relevant biological systems may not yet be at the appropriate developmental stage. Yet primates who genetically are very close to the human nonetheless lack this requisite spiritual component of personhood since even in the adult stage they are totally incapable of the distinctive human activities mentioned above. It is well to note here that neither the material component alone nor the spirit alone constitutes the person. But in the unique fusion/blend found in all members of Homo sapiens, they constitute the one existing being, the human person.

Subsequent to that ontological person are perhaps a legal person, a psychological person, and a moral person, but those are secondary terms and depend for their being on the first. As a consequence, what one often finds in discussions is that one group is really talking about psychological or legal personhood while the other group is talking about ontological personhood. Hence, when Professor Wikler raises the question, "Should the fetus be protected?" or, "Why should it be protected?" we are in the arena of values. But is the value of the right to life, for example, based on personhood in the legal sense? Is the right to life a value which society confers on a human individual? Or, is the right to life something which antecedes such a conferring and is rooted in the ontological person? Is it, as it were, standard equipment for all human beings? That perhaps, is the question, but there is no time now to discuss it any further except to assert that this is the position I hold.

I propose, then, that such a clarification regarding different uses of the term person might help to focus the issue and reduce, to some extent, the unnecessary acrimony which results because the conflicting groups are actually talking about different things even though the same word is used.

MARGERY SHAW: Dr. Grobstein, would you like to respond?

CLIFFORD GROBSTEIN (Conference Faculty): Well, I have a question. May I ask you, Father Moraczewski, when you refer to the ontological person, which you see as the substrate for the several others, do you conceive of that ontological person as having an ontogeny?

ALBERT MORACZEWSKI: Person in the ontological sense begins at a time when a new individual human diploid organism is constituted. The matter of continuity was raised, namely, that all life is a continuity from its inception on earth 3½ billion years ago. To a certain extent it is, but nonetheless, there is a discreteness or discontinuity at the time of fertilization when a new genetic individual organism has been constituted. I think that was one of the points made earlier at this meeting, that because of the fusion of the pronuclei of the male and female gametes there is, once that event has taken place, a new individual with a unique set of chromosomes.

A new biological entity has appeared and should that biological entity be a member of Homo sapiens, simultaneously a new human person (in the ontological sense, at least) is present. This begins the process of human development which proceeds until death. But it begins with an individual who had not existed before.

CLIFFORD GROBSTEIN: But that new genetic individuality, genome, or whatever you want to call it, which is established at that time, has with respect to all other matters, as we understand it scientifically, then an ontogeny before the characteristics of the fully developed organism appear. And my question is whether you distinguish person at the ontological level, which would have its initiation conceivably at the moment the genome is established. Is there, then, an ontogeny comparable to what happens with a limb, a head, or any other feature of that developing organism, or does it appear at the moment that that ontological person appears in toto and has no ontogeny?

ALBERT MORACZEWSKI: In its essence, person in the ontological sense is an all-or-none event, even though there is an ontogeny for its expression or manifestation. There is a gradual unfolding which is reflected by the biological development which takes place as further cell division and differentiation proceeds. But it is not, as such, a development of the ontological person. There is a development of its expression—eventually the psychological or phenomenological person is such an expression—but it is an all-or-none phenomenon at its very root. In other words, an individual is no more a person (in the ontological sense) as an adult than as a four-year-old, than as a fetus. But the observable and measurable manifestations of that person do develop just as the biological expression undergoes increasing complexity. My point is that the right to life is attached to that ontological person, and consequently the right to life is not a graded one; either the individual has it in full or he does not have it at all. It is an all-or-nothing phenomenon.

LEON ROSENBERG (Conference Faculty): Could I ask, if the right to life is as fundamental a right in a biological sense as you describe, why is it that it was discovered in a legislative or congressional sense in 1981?

ALBERT MORACZEWSKI: Well, I think what is of concern here is the principle of subsidiarity. In other words, individual rights are exercised and protected at the lowest possible organizational level. If a local jurisdiction is not able adequately to protect a right, then a higher jurisdiction has to step in. If the private sector is not able to protect a basic right, then the government needs to intervene. In the case of the right to life, our nation from its infancy recognized it, as is witnessed by the Declaration of Independence which asserts that all men are endowed by the Creator with certain unalienable rights such as the right to life. Clearly, as seen by the signatories this right was not conferred by court or legislative action but came from the Creator who had given life to each individual human. When that right has become so massively violated for the unborn human being, then the highest level of government needs to protect it through the provisions provided in its laws. That is what I see going on now; an effort is being made to protect that right by legislative means legitimately available to the people.

MARGERY SHAW: Thank you, Dr. Moraczewski. There are several comments that have been written down and passed forward to the panelists. The first one reads: "How can you talk about two "sides" (and by that I am sure the writer means pro-choice and right-to-life) whan A is trying to coerce B and force B to act according to A's norms, but B is seeking only to be let alone?"

DANIEL WIKLER (Conference Faculty): Well, we have discussed that several times. For example, slave owners could insist that they be let alone and so could civil rights abusers, but another group stood up and said, it doesn't matter what your conscience tells you. It doesn't matter whether you think blacks are people—the government has a legitimate role in protecting abused minorities and blacks happen to be one. So, if you accept that, and you can let your imagination stretch to the point where you can really imagine the fetus as being a person just the way you probably think of adult blacks and Indians as people, then this shouldn't be a question that's beyond answering.

MARGERY SHAW: Here is a question for Dr. Rosenberg. "Would Dr. Rosenberg comment on the recent British study which indicates that ingestion of folic acid prior to, and during very early pregnancy, dramatically reduces the incidence of neural tube defects."

LEON ROSENBERG: I have read the article and I think the statement is based on a very small clinical study. I think it is unfortunate that three human experimantation boards in England have ruled that, because the problem is such a large one, a controlled study cannot be done to determine whether the initial findings are valid. What that means is that the British, who certainly have the patient population large enough to have answered the question in a reasonable period of time, will not answer it. We will be faced with another major question about whether the limited sample size upon which the initial reports were based are sufficient to warrant extensive multivitamin supplementation for essentially all women of reproductive age. I don't know what should be done.

MARGERY SHAW: Our discussion time has run out. I would like to thank the members of the panel and the audience for a very stimulating discussion. We have raised more questions than we have answered but that is the nature of the topic of this symposium.

Chapter 18

Concluding Reflections

Bentley Glass

It would be quite impossible for me to summarize adequately in the 30 minutes allotted me all the stimulating and challenging things we have heard in the two and one-half days of this conference on the Concept of Person. It is particularly difficult for me because with advancing years my once keen hearing has begun to fail me badly. If I therefore slight some of the important things that have been said both by speakers and discussants, you should attribute that omission to my poor hearing. Yet I have been amply instructed and illuminated by what I have heard. Instead of a summary, I give you, therefore, my reflections on certain aspects of our conference.

As for the biological foundation of personhood, which arises so gradually and so mysteriously from the multiplication by mitosis and the differentiation into tissues and organs of the billions of cells all containing representatives of the same 46 chromosomes and the same genes with which the original fertilized egg was endowed, what can be said with assurance?

The persona, the personality of the individual, the awareness of selfhood, emerges even more gradually and mysteriously than the limbs, the facial features, the heart and brain of the human being. We know of genes, the mutation of which can impair these processes. We know of no genes that specifically *produce* an organ, or even a tissue. Somehow, in the course of human evolution over the past few million years, our DNA has diverged sufficiently from that of our closest living animal relative, the chimpanzee, to create the differences between us, even though many of our genes are still identical with those of the chimpanzee, as is indicated by DNA pairing. And our genes are presumably also largely identical in many cases with those of our forebears among the early hominid-australopithecine-line of descent. Were those forebears, still not fully human, possessed of selfhood? Were they "persons"? Should we not ask, too, whether a chimpanzee—especially one educated to speak several hundred words in sign language, to answer to its own name, to recognize its human friends as individuals—whether it also possesses the qualifications of selfhood, of being a "person"?

When I return home I will be welcomed by my beloved yellow Labrador dog, who will run circles around our living room in her joy at my return. Does she not recognize her own identity, as well as mine? Do the attributes of personhood not extend across the limits of species? Certainly, her senses are as keen as my own or better. Her joys and woes are as recognizable to me as those of any other friend, her memory as sharp. The human fetus lives in a warm darkness. Its eyes are unseeing, its senses poor until the later months of gestation, its memory negligible. Even a normal newborn infant must learn to focus its eyes, to direct each simple movement, to acquire slowly a set of memories and associations. From years of recent studies in developmental psychology we know that a young animal—and presumably likewise a human infant—if kept in a black box during its early weeks of life will grow and mature in size, but will remain a fearful, disoriented being that can never learn to play or adjust to life if its early learning experiences did not come at the right time. Senility reveals to us, too, that a person is a cluster of memories, and that as these fade, the personality fades, too, until it vanishes altogether. All of this is what Grobstein, Blandau, Milunsky and Rosenberg have been saying to you. There is more to a *person* than the biological foundation. That is a necessary, yet not sufficient, basis of personhood. It is a fallacy to suppose that the genotype of a person is a sufficient explanation of that person, even if the evolution of the human genotype, and the uniqueness of a particular person's combination of genes be included in the concept. But it is surely equally a fallacy to suppose that the genotype and the nature of developmental processes—yes, and the presence of a normal environment in which the development may proceed—are not an essential part of selfhood, awareness, and personhood.

So, I state my first important conclusion: *A person is not confined to what lies within the outer layer of his or her skin.* Each of us extends invisibly outward into the world of our experiences. That world supplies us with the stimuli to our senses, the experiences we remember, the objects we love or hate, that injure us or nourish us. John Donne, I suppose, was the first Englishman to apprehend this clearly when he penned those so familiar words, "No man is an island, but a part of the main, a part of the continent entire. So ask not for whom the bell tolls, it tolls for thee." Yet Donne seemingly thought only of his fellow-men. I would now extend the thought far more widely, in a second important conclusion. *Each man is a part of the world, and the world a part of him.* This is not just the vision of St. Francis, that all living things are God's creatures, our brothers and sisters. That, too, is true, says the evolutionist, but I say even more, that they are a part of you and you of them in so far as they sense and remember as do we. And even the inanimate creation, rocks and rivers, lakes and mountains, sea, air, sun and stars, are all a part of us, since we as persons are our experiences and our memories, our reactions, and our powers of reason about life and the universe.

I was greatly impressed by the analysis made by Robert Veatch. It seems so obviously true that definitions of death have much to tell us about definitions of the beginning of life and the generation of personhood. Clearly, as technology opens up new understandings, our concept of personhood will change yet further as it has been forced to change in the past in the light of gradual beginnings and of the gradual and unequal death of our tissues. A third major conclusion: *The person is not to be found simply in the living state of individual cells, but is a property of the whole.*

There are billions upon billions of cells in the brain, but when enough of them die the personality, the memory, the intelligence, the senses, all disappear. We must indeed continue the search for consistency in our interpretations or definitions of *life* and *death*, beginning and ending. The persona, the soul, is not, as Descartes thought, lodged in the pineal body in the center of the brain. It is a property of the whole body, abridged by loss of any part of it, even those parts not vital to continuance of life. If I deviate here somewhat from Veatch's superb analysis, I trust you will pardon me.

What is human life? There are different definitions, as Daniel Callahan rightly pointed out. Consider, I suggest, a culture of human fibroblasts. Are they human? Yes. Are they alive? Yes, alive and multiplying. Can they grow into a person? No, not as far as we know at present. Yet I point out that a culture of dissociated, undifferentiated carrot cells can be grown into a full carrot plant—root, stem, and leaves, and eventually flowers and seeds. Our technology in respect to human cell cultures may simply be inadequate, and some day the feat may become possible. Yet if we ask ourselves whether the carrot cell culture is truly a carrot and should be treated as a carrot plant, the scientist must answer: No, it is a carrot cell culture, *potentially* a carrot plant, yet not yet so. There is, then, a basis, apart from definition of carrot life, for a differing treatment of the culture, the seedling, or the mature plant.

The presentations of Golbus and Ryan predict further complications in our concept of the person if we confer the status of personhood on the unborn. But the gradual appearance, prenatal as well as postnatal, of signs of sensory activity, pain, and perhaps awareness make it difficult not to do so. The question remains: at what precise time in this gradual emergence of consciousness and awareness can we be sure that what we mean by personhood has arrived? The choice must be arbitrary, and it is not at all surprising that there are vigorous differences of opinion about it. These, as Sidney Callahan has shown, differ according to our religious beliefs and our preconceptions. As Ruth Macklin pointed out, there are also cases of two persons in a conjoined body, and other cases of multiple persona in a single body. I despair at present of the possibility of reconciling all such divergent opinions about abortion and the so-called right of a woman to eliminate her fetus. Is a third trimester fetus simply a parasite on the mother, of no human account? Are they not in actuality, if temporarily, two parts of the same person? I fear that our legal experts—Baron, Pilpel, Robertson, Westfall, and Dickens—can merely reveal to us the complexities of the law without answering our question. If we are to be simply pragmatic, then probably the Supreme Court decision in *Roe v. Wade* is, though quite arbitrary in setting a point in a continuum as a satisfactory dividing point, the best we can expect in a resolution of the conflict between the interests of the mother and the fetus.

Be sure, however, that advancing technology, as Leon Rosenberg has described, will steadily move forward the age of fetal viability outside the womb. Already, for the mouse, there has been developed in the laboratory an artificial placenta that can nurture the embryo from implantation to developed fetus. I am confident that the full process in a few years will be produced for other mammals and, yes, I think for humans, too. Oh, that we could go back to laying eggs like birds and reptiles, or even the platypus! But no, we are caught in the consequences of a once-marvelous step in evolution, the invention of the placenta.

The further reproductive separation of fetal development from the body of a woman may require, technologically, only a few more years. The whole process from in vitro fertilization using banked spermatazoa and banked ova, to the emergence of an infant at term is to be expected. Our present rage over abortion will then be a dead letter. Yet what will happen then to maternal and fraternal feelings, to the warmth of family relationships, as infants develop into persons in that brave new world? Unless we can protect the family from disintegration under those circumstances, our present conflict over abortion will seem a storm in a teacup in the gathering human calamity.

We are all of us—six billions of us—dependent for life and comfort, growth and joy, on the terrestrial environment in which we live and move and have our being. As I said earlier, that environment is actually a *part* of us, the oxygen we breathe, the food we eat, the pure water we drink, the pleasure we take in our motions and our senses. No duty rests on mankind more weightily than to see that world preserved for our descendents. We cannot survive without the green plants—the trees of the Amazon valley, the algae of the ocean—to restock our atmosphere with oxygen. We cannot survive without our crop plants and our animal proteins. We need the purity of our world in place of pollution, the preservation of each species of life—for we are all one inseparable ecosystem, one great symbiotic lifeform that vastly exceeds the human population alone. Even the inanimate parts of our environment must be preserved, lest we perish. For this, we require a *new ethic of trusteeship*—not simply of stewardship for some absentee owner—but a true trusteeship in the interest of all future persons and their world. If that ethic can be engendered and can prevail, we need not fear, I think, for the future of our family bonds or the resolution of our conflicts over abortion.

Table of Cases

Index

About the Editors

A. EDWARD DOUDERA is Executive Director of the American Society of Law & Medicine, Executive Editor of the *American Journal of Law & Medicine*, and Executive Editor of *Law, Medicine & Health Care*. He received his undergraduate degree from Boston University and his J.D. from Suffolk University Law School, and is a member of the Massachusetts and federal bars. Before joining the American Society of Law & Medicine in 1977, Mr. Doudera was Associate Administrator for Research at Tufts-New England Medical Center in Boston.

MARGERY W. SHAW is Interim Director of the Institute for the Interprofessional Study of Health Law, University of Texas Health Science Center at Houston and University of Houston College of Law, and Professor of Medical Genetics at the University of Texas Health Science Center in Houston. Dr. Shaw received her undergraduate degree from the University of Alabama, her M.D. from The University of Michigan, and her J.D. from the University of Houston. She is also Andrew D. White Professor-at-Large at Cornell University, President of the American Society of Human Genetics, and active in numerous professional associations, editorial boards, and committees of the National Institutes of Health and National Academy of Sciences.